# Take Heart

## GOOD PRACTICES IN CORONARY HEART DISEASE PREVENTION

A report prepared for the Health Education Authority
by Judy Berry with assistance from Nick Cavill and Helen King

Health Education Authority

Coventry University

© Health Education Authority 1990
First published 1990

Health Education Authority
Hamilton House
Mabledon Place
London WC1 9TX

ISBN 1 85448 118 5

Typeset by DP Photosetting, Aylesbury, Bucks
Printed and bound in Great Britain by
Biddles Ltd, Guildford and King's Lynn

# Contents

# Acknowledgements

Thanks are given to all the organisations that kindly allowed us to use their projects as case studies in the book or allowed us to reproduce their photographs and other materials as illustrations. There were many more examples of innovative work in CHD prevention which could have been included – the choice of which to include was difficult! Our thanks therefore to all who gave time to discuss their projects, including Stuart Ramsbottom, Rob Clarke, Robin Ireland, Michael Watson, Caroline Hawkridge, Amanda Killoran, Rosalind Eunson, Joan Corboy, Gill Combes, John Grigg, Vera Bolter, Lesley Shucksmith, Myra Garrett, Noel Olsen, John Gibson, Jo Harvey, and Ursula Miles.

Thanks are also due to Naomi Chambers, Jeanie McKenzie, Nick Cavill and Helen King for their research and editing of the book.

# Preface

The Look After Your Heart Community Projects Scheme was set up in 1987 to assist organisations and individuals trying to tackle the unacceptably high rate of coronary heart disease (CHD) in England. The job facing health workers at all levels was and is daunting – not only raising awareness in the community about CHD and how it may be prevented, but also helping people to change to a more healthy lifestyle. Since the Scheme was established Look After Your Heart (LAYH) has gathered a wealth of information about innovative CHD prevention projects which have been implemented around the country, including projects funded by other organisations. This information is important not only for the good ideas that have been generated but because it tells us how things were done.

The reports and evaluations produced at the conclusion of each project reveal that for every triumph there were irksome periods and a few failures. Either way we benefit from this first-hand experience and can apply these useful lessons in our own work.

To share this experience and to inspire you in developing your own CHD prevention programme, LAYH has brought together examples of different approaches to CHD prevention, and tried to distil from hundreds of projects some practical hints and guidelines to help minimise the problems and maximise the triumphs! We hope you will find it helpful.

Helen King
Programme Officer – Community Projects
LAYH
June 1990

# 1 Planning for success

# 1 Introduction

In England, heart disease is still the main cause of people dying prematurely. Much can be done to reduce the risk of heart disease and everyone has a part to play. Action can be taken at individual, community, regional and national level to tackle the problem.

This book is about good practices in heart disease prevention. It describes 16 case studies that vary in scale and ambition and which show how various organisations in England have worked with others to reduce heart disease. The book aims to provide inspiration and encouragement to those working in this field by showing what is possible and by identifying the ingredients of successful programmes.

The book has been prepared for the Look After Your Heart (LAYH) programme, the first national coronary heart disease education programme in England. Jointly funded and administered by the Department of Health and the Health Education Authority (HEA), the programme, since its launch in 1987, has successfully placed coronary heart disease prevention on the public and professional agenda and laid the foundation for a future programme of increased depth and diversity, which will involve nearly every organisation in society and reach everyone in England.

# Coronary heart disease in England

Coronary heart disease (CHD*) is the leading cause of death in England, killing 150 000 people every year. This represents over a quarter of all deaths. Research has shown that there is no single cause of heart disease, but that a number of factors may combine to increase an individual's risk. Some of these risk factors are unalterable, such as age and family history of heart disease, but many can be avoided or reduced. The main modifiable risk factors that the LAYH programme concentrates on are:

- smoking and tobacco use
- diet and nutrition, in particular a diet that is high in total fat, and especially saturated fat
- high blood pressure
- lack of exercise.

The prevention of CHD does not only involve the health service, it involves government departments, local authorities, mass media, industry and commerce, and community and voluntary groups working together. Adopting healthy public policies and practices at national and local level helps people who are already changing to a more healthy lifestyle to achieve and maintain changes. Conditions for both work and leisure also need to promote health and provide opportunities for making healthy choices.

* The term coronary heart disease (ischaemic heart disease) embraces a group of clinical syndromes including angina pectoris, acute myocardial infarction (fatal and non-fatal) and sudden ischaemic death. CHD is associated with atheroma, a build up of fatty deposits in the coronary arteries, and thrombosis or blood clotting.

# The Look After Your Heart programme

The Look After Your Heart programme is a national initiative that brings together a number of CHD prevention activities under one 'umbrella'. The main aims of the programme are:

1  To contribute towards a substantial reduction in the premature death caused by CHD. This will be achieved by contributing to a reduction in the major risk factors causing coronary heart disease by:

- promoting public awareness and understanding of the lifestyle changes required;

- equipping individuals with the knowledge and skills to make those changes;

- initiating, stimulating and supporting CHD prevention and health promotion activities through mass media, the workplace, local government, industry and commerce through joint activities between the HEA and the NHS.

2  To contribute towards a reduction in the variations in CHD mortality and morbidity between social groups, geographical regions and ethnic groups.

3  To contribute towards a reduction in the social and economic costs of CHD.

4  To promote healthy living.

One of the objectives of the Look After Your Heart Programme is:

to disseminate good practice through effective working partnerships with the NHS and other organisations in the field.

This is being achieved by funding innovative community projects under the Community Projects Scheme. Since 1987, this scheme has given awards to 270 small projects (funding up to £5000 per year), and six large demonstration projects. Most of the case studies described in this book have received funding through the Look After Your Heart Community Projects Scheme. They span a wide variety of activities that have taken place in different settings and with different target groups. They range from relatively small scale activities to more ambitious ones.

# Good practices in CHD prevention programmes

The criteria for 'good practices' that have been adopted for this book can be summarised under four main headings: careful planning; good management; special features; and impact.

Careful planning

To provide a broad context for developing action plans, many people find it useful to have a strategy and a statement of aims and objectives. Many of the projects described in this book are ones that have developed from within broader programmes; they have come about because the broader programmes were flexible and allowed space for development, as the opportunities arose.

The main aim of a strategy on CHD prevention should be to create a climate of professional and public commitment to promote heart health and prevent heart disease, allowing all effective measures to be used for this purpose.

Ideally, any CHD prevention strategy should stimulate action within the primary and secondary health services and within family, neighbourhood, community, public, voluntary and commercial settings. It should recognise the forces that promote the continued production and consumption of goods and services which affect heart health (such as manufacturers, or market forces), and be flexible to respond to these when the opportunity arises.

Specific projects and activities identified for action within the strategy for CHD prevention should have clearly defined objectives that are relevant and are stated in ways such that progress towards them can be measured. They should also be seen to be achievable. Early in the planning stage, it is important to develop a plan for the project, which should clearly set out:

- Who your project is aimed at.

- What activities you will be doing.

- Who will be doing them.

- Where they will take place.

- When they will happen.

- How much they will cost.

This will help to clarify the resources needed to make the project work, and will greatly aid the evaluation process.

The underlying reasons for particular patterns of behaviour are complex; many include social, economic, political and commercial factors beyond the immediate control of the individual. Action against heart disease needs community commitment and should not be confined to the health service. To bring about change often involves collaboration and co-operation with other sectors. The majority of the case studies in this book provide examples of how the processes of joint planning and inter-sector collaboration are working at local level.

Community heart health projects should be responsive to local needs. A few of the case studies show how the activity arose as a response to local demand (See the Women's 10km Run in Liverpool and the Men's Health Information Day in Lowestoft). Some involved local people in planning activities. (See Project Lionheart, East Dorset.) Too often 'professionals' decide what is to be done and how to do it without the necessary market research or feedback from the target group.

Good management

Successful activities do not come inevitably as the result of rational comprehensive plans and tight-reined management systems. Many thrive best where they have the right people in the right place at a particular point of time with the backing to get on with the job.

6

The case studies in the book highlight the different models for managing projects. Many had a working or advisory group to assist the project. This group can have two functions: firstly, to act as a sounding board for ideas; and secondly, to provide direct support to ensure that things happen.

All the case studies identified operational managers, and leaders or co-ordinators whose enthusiasm and hard work kept their programmes active and who steered them round all obstacles. A checklist for the successful management of projects can be found on pages 11–12.

**Special features**

CHD prevention activities should be planned according to the settings in which work is to be carried out. The case studies have been selected to illustrate innovative approaches to heart disease prevention activity in each of the following settings:

- provision of health information on coronary heart disease to the general public;
- screening, lifestyle advice and counselling in a primary health care setting;
- screening or promoting a healthy environment in the workplace;
- coronary heart disease education in schools or the youth service;
- coronary heart disease education activities with community groups;
- joint activities to promote healthy hearts with the commercial sector;
- activities in public places (e.g. restaurants) to reduce the risk of coronary heart disease.

In addition, case studies have been included which illustrate city-wide and region-wide programmes.

Programmes on CHD prevention can concentrate on one risk factor like lack of exercise, or smoking, others can be multi-factorial. Some of the case studies reported here were one-off events, although often coming under the umbrella of a wider heart-health programme. These one-off events have all resulted in further activity. For example the event has been repeated (see Ramadan Stop Smoking Posters) or it has been integrated into the existing work of the organisation (see Men's Health Information Day – Lowestoft).

Careful consideration should be given before deciding to run a one-off event as they usually involve a great deal of time to organise (see Chislehurst Health Week and Women's 10 km Run).

7

Many of the case studies obtained excellent coverage for their projects from their local media. This kind of support does not just happen. A plan on how to work with the media is very important. Local newspapers, radio and television reach a very large proportion of the general public and they are an important tool in creating a climate of awareness about the issue and they also show that something is being done.

In one project, there were 95 articles in the local press in one year. Some were part of a series that had been negotiated with the local paper on heart disease risk factors. However, the majority of articles were produced in response to a variety of local activities and events which were skilfully marketed to the journalists to capture their interest (see Project Health – Peterborough). Issuing a press release which finds a new angle on the topic and following up with a personal contact is always worth doing.

## Impact

The purpose of evaluating a particular project or activity is to compare what happened with what was expected to happen and to decide whether or not it was worthwhile. Many of the case studies in this book described what happened – the process – but not all were able to compare outcomes with the situation at the start of the project, as much valuable baseline information was not collected.

The case studies show that it is important that evaluation is not seen as something that is done after the project or activity is completed. A person responsible for monitoring progress or co-ordinating the monitoring should be identified at the planning stage. Programmes which carefully monitored their activities, carried out baseline surveys and produced regular reports which were fed back to funding organisations with plans for further developments, were more likely to attract substantial extra funding (see Look After Your Heart – Avon; and Project Lionheart – East Dorset).

Useful information which is often not collected is data on the activities of those interests that compete against heart health and which increase local risks.

The majority of the case studies received funding from a variety of sources including collaborative agencies and the commercial sector. Most projects whilst identifying the contribution of collaborative agencies or staff time and facilities, do not include this in their calculations of how much the project has cost to achieve the objectives. Support from commercial companies can be very valuable, but great care should be taken to ensure that the health interests are paramount. The HEA's commercial department have produced guidelines for those seeking commercial sponsorship, to help them to obtain the most agreeable sponsorship deal.

Evaluation reports provide helpful information to others wishing to carry out similar activities. Unexpected spin-offs might occur or problems might arise that were not foreseen. By recording what happened, useful lessons can be learnt. About half the case studies described their activities in their reports so that others could learn from them or repeat them. One project is producing a step by step guide to help others repeat the study in their own areas (see Healthy Meat in Hampstead).

# 2 Ingredients of success

Investigation of the case studies has revealed a number of factors that can affect the success of a project. These are listed below to provide a checklist for successful project management.

1  Projects need leaders who will make things happen and who can grasp opportunities as they arise.

2  Such leaders need time and delegated powers to get on with the job.

3  The best leader makes mistakes; what is important in the end is the balance of success and failure.

4  Projects need support from governing bodies and guidance from time to time; they do not want to be run by them.

5  The successful activities do not come inevitably as the fruit of rational comprehensive plans and tight-reined management systems; many thrive best where they have the right people, in the right place at a particular point of time with the backing to get on with the job.

6  An active multi-sector working group is often helpful for assisting the project workers. Collaboration with others outside the health service is important.

7  The project cannot do all the work. Transferring responsibility for action from the group to others with the power to act is a key element in success; sometimes this is done through training in new skills, sometimes by stimulating other individuals or groups to take up the action themselves using their own powers and resources.

8  Successful projects learn from their mistakes and use the best ideas from others; their secret is building on success, maintaining sparkle, freshness and enjoying the work. They are happy to pass on what they have learnt, they are not jealous of their own knowledge.

9  Working with the media and using their skills at presentation ensures that the project reaches a large audience.

10  Involving the local community, accepting the contribution of all people and not limiting participation to those with professional qualifications is a common feature of the successful projects. This requires clear documentation so that everyone knows what is happening.

11  Projects can get too complex; the best keep their activities direct, simple and relevant and prune out the unnecessary; their staff are protected from other vicarious activities.

12  Using existing powerful networks to work with a project can enhance the capacity for achievement.

13  To work with others you need to know what motivates them and why they may want to work with you.

14  Successful projects are willing to try out new methods of working, but they also keep a check on whether the new methods are effective.

# **3** Case studies

The case studies show that there is no one model for CHD prevention that works for everyone. There are principles for 'good practices' which emerge from the case studies, and there are ingredients for success. The next section provides information on both of these.

Not all of the projects described in this book exhibit all of the 'good practice' criteria. Nor are these the only heart disease prevention projects which are examples of 'good practice' – many others could have been included.

The projects that have been selected cover a variety of activities that have taken place in different settings, and with different target groups. They range from relatively small scale activities to more ambitious ones.

Table 1 shows the main criteria of 'good practice' illustrated by the case studies, and Table 2 summarises the main characteristics of the case studies.

Planning for success

TABLE 1   Main criteria of 'good practice' illustrated by the case studies.

| Criteria | Walks in 1066 country | Men's health information day – Lowestoft | Liverpool women's 10 km run | Project Health – Peterborough | LAYH – Avon | Chislehurst health week |
|---|---|---|---|---|---|---|
| Background research baseline data | | | | | • | |
| Steering/Group | | • | • | • | • | • |
| Objectives identified | • | • | • | • | • | • |
| Progress & planning & implementation reports | • | | | | • | • |
| Evaluation/research report | | • | • | | • | |
| Joint planning | | • | • | • | • | • |
| Local community involved in planning | | • | • | | | • |
| Joint funding | • | • | • | • | • | • |
| Cost identified | • | • | • | • | • | • |
| Good press coverage | • | • | • | • | • | • |
| Described so others can repeat | • | • | | | • | • |
| One off activity stimulated further action | | • | • | | | • |
| Part of wider programme | • | | • | • | • | |

14

| Look After Your Heart in the workplace – ICL | Schools project – Birmingham | Healthy eating guidelines for school caterers – Hereford & Worcester | LAYH campaign – Newcastle upon Tyne | Project Lionheart – East Dorset | Ramandan stop smoking posters – Tower Hamlets, London | Healthy meat in Hampstead, London | Heartbeat award – North Kesteven D.C. and the Boundary cafe, Lincolnshire | Birmingham LAYH Campaign | Yorkshire Heartbeat |
|---|---|---|---|---|---|---|---|---|---|
|  | • |  |  | • | • | • |  |  |  |
|  |  | • | • |  |  |  |  | • |  |
| • | • | • | • | • | • | • | • | • | • |
| • |  |  | • | • | • |  |  |  |  |
|  | • |  |  | • |  |  |  |  | • |
| • | • | • | • | • | • |  | • | • | • |
|  | • |  | • | • | • |  |  |  |  |
|  |  | • | • | • | • | • |  | • | • |
| • | • | • | • | • | • | • | • | • | • |
|  | • | • | • |  | • | • | • | • | • |
|  | • |  |  | • | • | • |  |  | • |
|  | • | • |  |  | • | • |  |  |  |
| • |  |  | • | • |  | • | • | • | • |

*TABLE 2   Main characteristics of the case studies.*

| PROJECT | SETTING | DESCRIPTION | LOCATION | TIMESCALE |
|---------|---------|-------------|----------|-----------|
| Walks in 1066 country | Public information and promotional activity | Package of town and country walks | Hastings | 1987/88 1 year from planning to launch |
| Men's health information day – Lowestoft | Public information and promotional activity | Day-long programme of health events aimed at men | Lowestoft | 1988 6 months from initial planning to event |
| Liverpool women's 10 km run | Public information and promotional activity | 10 km race for women, to encourage more women to enjoy sport | Liverpool | Yearly event Takes 1 year to plan |
| Project Health Peterborough | Public information and promotional activity | Health bulletins and promotional material | Peterborough and Fenland | April 1989 – first bulletin; issued every two months. Promotional material continual development |
| Look After Your Heart – Avon | Region-wide | Inter-agency co-ordinated programme of heart disease prevention activities | County of Avon covering Bath and Bristol | Originated 1987 and continuing |
| Chislehurst health-week | Primary health care | Health week organised by a GP medical receptionist | Chislehurst | 21 months to plan – 6 day event |
| Look After Your Heart in the workplace – ICL | Workplace | Look After Your Heart campaign at ICL | ICL offices throughout the country | Started 1987 and continuing |
| Schools project Education about CHD – Birmingham | Schools and youth service | Education about coronary heart disease | Three inner city multi-racial primary schools Birmingham | 1988–89 |
| Healthy eating guidelines for school caterers – Hereford & Worcester | Schools and youth service | Guidelines and menus for school caterers | County of Hereford & Worcester | 1989–90 |
| LAYH Campaign – Programme of community initiatives, Newcastle upon Tyne | Community | Community based LAYH initiatives targeted at adults in high risk wards | Newcastle upon Tyne | Since 1987 and continuing |
| Project Lionheart – East Dorset | Community | Community action programme to reduce deaths from coronary heart disease | 1st Stage – Wool rural community 2nd Stage – Canford Heath – suburban Both in East Dorset | Wool started 1987 Canford Heath started 1989 |

| COST | SOURCES OF FUNDING | MANAGEMENT | TARGET GROUP |
|---|---|---|---|
| £3200 | Health Promotion Unit LAYH Community Projects Scheme | Health Promotion Officer as an activity for the Unit's 'Action Heart Programme' | Local people and holiday makers |
| £550 | LAYH Community Projects Scheme; donations; Time without charging from Community Education; Health Promotion & College | 15 member multi-disciplinary, inter-agency planning group, co-ordinated by the Health Promotion Officer | Men in Lowestoft |
| In 1989 £25 000 | Commercial Sponsorship Entry fees Regional Health Auth. City Council | Race director (who is a Regional health promotion officer) co-ordinates the planning & implementation in close collaboration with the City Council | Women |
| £270 per issue £2244 for promotional material | LAYH Community Projects Scheme; sponsorship and staff time by participating agencies | Managed by District health promotion officer supported by multi-agency advisory group | 'Key' people in the community |
| £7000 for events to date £20 000 p.a. for 3 years for co-ordinator 1990-93 £50 000 p.a. for 3 years localities project 1990-93 | LAYH Community Projects Scheme – categories 1 & 2; Participating agencies; Sports Council | Multi-agency steering group meets every 6 weeks. Co-ordinating activity responsibility of District Health Promotion Officer, Frenchay Health Authority | General public but now with special emphasis with communities in two localities |
| £2938 | Local fund raising Rotary Club LAYH Community Project Scheme | Co-ordinated by GP's medical receptionist from local health centre, supported by steering group | Children and young adults |
| No substantial additional costs | Met from existing occupational health budgets with assistance from local health promotion units | Organised by Occupational Health Department | Workforce company-wide |
| £4995 | LAYH Community Project Scheme | The 2 researchers worked together supported by their agencies – the Health Authority and Community Education | Children aged 6 and 10 and their parents |
| £5000 | LAYH Community Projects Scheme. Health Education Units involved | District Health Ed. officer chairs monthly meeting of planning consortium. Members of group play active role at different phases of programme | School caterers |
| £5000 in 1987–88 £4900 in 1989 | LAYH Community Projects Scheme; Staff time & facilities provided by participating agencies | Co-ordinating group with different schemes being the responsibility of different members of the group | Adults in deprived city wards; the Asian community; relatives and sufferers from heart disease |
| Wool £24 000 Canford Heath £40 000 | East Dorset Health Auth. British Heart Foundation LAYH Community Project Scheme, TVS Trust | Specialist programme linked to E. Dorset Health Promotion Unit & Dept of Public Health Med. Project Director & Project Officer | Needs related action based on community profile |

# Planning for success

| PROJECT | SETTING | DESCRIPTION | LOCATION | TIMESCALE |
|---|---|---|---|---|
| Ramadan stop smoking posters – Tower Hamlets, London | Community | Ramadan fasting timetables with messages encouraging people to give up smoking | Tower Hamlets London | 1989 Took three months to plan |
| Healthy meat in Hampstead, London | Activity with the commercial sector | Project to monitor fat content in mince | Hampstead London | Main study Nov. 1987 – May 1988 Follow-up – June 1989 & Feb. 1990 |
| Heartbeat Award – North Kesteven D.C. and the Boundary Cafe, Lincolnshire | Public places | Implementation of Heartbeat Award in eating places | North Kesteven District Council and transport cafe on A15 Lincoln to Sleaford Road | Scheme started by Environmental Health Department 1988 |
| Birmingham Look After Your Heart campaign | City-wide | Programme of city-wide activities under LAYH banner | Birmingham | Started 1987 and continuing |
| Yorkshire Heartbeat | Primary health care | Collaborative training programme for primary health care teams | Yorkshire Region | Yorkshire Heartbeat co-ordination began September 1988 – continuing activity |

| COST | SOURCES OF FUNDING | MANAGEMENT | TARGET GROUP |
|---|---|---|---|
| £3335 | LAYH Community Projects Scheme | Managed by community Health Campaign in consultation with the Health Promotion service | Muslim smokers |
| £2500 | LAYH Community Projects Scheme; Hampstead Public Health Medicine Dept. | Project devised and supervised by Hampstead's Director of Public Health Medicine. Implementation by senior scientific officer | Retailers selling mince |
| No additional cost | LAYH Heartbeat Award materials from HEA Staff time – North Kesteven D.C. | Implemented by senior environmental health officer with support from chief officer and District council and advice from community dietitians | Small eating places most frequently used by the general public , e.g. transport cafe |
| 1989–90 £15000 on LAYH activities. £400000 on City's schools Health Ed. Prog. | City Council Ed. Dept; Joint Financing; Env. Health Dept; LAYH Community Projects Scheme; Commercial sponsors | LAYH Campaign committee meets every 6 weeks. Members take responsibility for action. Serviced by Environmental Health. Initiatives in school led by schools adviser on Health Education | Main emphasis – school children & young people and City Council employees |
| £30600 per year | Yorkshire Hearbeat Health Education Authority Family Practitioner Committees | Co-ordination of training in the Region by co-ordinator of Yorkshire Hearbeat | Primary Health Care teams |

# 2 Good practices

# 1 Walks in 1066 country

## Setting – public information and promotional activity

A package of town and country walks in the Hastings area was produced and promoted in this project which formed part of the Health Authority's Action Heart Campaign.

The six guides are extensively used by local people and holidaymakers alike. A second series is being planned as a result of their popularity.

**Key facts**

| | |
|---|---|
| **Location:** | Hastings area<br>Population 170 000 |
| **Timescale:** | 12 months |
| **Costs:** | £3200 |
| **Sources of funding:** | Health Promotion Unit and LAYH Community Projects Scheme |
| **Initiator:** | Health Promotion Officer |
| **Implementation led by:** | As above |
| **Special features:** | • Promotion of walking as healthy and fun.<br><br>• Identified six local walking routes.<br><br>• Produced leaflets describing the walks (Fig. 1.1). |
| **Contact:** | Stuart Ramsbottom<br>Health Promotion Adviser<br>Hastings Health Promotion Unit<br>Eversfield Hospital<br>Westhill Road<br>St Leonards on Sea<br>East Sussex TN38 0NG |
| **Documentation:** | 1066 Walks Pack. A pack containing six different walks within Hastings Health Authority available from the above address.<br><br>Project evaluation report to the Health Education Authority |

**Good practices**

- Objectives identified
- Project could be repeated by others
- Resources identified
- Implementation report provided
- Participation by Community Programme workers
- Long-lasting effects
- Part of an agreed local heart health promotion programme
- Simple idea using attractions of locality

# Origins

In the Hastings Health Authority, coronary heart disease accounts for about a quarter of all deaths each year. In response to this problem, the health promotion unit developed the Action Heart Project, which encompasses a variety of ideas designed to make people more aware of the risk factors leading to the disease, and to encourage them to recognise that healthy activities can also be fun.

The Project includes Look After Yourself (LAY) courses, Smoke Stop courses and the 1066 Walks pack. Acknowledging that lack of exercise is one of the major contributory risk factors in relation to coronary heart disease, the idea behind the pack was to promote walking in the locality.

# Objectives

- To promote walking as an activity which will enhance health and is fun for all ages and abilities.
- To provide the public with an easy to follow map and guide to walks around the town and countryside within the Hastings Health District.
- To produce a comprehensive package of walks within the district, containing six different routes.

# What happened

Six routes were chosen, which varied in length from two to five miles, with recommended walking times from one to two and a half hours. The routes were walked by a Community Programme workforce and health promotion staff, and the details checked.

Then followed the actual writing of the guides, which include a simple map, written description of the walk, key landmarks and useful information (for example, location of toilets, car parks, and refreshments). The maps and folders both carry the LAYH logo (Fig. 1.1).

Effective promotion of the packs was an essential element in the success of the project. The walks were featured on local television and radio, and in the press. Packs were distributed to public libraries, the Sports Centre and to tourist information offices. They were also handed out at the Hastings Town and Country Fair and various local health fairs and by LAYH/LAY tutors.

**Fig. 1.1** The 'Walks in 1066 Country' pack and one of the maps

# Impact

Letters have been received from members of the public praising the pack. In one letter the 'excellent presentation' was complimented.

Two thousand leaflets were distributed in 10 months.

Because of the large response, a second series, with six new routes, is being planned and funding is being sought to cover the printing costs.

It has not, however, been possible to identify how many of the packs have been used, nor, indeed, how many miles have been walked. In future series, the Health Promotion Unit have decided that they would place a questionnaire inside each pack inviting a response regarding usage.

# Management

The Project has been managed by the Health Promotion officer, responsible for Action Heart, in the Health Promotion Unit.

# Resources

The cost of the project was as follows:

| | |
|---|---|
| Travel | £116 |
| Human resources | £1903 |
| Printing | £1153 |
| Other | £30 |
| Total | £3202 |

# 2 Men's health information day – Lowestoft

## Setting – public information and promotional activity

A number of men in the Lowestoft area inspired by the success and frequency of health initiatives directed at women decided to organise a health event for men. A planning team comprising individuals from voluntary and statutory organisations working in and for the community was set up in May 1988 and members of the public were invited to attend planning meetings. A full programme of events was planned and the Men's Health Information Day took place in October 1988. Evaluation showed strong support for the day and highlighted areas for improvement. Since then a men's health initiatives group has been formed and a variety of follow-up activities and information mornings have taken place.

**Fig. 2.1** The programme for Lowestoft's Men's Health Information Day

**Key facts**

| | |
|---|---|
| **Location:** | Lowestoft<br>Population 55 000 |
| **Timescale:** | Planning May 1988 leading up to the event in October 1988 |
| **Cost:** | £550 |
| **Sources of funding:** | LAYH Community Projects Scheme<br>Donations<br>Extra resourcing without charging from Community Education, District Health Promotion Services, Lowestoft College |
| **Initiator:** | Planning group |
| **Implementation led by:** | Senior Health Promotion Officer |
| **Special features:** | • Information and advice day aimed at men, inspired by frequency of health initiatives aimed at women<br><br>• Information stands, advice, free health MOT, group discussion sessions<br><br>• Evaluation showed positive support from the participants, who also suggested areas for improvement<br><br>• Series of health initiatives resulted e.g. stop smoking group, self-help men's group. |
| **Contact:** | Rob Clarke<br>Senior Health Promotion Officer<br>Gt Yarmouth and Waveney Health Authority<br>Health Promotion Centre<br>Northgate Hospital<br>Northgate Street<br>Lowestoft<br>Norfolk NR30 1BU |
| **Documentation:** | Men's Health Information Day evaluation report.<br>R. Clarke, Gt Yarmouth & Waveney Health Authority, 1989. |

**Good practices**

> - Objectives identified
> - Resources identified
> - Joint planning multi-agency collaboration
> - Involvement of public in planning
> - Careful planning
> - First such event in East Anglia
> - Although one-off event, follow-up activities resulted
> - Will become integrated into existing health programme
> - Evaluation report describes activities so others could repeat

# Origins

A number of men in the Lowestoft area inspired by the success and frequency of health initiatives directed at women began to assess the feasibility of holding an event for men. A planning team was formed in May 1988 with the aim of staging a Men's Health Information Day in October 1988.

The planning group included teachers, general practitioners, paramedical staff, sports officer, health promotion officer, community development and liaison officers, and representatives of voluntary groups.

The planning meetings were open. Group members were encouraged to share ideas with others who had an interest in men's health. Anyone interested was encouraged to attend future meetings or to be involved on the day. Posters were displayed with a contact name for further information or involvement.

These open planning meetings were an essential element in making certain that the event was tailored to people's needs. The main subjects of interest to emerge were:

1. Prevention of coronary heart disease
2. Sports and fitness
3. Mental health
4. General practitioner profile
5. Men's groups/clubs
6. Disabled and advice services, e.g. CAB, Relate

Co-ordinators were appointed for each subject area and given responsibility for seconding appropriate people and organisations to help.

# Objectives

- To raise consciousness of factors which affect health.
- To introduce men to the means of monitoring a healthy lifestyle.
- To explore feelings and attitudes in relation to health issues in order to make personal decisions regarding health behaviour.

# What happened

Before the event

The Planning group met six times between May and the Information Day, which took place on Saturday 15 October 1988. In June, a press release was issued to all local newspapers inviting those interested to the planning meetings. In August, photocopied posters advertising the event were distributed throughout the Health District.

Press releases sent out in August and September resulted in substantial local media coverage and one local paper carried half page feature articles in three separate editions in October. This paper and another local paper carried half page advertisements about the event in October.

The local college of further education reproduced information leaflets for the event and these were widely distributed throughout the area using existing network systems. In addition, there was door to door distribution, and snooker clubs and local petrol stations were supplied with leaflets to distribute to members and customers.

The event

The Men's Health Information Day took place in a local school and the facilities were provided free of charge. One common-room was transformed into a bar selling non or low alcohol beers and wines and soft drinks. Crèche facilities were available and older children were entertained by staff trained in operating play schemes for 5–14-year-olds.

Advice stands were set out in the main hall; screening services were in a separate room; the gymnasium was used for coaching sessions in badminton and T'ai-Chi; a classroom served as a 'film studio' with a continuous programme of videos, networked for viewing in the bar and screening room.

Group sessions were held throughout the day in different classrooms and included 13 different topics.

# Impact

Of the 331 people who attended, 261 were men and of these 95 were screened. The results were recorded on screening forms and 69 completed forms were handed in. In addition, an evaluation form was given to every man attending the event with the request that it be completed and returned before he left. Only 54 forms were handed in. However, the views expressed by those who did complete questionnaires proved most helpful.

Participants felt that there were two main areas where improvements could have been made. Many felt that they had to queue for too long for fitness testing and cholesterol screening. The organisers were overwhelmed by the interest in screening and existing staff had difficulty keeping up with the demand. This was compounded by the fact that staffing levels were unavoidably lower than anticipated. To try to avoid queuing problems a numbering system was in operation, but despite this many men insisted on queuing. Examples of comments received:

Too long to wait for fitness testing.
Not enough equipment and staff on MOT.
More staff and equipment in MOT/fitness area.

**Fig. 2.2** A cartoon in the local press following the Men's Health Information Day (reproduced by courtesy of the *Lowestoft Advertiser*)

There was much interest in the group sessions, but those who attended felt that only allowing 30 minutes for each session was too short.

The majority of the feedback was positive. For example:

> A most useful and helpful day.
> Make it an annual event.
> More free MOTs clearly needed.
> Repeat it.

The day helped sharpen the focus on men's health issues. Following the event a self-help men's group was set up and a stop smoking group was run. A men's health initiatives group was formed and a series of information mornings have been run. These have had a health education emphasis and have included clinical screening with the omission of cholesterol testing.

The planning team is now designing a suitable questionnaire on coronary heart disease prevention for use at future events.

# Management

Fifteen-member multi-disiplinary, inter-agency planning group co-ordinated by the Senior Health Promotion Officer.

# Resources

The main resource involved in planning and running this event was people. The staff involved were mainly from the school where the event took place, Community Education, the District Health Promotion Service, the voluntary sector and general practitioners and health authority staff.

Leaflets were produced by Lowestoft College, and posters, screening forms and questionnaires came from the District Health Promotion Service.

The main expense was newspaper advertisements – £400. Small donations of £20 were made to a few of the organisations who took part, particularly those involved with the crèche and play scheme.

Two commercial organisations gave sponsorship totalling £65. The main funding came from the LAYH Community Projects Scheme.

# 3 Liverpool women's 10 km run

## Setting – public information and promotional activity

This event aims to encourage more women to enjoy sport, especially running. It is known that fewer women than men participate in sporting activities. It is also clear that regular exercise reduces the risk of coronary heart disease for everyone. The 'women only' run has been organised by Mersey Regional Health Authority and Liverpool City Council annually since 1987. It is part of a continuing programme of heart disease prevention activities organised by Mersey Regional Health Authority. The run has become a bigger event each year. In 1988 the LAYH Community Projects Scheme assisted with funding. Since then, the costs have been met from commercial sponsors, the Regional Health Promotion Unit, and the City Council. The event attracts participants from all over Britain and abroad, and national as well as local media attention.

**Fig. 3.1** Participants in the 1989 Liverpool Women's 10 km Run

**Key facts**

| | |
|---|---|
| **Location:** | Liverpool<br>Population 500 000 |
| **Timescale:** | Each run takes 12 months to plan |
| **Cost:** | £25 000 in 1989 plus administrative support from Regional Health Authority and City Council |
| **Sources of funding:** | Commercial sponsorship<br>Entry fees<br>Regional Health Authority<br>City Council |
| **Initiator:** | Health Promotion Officer, Mersey Regional Health Authority. |
| **Implementation led by:** | As above |
| **Special features:** | • Stimulated by local public demand<br><br>• Annual 'women only' run<br><br>• Produced simple training guide for the run<br><br>• High profile sporting event – wide media coverage<br><br>• Commercial sponsorship<br>• City-wide event involving multi-sectoral collaboration<br><br>• Local charity benefits<br><br>• Now recognised as a national event by Women's Cross Country and Road Racing Association and by British Sports Association for the Disabled |
| **Contact:** | Robin Ireland<br>Health Promotion Unit<br>Mersey Regional Health Authority<br>Hamilton House<br>Pall Mall<br>Liverpool L3 6AL |
| **Documentation:** | Evaluation of 1987 Run available from:<br><br>Malcolm Tungatt<br>Senior Research Officer<br>Sports Council Research Unit<br>Astley House<br>Quay Street<br>Manchester M3 4AE |

**Good practices**

- Substantial sponsorship
- Part of a Region-wide heart health promotion programme
- Could be repeated elsewhere
- Innovative idea
- Project evaluated
- Joint planning with the commercial sector, voluntary organisations, running clubs and the City Council
- Wheelchair entrants welcomed
- Grassroots activities stimulated
- Impact on women who have not previously taken part in sport
- Significant coverage in local and national media

# Origins

The idea for a women's run in Liverpool began with a telephone enquiry to Mersey Regional Health Authority's Health Promotion Unit. A small group of women runners were interested in the possibility of the city-wide run for women. They had spotted a newspaper report about a health promotion initiative to encourage exercise as a way of keeping healthy. The health promotion officer concerned, Robin Ireland, planned the first run and has been race director ever since.

# Objectives

- To present women with the opportunity of running in a 'women only' event.
- To stimulate local fitness programme initiatives.
- To encourage women to take up running as a way of keeping healthy.
- To promote women's sport in a positive and progressive manner.
- To fund-raise for a relevant charity.

# What happened

Planning

The run takes 12 months to plan. Approaches need to be made to potential sponsors early on in order to finance the project. The charity, which will be the beneficiary of sponsorship monies obtained by the runners, has to be chosen. An organising committee is set up with three to four people, including the race director, with each member having clear responsibilities. The Health Promotion Unit organises the marketing of the event, including press and publicity, and the City Council Sport and Recreation Division is responsible for administration, in particular the processing of entry forms. The City Council maintain close liaison with the police and city engineers with regard to the route. Nearer the actual day, a further eight or nine people are recruited to undertake specific tasks, such as public relations, administration and marshalling.

On the day

In the first year (1987) over 1800 women took part. In the subsequent years this figure increased to nearly 3000. This large scale type of event requires careful management on the day itself, in addition to the months of planning beforehand. Individuals are appointed to 'manage' the start, the course, facilities for the participants, including a crèche, and general enquiries. Overall around 250 volunteers are required. The run is now officially recognised as a national event by the Women's Cross Country and Road Racing Association and by the British Sports Association for the Disabled, which means proper arrangements for refereeing and timekeeping. It also means that the event welcomes and caters for runners of all abilities.

Media coverage

In 1989 there were over 30 reports about the run in newspapers, including three articles in the national press, and five minutes coverage on television. In the first year, the press was a principal source of information for those interested in taking part. The Health Promotion Unit, which also enlisted the support of the Regional Health Authority's public relations office, encourages considerable press coverage by circulating details of 'personal interest' stories. In 1989, these included the story of two runners with cystic fibrosis, who had heart and lung transplants, and the story of the eight sisters from one family who all took part.

# Impact

The 1987 run has been comprehensively evaluated by the Sports Council. A report will be available as part of the Sports Council's overall evaluation of Mersey's Health and Recreation Team Project. The following figures give an indication of the profile of the runners in 1987:

a) 30 per cent were taking part in their first ever run

b) 23 per cent took up running as a result of the Liverpool Women's Run

c) 38 per cent ran again in the 1988 Run

d) 50 per cent came from Merseyside

e) 40 per cent were aged between 25 and 35

In addition, the evaluation suggests that one of the most popular reasons for taking part was the opportunity to run in a 'women only' event. The runners were also attracted by the challenge presented and by the fact that the run was also to raise money for charity.

Each entrant was given a training programme with the entry application. The programme gives suggestions for gradually increasing running distances in order to prepare sensibly for the run, and has different schedules for beginners, improvers, and experienced runners. The evaluation identified that the programme was used by over half of the 'new' runners and by a quarter of all participants.

There was not such a comprehensive evaluation of the run in the subsequent year, but the analysis which has been carried out indicates a remarkable similarity in the age group profile of the runners, and a similar proportion coming from Merseyside as in the first year. One difference appears to be how the participants hear about the race. Now that it is an established event, more people hear about it from either running in previous years, or from friends, than from reports in the press.

# Management

The project is managed by the health promotion officer from Mersey Regional Health Authority in close collaboration with the City Council. When the first race was planned there was a large advisory group with key people throughout the city. There is now a much smaller implementation group of four people – two from the City Council and two from the Regional Health Authority. Briefing meetings are held with volunteers and marshalls before the event takes place.

# Resources

(1990 estimate)

| Expenditure | £ |
|---|---|
| Advertising, printing and stationery | 4 000 |
| Equipment (inc. marquees, clocks, radios, gantries) | 12 000 |
| Toilets | 2 000 |
| Parks staff | 4 000 |
| Other expenses | 3 000 |
| | 25 000 |
| Income | |
| Main sponsor | 10 000 |
| Secondary sponsor | 2 000 |
| Entry fees | 9 000 |
| City Park staff costs | 4 000 |
| | 25 000 |

In addition, the Regional Health Promotion Unit and the City Council jointly provide the administrative support required.

# 4 Project Health –

## Peterborough

### Setting – public information and promotional activity

Project Health is a joint initiative to promote healthy lifestyles, involving the health authority and the two local councils (Peterborough and Fenland). As part of this project regular health bulletins are produced aimed at key people in the community who are, or who could be, involved in coronary heart disease prevention. A variety of promotional materials has also been developed and there has been much coverage about coronary heart disease prevention in the local media.

**Key facts**

| | |
|---|---|
| **Location:** | Peterborough and Fenland<br>Population 200 000 |
| **Timescale:** | Health bulletins and promotional material begun 1989 and continuing |
| **Cost:** | £270 per issue of Health Bulletin<br>£2244 – Resources |
| **Sources of funding:** | LAYH Community Projects Scheme for bulletins and materials.<br>Small scale sponsorship by local companies.<br>Staff time provided by participating agencies |
| **Initiator:** | District Health Education Officer |
| **Implementation led by:** | District Health Education Officer as Project Health Co-ordinator |
| **Special features:** | • Bi-monthly Health Bulletins giving latest news on CHD prevention locally and nationally<br><br>• Distribution in Peterborough Health Authority<br><br>• Other materials include: leaflets, stickers, table mats, signs, bags, folders, fact cards and book marks<br><br>• Target audience key people in community<br><br>• Considerable local media coverage with 92 articles on CHD in past year<br>• Part of wider project including health policy development, e.g. food policy training courses for professionals. |
| **Contact:** | For further information contact:<br><br>Michael Watson<br>District Health Education Officer<br>Health Education Service<br>City Health Clinic<br>Wellington Street<br>Peterborough PE1 5DU<br>Tel: 0733 312931 |
| **Documentation:** | Project Health bulletins |

**Good practices**

- Objectives identified
- Multi-agency collaboration
  Health authority and two district councils
- Well produced material and information for key people in community
- Extensive media coverage ensures information reaches the general public
- Evaluation report on media coverage

# Pr♥ject HEAL♦H   BULLETIN 1

APRIL '89

### WELCOME TO THE FIRST PROJECT HEALTH BULLETIN

This is going to be a bi-monthly production from Peterborough's Health Education Service

   -giving you the latest news and developments on the prevention of coronary heart disease, locally and nationally

   - giving you the chance to share your ideas and views on coronary prevention

   - volunteers step forward please!

**Pr♥ject HEAL♦H** wants your news, your views.

Please put pen to paper and we look forward to your contributions in future editions.

**"CORONARY HEART DISEASE - REDUCING THE RISK"**

**A teaching pack produced by the Open University for primary health care teams - reviewed by Dr. L. Jacobs**

Coronary Heart Disease is the greatest single cause of death in Britain, yet we have made little impact on the high level of this problem in the community. In fact here in England, we are in the unenviable situation of having one of the highest death rates from heart attacks in the world - second only to Scotland!

This Open University pack is a collection of data presented in video and audio cassette and also in "book" form. It takes a detailed look at the causes of Coronary Heart Disease - the main ones being smoking, high cholesterol, high blood pressure and overweight - and discusses the various ways the primary health care team (i.e. doctors, nurses and health educators) can best tackle these difficult areas.

The pack describes various ways to screen for risk factors and whether we should aim not just at individuals but also at the general population by involving schools, the "media", adult education classes, etc. The details of these various schemes are described, showing how screening programmes can be set up in most situations, to gain maximum benefit. The pack should also be essential reading for those with responsibility for funding, so that proper resources can be channelled where they are really needed.

What we are all looking for is some improvement in our outlook for heart disease in the future, and on reading the pack it certainly gives us encouragement. For instance, in the USA for the past 10 years they have been following the broad preventative approach to Coronary Heart Disease - with less smoking, less fat in diet and more exercise, and they have achieved a 25% reduction in coronary events.

**Dates For Your Diary**

**Friday 21st April**
11.00 - 6.00
Health Fair incorporating BBC
Radio 2 live broadcast 3.30 - 5 pm
with Adrian Love
Cathedral Square, Peterborough

**Friday 26th May**
10.30 - 2.30
Women and Sport
Cathedral Square, Peterborough.

**FRIDAY 5th MAY**
Deadline for contributions to the
next **Pr♥ject HEAL♦H**
BULLETIN

**Fig. 4.1** Project Health bulletins bring together both local and national heart information

# Origins

Project Health was launched as a joint initiative between Fenland District Council, Peterborough City Council and Peterborough Health Authority with the long term aim to reduce the incidence of coronary heart disease in the district.

In Peterborough there were a number of people working in the field of coronary heart disease prevention and a variety of key people in the community who could be involved.

It was felt that a newsletter or bulletin (Fig. 4.1) would be useful in co-ordinating information about local and national activities. It was hoped that the newsletter would bring together those working in the area under the campaign umbrella of Project Health. Early market research showed that there was a positive interest and support for this initiative.

# Objectives

- To raise awareness and increase knowledge of key people about the:
    - extent of coronary heart disease
    - factors leading to coronary heart disease
    - ways in which coronary heart disease could be prevented
    - good initiatives in the District
    - resources available.

- To promote thought and discussion about coronary heart disease.

- To increase the commitment of key people to work on prevention of coronary heart disease.

- To unify the information given to the general public via key people.

- To make the national LAYH campaign relevant to people working in Peterborough Health Authority.

- To promote changes in the environment to make healthy choices more available.

# What happened

The first bulletin was produced in April 1989 and by April 1990 seven will have been produced. 1500 bulletins are printed each time and are distributed to key people in the local community. For example, local council officers, teachers, health workers, general practitioners, LAYH/Look After Yourself (LAYH/LAY) tutors, work-place managers and restaurant owners.

Information for the bulletins is collected by a health education officer who discusses with the District Health Education Officer the focus of each issue and what items to include. The material is then sent to a local printer who does the layout as well as printing the bulletins.

The four-page A4 bulletins focus on a different aspect of coronary heart disease prevention in each issue. In addition, they include diary dates for the next two months; information on recent reports and research; nutrition news; LAY courses and information on local and national initiatives.

The publicity materials and resources are produced by the Health Education Unit often adapting ideas that have been found to be useful elsewhere in the UK and building on the work of Project Smoke Free, a smoking education campaign run in the North West of England in the mid-eighties.

The District health education officer managed to negotiate with a local newspaper for regular half-page feature articles on aspects of coronary heart disease prevention (Fig. 4.2). Project Health issues regular press releases which are followed up by personal contact and this has resulted in substantial local media coverage in the past year.

**Fig. 4.2** Typical press coverage and promotional material for Peterborough's Project Health

# Impact

A report has been produced about the media work and the press coverage received by the Project. Feedback from training days indicated that the bulletins and promotional material have encouraged more key people in the community to become involved, but no formal evaluation has yet been completed.

# Management

The District health education officer acts as Project Health co-ordinator, and coronary heart disease prevention is one of the main priorities of the Health Education Unit.

The co-ordinator is supported by a multi-agency advisory group which meets once every two months to plan and evaluate Project Health activities. The group consists of representatives from the local councils and the community health council. There is also a LAYH/LAY tutor, a dietitian and an ethnic minority adviser. Action groups are set up for specific tasks bringing in other enthusiastic experts to the project, for example the food policy action group.

# Resources

The production costs for the bulletin are funded by the Health Education Authority under the LAYH Community Projects Scheme. A sum of £2750 has been allocated to the Project for this purpose. Each issue costs approximately £270 to produce.

A further grant of £2244 from the LAYH Community Projects Scheme was allocated for the production of a variety of promotional material.

A small amount of local sponsorship was obtained for competition prizes and specific leaflets.

The staff of the health education unit worked on producing the newsletter and the development of resources as part of the work of the unit. The LAYH award did not include an allowance for staff time but was entirely used for materials.

The production of news bulletins and promotional materials is only one element of Project Health. Other activities which come under the umbrella of Project Health are funded in a variety of different ways. For example, Henry the Heart Beatle is funded by the City Council, the mobile fitness testing unit is staffed by health professionals and the food policy conference was funded by Peterborough Health Authority.

# 5 Look After Your Heart –
## Avon

### Setting – region-wide

Look After Your Heart – Avon (LAYH – Avon) is a 12-member inter-agency programme, to co-ordinate and stimulate an inter-sectoral approach to heart disease prevention activities in the County of Avon. Officially launched in April 1988, the activities have included a training programme for health educators in group work skills, healthy eating, stopping smoking and stress management, a lifestyle survey of 1 in 50 adults in Avon, 'heart weeks' fitness testing and collaborative work for National No Smoking Days and other smoking prevention initiatives. In addition members promote activities within their own organisations. The programme has been successful in reaching the policy-makers in the participating agencies and involving field staff with a health promotion role in LAYH activities. The steering group is now concerned to increase community participation in LAYH – Avon, and a localities project is being funded that involves community health workers in two localities using a community based approach. The participating organisations are demonstrating their commitment by funding an assistant co-ordinator for the programme from 1990.

**Key facts**

| | |
|---|---|
| **Location:** | The County of Avon<br>Population one million |
| **Timescale:** | Originated 1987<br>Officially launched 1988<br>Ongoing |
| **Cost:** | £7000 for events to date<br>£50 000 per annum for three years for localities project commencing 1990<br>£20 000 per annum for three years for co-ordinator commencing 1990<br>Staff time provided by member agencies |
| **Sources of funding:** | LAYH Community Projects Scheme category 1 – 1989<br>LAYH Community Projects Scheme category 2 – 1990<br>Participating agencies<br>Sports Council |
| **Initiator:** | Avon Joint Care Planning Team |
| **Implementation led by:** | Frenchay Health Authority's District Health Education Officer |
| **Special features:** | • Intersectoral approach to heart disease prevention activities<br>• Project supported by 12 statutory agencies in Avon, under the auspices of Avon Joint Consultative Committee<br>• Official launch began process of raising public and professional awareness which also included:<br>– Production of publicity material and local media coverage<br>– Fitness testing<br>– 'Heart' weeks with a wide variety of activities<br>– Training programme for health educators involved in LAYH – Avon<br>– Collaborative work on smoking prevention initiatives<br>– Collaborative work with LEA and University in targeting schools |

- In addition members of the steering group promote LAYH activities in their own organisation
- Localities Project to develop greater community involvement

**Contact:** Ursula Miles, Chairperson
Look After Your Heart
Avon Steering Group
Frenchay Health Education Service
Beckspool Road
Frenchay Common
Bristol BS16 1ND
Tel: 0272 701070

**Documentation:** *Look After Your Heart – Avon*
*Heart week evaluation report 1989*
*Avon lifestyle survey report 1989*
*The CAFE Project, Yate*
*Progress Report June 1989*
Frenchay Health Education Service
Frenchay Health Authority

*Hartcliffe Healthy Eating Community Project*
Bristol Weston Health Authority
November 1989

LAYH – Avon report on activities 1989

LAYH – Avon publicity pack

*LAYH – Avon heart week schools report*
(In press)

*LAYH – Avon Constitution 1990*

**Good practices**

- Objectives identified
- Inter-agency collaborations
- Joint funding – LAYH
      Sports Council
      Participating organisations
- Staff and resource commitment from member organisations
- Avon – lifestyle survey provides useful planning information and baseline data
- Evaluation reports produced on each element of the programme supported the development of a larger more comprehensive programme
- LAYH – Avon managed by steering group which takes overall responsibility for policy, planning management and evaluation; members are high ranking in their organisations.
- Project has developed from modest beginnings. There is now a core team of assistant co-ordinator, two project workers and administrative staff. They are based in one health authority but work across the County of Avon.

# Origins

The County of Avon consists of four health districts and six local authorities with no shared boundaries. It has a population of nearly one million inhabitants in localities as diverse as seaside towns, rural villages, expanding housing developments and inner city populations. It poses particular challenges for health promotion especially around Bristol which is well-known for its large tobacco and wine industries.

LAYH – Avon originated in 1987 when the Avon Joint Care Planning Team under the Chairmanship of Frenchay Health Authority's District General Manager, Dr Paul Walker, discussed the WHO 'Health for All by Year 2000' issues, and focused particularly on ischaemic heart disease and its effect in Avon.

It was agreed that those organisations involved in the prevention of disease should meet and look at the feasibility of an Avon prevention programme. The District Health Education Officer at Frenchay Health Authority convened and chaired this meeting which led to setting up the LAYH – Avon Steering Group and the LAYH – Avon programme.

## Aim

To co-ordinate and stimulate an inter-sectoral approach to heart disease prevention activities and to monitor the progress of these activities.

## Objectives

Objectives have been defined for each of the various activities which comprise the LAYH – Avon Project.

## What happened

During the first year a number of activities took place under the heading of LAYH – Avon. People from a number of participating organisations allocated a percentage of their time to these initiatives. This amounted to the equivalent of three full-time staff. The official launch of LAYH – Avon was attended by member agencies' officers, members, chairmen and civic dignatories. This demonstrated political commitment to the

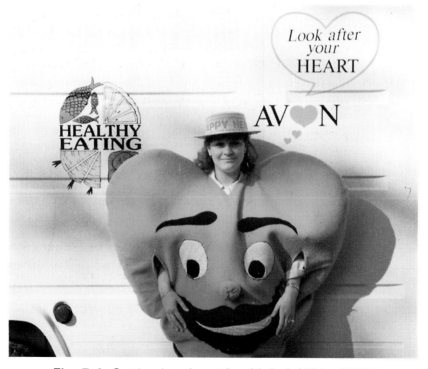

**Fig. 5.1** Getting into heart health in LAYH – AVON

programme and began the process of raising public and professional awareness. TV coverage of the event was estimated to be worth £12000. Since then commitment to the programme has increased the workforce from the participating agencies. Below is the programme of activities for Avon Heart Week October 1989.

A Lifestyle Survey carried out in April 1989 with 1 in 50 adults in Avon provided baseline data and information for planning.

Schools involvement is being initiated in two ways. Avon Heart Week gave opportunities for a variety of activities some of which are continuing. The Physical Education adviser, the University, two teachers and two members of the steering group are designing ways in which LAYH and exercise can combine in the Physical Education curriculum.

All Councils now run healthy eating schemes.

# Impact

Each element of the programme is evaluated and the lifestyle survey will provide useful baseline data. This survey will be repeated within the near future to monitor changes in knowledge and behaviour.

Joint activities and planning workshops have led to a firm commitment to the LAYH – Avon programme by the Steering Group and a belief that this method of working is a positive way forward for the promotion of good health in Avon.

Evaluation reports have shown that LAYH – Avon is successful in reaching the policy-makers in the participating agencies and involving field staff with a health promotion role in LAYH activities such as National No Smoking Day and LAYH – Avon Heart Week.

However, few community groups have responded to invitations to be involved, so in 1990, two community health project workers are being recruited to develop a community based approach in two different localities in the county.

There is now an established LAYH-Avon Training Programme which offers training on risk factors subjects to those interested in setting up groups in support of LAYH-Avon.

# Management

The steering group consists of senior officers from the Health Authorities and Councils as well as a representative from the Family Practitioner Committee and Public Health Medicine. It meets on average every six weeks and has overall responsibility for policy, planning, management and evaluation.

Chairing the Steering Group, co-ordinating activity and day to day management is the responsibility of the district health education officer for Frenchay Health Authority, who was appointed to this task by Avon Joint Consultative Committee in 1987.

By 1989, the co-ordination of this work became so time-consuming that the level of work could not be sustained. An application was supported by Avon Joint Consultative Committee for an assistant co-ordinator with effect from April 1990. The postholder will be directly managed by the Frenchay's district health education officer and will be located in Frenchay Health District to enable easy communication. However, the assistant co-ordinator will work right across Avon and this is totally acceptable to all member organisations.

The assistant co-ordinator will manage the two community health workers for the localities project.

# Resources

In the first two years LAYH–Avon has been financed in the main by member agencies, who contributed varying amounts of staff resources. Non-recurring finance has been allocated from participating agencies, budgets for specific events such as the programme launch in 1988 and LAYH–Avon Heart Week in 1989. This is likely to continue.

Awards have been secured for specific events from the Health Education Authority and Sports Council.

Sponsorship is being actively sought.

Funding for the assistant co-ordinator comes from the member agencies, each of which is contributing a share based on the size of its population. This formula is in accordance with the recommendation of the Avon Joint Consultative Committee.

The localities project is being funded for three years from the Health Education Authority's LAYH Community Projects Scheme.

# 6 Chislehurst health week

## Setting – primary health care

This health week, focusing on preventing heart disease in the Chislehurst area, was organised by a team of local health professionals and interested lay people. The project was co-ordinated by a General Practice medical receptionist. Events included talks on health topics with schoolchildren, youth and community groups, and an exercise club. The culmination of the week was a health fair on the Saturday (Fig. 6.1) which was very well attended. The fair consisted of a number of stands and exhibits, demonstrations, children's entertainments and a Fun Run (Fig. 6.2). Many visitors to the fair completed a health questionnaire, which produced a collective picture of their health status.

**Fig. 6.1** Fitness testing at the health fair during Chislehurst's health week

**Key facts**

| | |
|---|---|
| **Location:** | Chislehurst, Kent Population 16 000 – mainly commuters and their families |
| **Timescale:** | 21 months to plan; 6 day event |
| **Cost:** | £2938 |
| **Sources of funding:** | Local fund-raising Rotary Club LAYH Community Projects Scheme |
| **Initiator:** | General Practice |
| **Implementation led by:** | General Practice medical receptionist |
| **Special features:** | • Provision of health information to the general public

• Community run

• Large number of volunteers assisting

• Health questionnatire

• Children and young adults participated

• GP involvement

• Multi-sectoral collaboration |
| **Contact:** | Rosalind Eunson 38 The Ridge Orpington Kent BR6 8AQ |
| **Documentation:** | Project evaluation report submitted to the Health Education Authority |

**Good practices**

- Objectives identified
- Younger age group targeted
- Report on planning and implementation
- Ideas or format could be used elsewhere
- Resources identified
- Collaboration between health professionals and local community
- Attracted popular support

**Fig. 6.2** Waiting for the starter before the Fun Run during Chislehurst's health week

# Origins

A medical receptionist undertook the local health week as part of an academic project. This project had the support of the GPs who were keen to develop heart disease prevention work. The aim was a framework for transmitting a number of important health messages in an effort to reduce local rates of coronary heart disease.

# Objectives

- To reduce the number of people suffering heart attacks in Chislehurst.
- To raise awareness of the ways in which people can improve their health.
- To highlight the effects on health of smoking, diet, exercise, alcohol and stress.
- To attract people not normally in receipt of preventative health education.
- To encourage as many local people as possible to become involved in the week.

# What happened

It was initially decided that there would be two main elements to the week: a series of health talks to various groups during the week and a Health Fair on the Saturday. The two other practices in Chislehurst were invited and agreed to participate. A formal Steering Committee was established to guide the planning. The Committee members included GPs, the District Health Education Officer, a councillor, Townswomen's Guild representatives, a member of the Community Health Council and of the local Chamber of Commerce and the medical receptionist (see Key facts).

The first major task was to finance the venture. A letter to 200 organisations inviting donations raised £1025. The Rotary Club gave £1000 and the LAYH programme of the HEA made an award of £1500 available. Entry to the fair was free and all participants gave their time voluntarily.

Health talks led by a doctor and a nutritionist were arranged for local schools and community groups.

Health professionals and voluntary groups were invited to organise stands and various activities for the Health Fair.

To attract as many as possible, the event was well publicised:

a) a student from the local art college designed the publicity material

b) local newspapers were given details and reported both the planning and the event itself

c) a banner was displayed across the High Street during the week

d) schools were circulated with entry forms for the Fun Run

e) publicity material was distributed to surgeries, shops, library, halls, schools and the local clinic

f) programmes giving full details of the events at the Health Fair were circulated with the local free paper.

The health week itself

One local school did a painting project on dental health and one school devised a dice game, and prepared posters on healthy eating.

A total of 208 children participated in talks in school. In addition, there were sessions on health topics at meetings of the Boys Brigade, Scouts, Guides, Cubs and Brownies, Townswomen's Guild, Rotary Club, exercise club and school Parents Associations.

The fair lasted from 11 am to 4 pm. It was estimated that between 1000 and 1500 people attended. Each visitor was given a health questionnaire to complete, asking for information about lifestyles and screening histories; 418 questionnaires were completed.

The many health checks on offer were the most popular attractions. These included tests on blood pressure and fitness. There were queues all day for these stands. Some people were referred to their GP for follow-up checks.

Other busy stands included those on dental health, stress, vision screening, alcohol consumption, and those staffed by the Red Cross, health visitors, the Family Practitioner Committee and Age Concern. Less busy stands, partly because of their location, were those on Women's Health, yoga and Lifestyles.

There was also a dance display, a disco-dance session, keep fit to music, library and children's bouncing castle (450 children had a go).

The two-mile Fun Run was started by Dr Alan Maryon-Davis. There were over 1000 entrants. Babies in pushchairs and dogs on leads were allowed.

# Impact

This was a popular venture with almost 2000 local people participating in some event connected with the Health Week. The Fair was particularly well thought of. Many visitors made favourable comments and expressed gratitude at having the opportunity to obtain information or have a test without going to their doctor.

The health questionnaire was completed by 418 visitors to the Fair, of whom 245 people came from Chislehurst. The questionnaires from this group of respondents were analysed. The results showed that these people followed a broadly healthy lifestyle, particularly in relation to drinking, smoking and diet. However, just under half did not have regular screening checks and very few took sufficient regular exercise. These two results have implications for the orientation of the work of the local health professionals.

The week was also a success from the point of view of collaboration between health professionals and representatives from the local community.

The Steering Committee is considering holding another Fair in three years time. The kinds of improvements which they would make include: more frequent reporting to the press, more managers to enable delegation, a larger hall to accommodate all the stands in one area and earlier Fun Run publicity.

In 1990 follow-up questionnaires are being sent out to 100 randomly selected respondents to the original questionnaire. The aim is to identify what effect the Health Week had on lifestyles and subsequent presentation for screening.

# Management

The Health Week activities were co-ordinated by the medical receptionist from a local group practice, who was supported by a formal steering committee. Planning started 21 months before the event took place.

# Resources

The cost of this project was as follows:

| | |
|---|---|
| Administration | £311 |
| Publicity | £1192 |
| Fair and Fun Run | £1355 |
| Miscellaneous | £80 |
| Total | £2938 |

The time of the organiser, health professionals and others was given freely.

# 7

# Look After Your Heart in the workplace – International Computers Limited

## Setting – workplace

Employers in England are becoming increasingly aware of the benefits of having a healthy workforce. At least 25 million working days are lost every year and 21 per cent of all male absence from work is caused by heart and circulatory disease. Heart disease is an expensive illness.

The LAYH Programme is encouraging employers to agree to undertake measures to combat heart disease in their workplace. Those that do sign a Look After Your Heart Charter.

ICL (International Computers Limited) signed up in April 1987 and since that time an ongoing series of wide ranging activities have taken place to improve staff fitness and provide a work environment conducive to good health.

**Key facts**

| | |
|---|---|
| **Location:** | All ICL sites<br>Total workforce in the UK is 15 000 based at 90 office and manufacturing locations |
| **Timescale:** | Ongoing activities since LAYH charter signed in April 1987 |
| **Cost:** | No substantial additional costs |
| **Sources of funding:** | Met from existing occupational health budgets<br>Leaflets and assistance provided by local health promotion units |
| **Initiator:** | Chief occupational health nursing officer |
| **Implementation led by:** | ICL occupational health service |

**Special features:**
- Healthy eating promoted on all sites
- Most occupational health nurses trained as Look After Yourself tutors
- Occupational health nurses routinely check blood pressures
- LAYH displays on different sites
- Sponsored slimming
- Occupational health nurses run smoking cessation classes
- Stress control, aerobic and yoga classes held in the lunch break
- Prevention services available to local community around some ICL sites

**Contact:**
Joan Corboy RGN
Chief Nursing Officer
ICL Occupational Health Unit
Carlton House
27a Carlton Drive
London SW15 2TE
Tel: 071-788 7272

**Good practices**

- Objectives identified
- Project could be repeated and adapted according to location needs
- Minimal resources required
- Minimal time away from work
- Used as part of company quality programme

# Origins

When the company agreed to sign the LAYH charter in April 1987, they examined ways in which they could fulfil the criteria for joining. The occupational health department developed a programme which would have maximum impact and minimum expenditure. Participation by employees was to be voluntary.

# Objectives

- To enable employees to understand and improve their own and their families' lifestyles.
- To minimise the cost of ill health to the company.
- To improve staff morale.
- To raise the profile of the occupational health service.

**Fig. 7.1** Fitness testing – one of the wide variety of activities available to promote health within ICL

## What happened

A wide variety of activities have taken place in sites throughout the company. To date:

- 9320 employees have been seen on 45 locations at LAYH events. These events include fitness testing and blood pressure screening and are offered on an annual basis

- 4000 employees have been seen for blood pressure screening

- 2500 employees have been seen for individual 'MOT' sessions

- 500 employees have been seen for fitness testing using static equipment and a computer

- 500 senior management employees have received annual health checks

## Impact

The programme was successful in generating much activity and interest without extra funds.

Evaluation forms received after LAYH events were positive and employees were appreciative of the efforts of the occupational health nurses.

ICL have now helped other firms set up workplace programmes.

The occupational health staff have also benefited from implementing the scheme.

## Management

The programme has been managed by the occupational health service of ICL with the support of senior management and with help from local health promotion units.

## Resources

The ICL Look After Your Heart programme has been achieved by re-arrangement of the duties of the occupational health nurses. Small additional costs were incurred:

1 Purchases of necessary equipment, including the Look After Yourself Display

2 Additional travel and subsistence costs incurred in running LAYH events at remote locations.

These costs were absorbed within existing occupational health budgets. Free leaflets and assistance were provided by local health promotion units.

# Schools project –

## 8

# education about coronary heart disease, Birmingham

## Setting – schools and youth service

Working in three inner-city, multi-racial primary schools in Birmingham, the study showed how parents and young children perceived and understood illness and health, and how this related to their views of coronary heart disease (Fig. 8.1). New strategies for the development of work in this field were recommended. Based on this work the LAYH programme is now supporting a project to develop effective ways for professionals to work in partnership with parents' groups on coronary heart disease prevention.

**Key facts**

| | |
|---|---|
| **Location:** | 3 inner-city multiracial primary schools in Central Birmingham |
| **Timescale:** | 1988–89 |
| **Cost:** | £4995 |
| **Sources of funding:** | LAYH Community Projects Scheme |
| **Initiator:** | Dr Gill Combes<br>Schools Health Education Adviser<br>Central Birmingham Health Authority<br><br>Dorit Brown<br>(then) Development Officer<br>Family Education Unit<br>Community Education Development<br>Centre, Coventry |
| **Implementation led by:** | Joint research work between initiator and Development Officer in the Family Education Unit, Community Education Development Centre in Coventry. |

**Special features:**
- Explored perceptions of health and illness with groups of children aged 6 and 10 years
- Discussed children's work with their parents and looked with them at key questions on health
- Recommended development of appropriate health education strategies based on findings

**Contact:**
Gill Combes
Development Officer
Family Education Unit
Community Education Development Centre
Lyng Hall, Blackberry Lane
Coventry CV2 3JS
Tel: 0203 638660

**Documentation:**
Combes, G. and Braun, D. (1989). *Everything gives you heart attacks these days.* Children's and parents' experiences and understanding of health and illness in relation to coronary heart disease prevention in three primary schools in Central Birmingham. Report to the Health Education Authority (LAYH Programme)

**Good practices**
- Objectives identified
- Exploring need for appropriate health education from children and their parents' point of view
- Report sets out clearly how research was carried out. Others could repeat
- Resources identified
- Research report provided
- Recommendations for improved provision of health education to this age group
- Report used to stimulate further work building on findings – looking at effective ways for professionals to work with parents on CHD prevention

# Origins

Health educators are being encouraged to work with primary school children in the area of coronary heart disease prevention. Very little information exists about how young children perceive and understand heart disease or the links between their lifestyle and health.

In addition, parents are a major influence on the ideas and views of young children. They make many decisions for them which directly affect their health. Information about parents' perceptions and understandings is also important when determining what an appropriate health education strategy might be.

As both researchers had local and national experience of curriculum development and of research in health education, they felt that a collaborative project between the Health Authority and the Community Education Development Centre would provide useful information for planning and delivering 'healthy heart' education about coronary heart disease in schools.

To develop appropriate work in schools on coronary heart disease perception, the researchers felt it was necessary to work with groups of children and their parents to explore experiences and understandings of coronary heart disease, in the context of health and illness.

The focus of the research was in inner city schools with high proportions of pupils from ethnic minorities. Three schools in central Birmingham were selected. In two of the schools the majority of pupils were of Asian origin and in the third school there were fewer Asian and more Afro-Caribbean pupils.

# Objectives

- To work with small groups of children aged 6 and 10 years, to explore their perceptions of health and illness.

- To invite parents to meetings two to three weeks after the work with their children to discuss key questions on health.

- To look at the implications of the research for the development of an appropriate health education strategy.

# What happened

Method

In each school the researchers worked with small groups of children aged 6 and 10 years (usually six in a group) for around 30 minutes, to explore their perceptions of health and illness. They also worked with the children's parents to discuss with them their children's ideas and their own views of health and illness.

The discussions with the children were structured very carefully in order to ensure that the approach was child-centred and the questions were open-ended. In each school the first group of children were used as a pilot for the questions which were then revised in the light of that group's response. The researchers asked the same questions of children in both age groups.

**Fig. 8.1** Two of the drawings produced by children during Birmingham's CHD school project – making vegetable soup and parts of the body

Both researchers were in the room with the children and took it in turns to lead the discussion or keep a record of the children's ideas. They chose not to tape record discussions because they felt it might be off-putting to children and inhibit discussion.

A different approach was taken in each school to explore the potential of different health education approaches. In School 1 the starting point was illness; in School 2 it was lifestyles and in School 3 it was body awareness.

In all the schools the researchers and children sat in a circle and after introductions the children were asked to do a drawing. This allowed them to settle down and gave each child an opportunity to express their ideas.

Discussions with parents took place in two of the schools. At the third school the parents' meeting that was arranged was not supported by the parents invited.

**Summary of findings**

Open-ended discussion groups revealed a wealth of complex understanding and experience related to health. The breadth of issues raised contrasted sharply with the relatively narrow set of health topics on the schools' curricula. Many children had apparent high levels of knowledge about topics such as smoking, nutrition and hygiene, but this was rarely grounded in understanding and bore little relation to their own experiences.

Parents had complex and realistic views about their role in their child's health. However, they were commonly seen by the schools as in need of advice or health education themselves, particularly concerning stress and the difficulties they experienced in using the Health Service.

The study showed that a topic based approach to the health education curriculum falls far short of either meeting children's needs or constructively relating to their existing understanding and experiences. The children and parents in the study did not experience the world in compartments or topics, such as nutrition, exercise or smoking. In addition they raised a number of issues as crucial to their health which rarely or never feature on a topic-based curriculum – bullying, environmental concerns, life changes, loss and death.

The study showed clearly how parents' and children's needs and experiences are intertwined. Child health cannot be divorced from family health and parental involvement is therefore not an option or added extra.

# Impact

The researchers originally intended to develop teaching material based on the outcomes of the action-research. However, this was felt not to be appropriate once the research had been completed. The research method did itself suggest useful classroom approaches which could have been translated into teaching materials but the key issue which emerged was about changing the basis for health education work in schools.

It was decided to invite teachers from the three schools involved in the research to a pilot in-service day. This was attended by eight teachers from the three schools and one health visitor. Although school nurses were invited none were able to attend. The day provided participants with a structured opportunity to re-think their understanding of the schools' role in health education.

Recommendations

Teachers and health workers need to re-think their role in a number of respects. They need to come to terms with the complexity of issues surrounding a broader concept of health and to acknowledge that a medical view of health issues is both limited and limiting.

Professionals need to recast their role from being experts who 'know' all about health to being facilitators who can support individuals, families and communities in improving their own health. This will mean providing support and resources on people's own terms and starting from their identified needs. This shift in role requires training and support.

The research highlights the need for all those professionals with a health promotion and education role to support the development of community based approaches to health education.

Development of this work

Arising from the recommendations of this study the Community Education Development Centre has started a project funded by the LAYH Community Projects Scheme exploring new approaches to developing partnerships with families on coronary heart disease prevention. This project is being developed in conjunction with a larger project on working with parent groups, funded by the Bernard Van Leer Foundation.

# Management

The school project was managed by the District Health
Education Officer for central Birmingham, supported by the
researcher from the Community Education Development
Centre, with agency support.

Timescale

| | |
|---|---|
| Planning and setting up work | – September–October 1988 |
| Work with children | – November–December 1988 |
| Parents' meetings | – January 1989 |
| Review of progress and preliminary report | – February–March 1989 |
| Planning training | – April 1989 |
| Pilot training | – May 1989 |
| Final report | – June 1989 |

# Resources

The cost of the project was as follows:

| Funding | £ |
|---|---|
| Travel | 250 |
| Hire of interpreters and crèche workers | 150 |
| Refreshments for Parents' meetings | 50 |
| Research service costs to collaborating organisation | 3295 |
| Production costs for mounted display of children's work | 50 |
| Costs of running pilot in-service training (teachers cover costs, lunch, training materials) | 900 |
| Materials, photocopying, report production | 300 |
| Total | 4995 |

# 9

# Healthy eating guidelines for school caterers –
## Hereford and Worcester

## Setting – schools and youth service

A consortium of District Health Authorities, the local education authority and the environmental health departments in the county of Hereford and Worcester has been formed to improve the nutrition standards of school meal provision. As part of this programme, healthy eating guidelines for school caterers are being produced. These will be mailed to each school caterer and head teacher simultaneously. School caterers will be invited to launch days in various localities and a training programme will be established.

**Key facts**

| | |
|---|---|
| **Location:** | The county of Hereford and Worcester |
| **Timescale:** | Planning meetings started Autumn 1989<br>Guidelines and menus piloted Spring 1990<br>Launch proposed for Autumn 1990 |
| **Cost:** | £5000 |
| **Sources of funding:** | LAYH Community Projects Scheme<br>Health Education Units |
| **Initiator:** | Hereford and Worcester Consortium on Healthy School Meals |
| **Implementation led by:** | District Health Education Officers of Kidderminster and District Health Authority and Worcester Health Authority |
| **Special features:** | • Guidelines to include set of menus to cover three weeks, which translate the advice to caterers into practice |

- The information in the guidelines will be nutritionally sound, have customer acceptability and be profitable

- A dissemination and training programme has been planned

- Monitoring by school nurses using standardised assessment form

**Contact:**  John Grigg
District Health Education Officer
Kidderminster & District Health Authority,
6 The Crescent
Cookley
Kidderminster DY10 3RY
Tel: 0562 851677

**Documentation:**  Guidelines in production

**Good practices**

- Objectives identified

- Careful background research

- Co-ordinated approach adopted

- Practical approach translating philosophy into costed menus

- Involves joint planning

- Target group – school caterers

- Forms part of wider CHD prevention programmes which included education of children about healthy choices

# Origins

Following the Education Act of 1980, Hereford and Worcester County Council stopped its school meals service to primary schools and its service to middle and high schools ceased in 1984.

Private contractors at present provide the majority of the school meals and local research has shown that overall healthy eating choice has declined to a low ebb. Previous attempts to improve school meals have not been successful because of lack of guidance and co-ordination between caterers.

A number of documents including the Coronary Prevention Group's *Diet or disease, the case for school meals guidelines* and the Community Nutrition Group's *Nutrition guidelines for school meals* have highlighted the great need for concentrated effort to raise the standard of school meals. It was decided that realistic help should be offered to caterers, bearing in mind the profit motive constraint of the majority of services.

# Objectives

- To increase awareness amongst those responsible for the production of school meals, of the need to provide a healthier food choice for children.

- To develop a set of guidelines for school caterers widening the healthy eating choices within realistic budget limits. Guidelines based on NACNE, COMA, Coronary Prevention Group and Community Nutrition Group, diets of British schoolchildren.

- To develop a set of interesting three one-week menus which translate healthy eating guidelines into practice.

- To disseminate the project to school governors, head teachers and school caterers through a series of workshops.

- To co-ordinate the dissemination with a newly developed *Healthy eating for life* schoolchildren's education pack.

- To work closely with the Local Education Authority to ensure that the guidelines for school caterers become a policy document to be issued to prospective competitive tenderers for the School Meals Service.

# What happened

The project began in January 1990 and is still in the early days of development. Draft guidelines and suggested menus have been produced by the dietitian member of the consortium and these will be piloted in a variety of different schools throughout the county. It is planned that the guidelines will be launched in the autumn.

# Management

The monthly meetings of the consortium are chaired by Worcester's District Health Education Officer. The guidelines are being prepared and piloted by Worcester's District dietitian. Other members of the consortium will play a more active role at different phases of the development, dissemination and training.

# Resources

An award of £4500 from the LAYH Community Projects Scheme was made for the production of the guidelines including printing, promotions and publicity. This sum will also contribute to the cost of training and dissemination and evaluation.

A total of £500 has been contributed by the Health Education Units.

These figures do not include the staff time of officers from the health authorities and local authority.

# 10

# Look After Your Heart campaign – programme of community initiatives, Newcastle upon Tyne

## Setting – community

The Northern Region has the highest incidence of heart disease in the country and within the Region there are pockets of longstanding ill health and deprivation. The campaign was co-ordinated by the Secretary of Newcastle Community Health Council acting as voluntary co-ordinator of the city's Community Initiatives. It was targeted at adults in Newcastle, in wards with a concentration of socio-economic groups including a high proportion of unemployed, who were likely to be at risk from coronary heart disease (CHD). Other target groups were the Asian community and relatives of sufferers from heart disease. A variety of community based initiatives were carried out, commencing in 1987 and continuing to the present day.

**Key facts**

| | |
|---|---|
| **Location:** | Newcastle upon Tyne<br>Population 192 000 |
| **Timescale:** | Commenced Summer 1987<br>Still continuing |
| **Cost:** | £5000 in 1987<br>£4900 in 1989 |
| **Sources of funding:** | LAYH Community Projects Scheme<br>Staff time<br>Facilities provided by participating agencies |
| **Initiator:** | Secretary, Newcastle Community Health Council in liaison with the Health Education Unit and Newcastle Community Health Projects |
| **Implementation:** | Voluntary Co-ordinator Community Initiatives |
| **Special features:** | • Information about CHD prevention at summer events in inner city neighbourhoods<br><br>• Newsletter on LAYH circulated in inner city areas<br><br>• Promotion of health days on LAYH at community health projects<br><br>• Use of theatre group to support the campaign<br><br>• Events for Asian communities<br><br>• Self-help group for relatives of sufferers from CHD<br><br>• LAYH information and screening at unemployment benefit offices (Fig. 10.1) |
| **Contact:** | Vera Bolter<br>Community Initiatives<br>48 Osborne Road<br>Jesmond<br>Newcastle Upon Tyne NE22 2AL<br>Tel: 091-281 6311 |
| **Documentation:** | Progress reports to Health Education Authority |

**Good practices**

- Objectives identified
- Joint planning/multi-agency collaboration including Health Authority, City Council, voluntary and community groups
- Organisation of the pooling of facilities and resources by the co-ordinating group
- Targeted at certain high risk groups
- Regular progress reports provided
- Expenditure identified
- Innovative activity using a theatre group
- Initial activities stimulated further action
- Co-ordinated approach highlighted the value of liaison and collaboration in a city where many different initiatives are developed.

# Origins

The co-ordinating group representatives of community health projects in Newcastle felt that publicity through the media and the approaches from the statutory authorities might not be reaching those most at risk. They submitted proposals for a community based project targeted at wards in Newcastle with a concentration of unemployed people and those suffering from longstanding ill health and deprivation.

The co-ordinating group had the support of the Health Authority and the local authority plus access to local events and to premises based in the relevant areas of the city. All the community health projects and the self-help project would be able to include aspects of the campaign into their regular activities. The Health Authority's Health Education Unit and the Priority Area teams network of the Local Authority would also support the campaign.

# Objectives

- To enable the LAYH campaign to reach high risk groups in priority areas of the city.
- To initiate 'fun' activities and materials in a style and language relevant to the communities in the priority areas.

- To build on existing group activities and to extend support groups and self-help initiatives.
- To increase the uptake of LAYH/LAY courses and 'Save a life' demonstrations.

# What happened

A variety of community initiatives have taken place since 1987.

| | |
|---|---|
| Festivals and fun events | The Health Education Unit's caravan containing an LAYH display and stocked with campaign material visited five inner city neighbourhood festivals or fun events each summer. The van was staffed by a LAY tutor, a health education officer and a health visitor. Visitors were given a health check and were presented with an LAYH information pack |
| Health Matters – newsletter | A special LAYH issue of Health Matters, a newsletter circulating in inner city areas, was published by the information worker of Newcastle CHC and distributed. |
| Community health projects – promotion of health days on LAYH | Health days have been run in conjunction with community health projects using the caravan and the services of a theatre group. Drama Works were commissioned to write and perform a series of short sketches around the LAYH theme and suitable for a wide range of audiences. The show, 'Heart to Heart', was performed in local shopping centres, luncheon clubs, pop-ins and toddler groups. A video recording of a performance at a Community Health Project was commissioned and is available on loan or sale. |
| Work with Asian communities | A series of discussions with workers with ethnic minority communities and community leaders at the Community Relations Council was helpful in exploring the opportunities to reach out to people of Asian background. A keep fit course linked to LAY was organised for a group of Bangladeshi women meeting at a playgroup centre and a LAY course was organisd for community workers with ethnic minorities. The Community Relations Council jointly sponsored a seminar on 'Heart-health and Asians on Tyneside', and a further seminar was organised which brought together Asian women and health workers in October 1989 on the topic 'Asian Communities and Changing Lifestyles'. |
| Development of self-help | The idea of a self-help group for the relatives of sufferers of heart disease is being slowly developed by the self-help project of Newcastle CVS. |

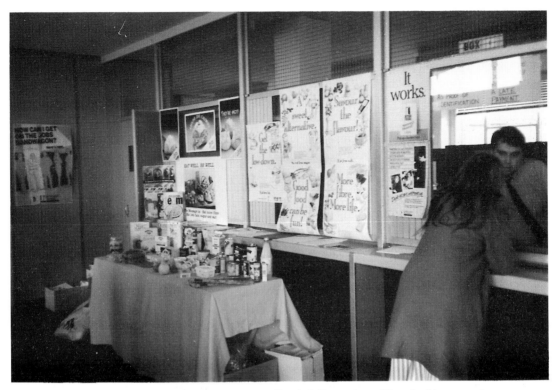

**Fig. 10.1** The LAYH display in a Social Security office in Newcastle

Work with unemployed people

During 1989, emphasis was given to work with unemployed people. Two unemployment benefit offices were selected and the LAYH exhibition and a simple screening service were provided over a two-week period (Fig. 10.1). This initiative was the idea of the manager for community nursing services, whose staff were involved in this project, in addition to LAYH/LAY tutors. The community nursing services won the Health Authority's first 'Achievement Award' for this scheme.

# Impact

The project was evaluated by recording the numbers of people reached by each community event; by the uptake of health promotion facilities resulting from the campaign and by providing a descriptive account of each initiative and a commentary on its effectiveness based on the subjective assessments of the organisers and participants. The campaign organisers felt that an outside objective assessment although desirable was beyond their means.

Regular progress reports were produced which provided the information outlined above.

## Assessment of community festivals and fun events

All the staff involved felt the occasions were worthwhile and were pleased with the quality of the events as well as the numbers of contacts. The organisers feel that it is a myth that inner-city residents do not want information. Their evidence was that they need more information rather than less; but they also require opportunities to discuss the information they have before deciding to act on it.

Valuable lessons were learnt about the choice of locations and the best method of attracting public attention.

## Assessment of health days and the theatre group performances

Feedback from the workers involved was positive in that they felt they reached out to people who would not otherwise have been aware of the campaign. The best location for the caravan was in the car park near to the entrance of a supermarket.

The theatre group was very popular. Audiences felt that this was a novel way of presenting health messages and was enjoyable and not off-putting. The friendly and informal approach of the actors was appreciated wherever they went. The theatre company produced their assessment of the performances. They felt that theatre can provide a very special means of communicating feelings and reactions, but they thought that the brief for future projects should be less ambitious about the variety of different audiences. Specific performances for certain client groups might be better.

## Work with Asian communities

The seminar proved helpful in gaining interest and commitment to further activities. For example, the Community Relations Council is now committed to organising talks, events and exhibitions at centres used by the relevant communities, and materials are being translated into the relevant languages.

The seminar illustrated how stress and heart disease and stress and racism are areas that are least understood, and the campaign is involved in further work in exploring these issues. In particular, the LAYH video in Asian languages is being shown to small groups in their own homes, with community workers using a questionnaire to assess effectiveness.

# Management

The first award was made to Newcastle Community Health Council as the secretary was in close liaison with the Health Education Unit and Newcastle Community Health Projects. The co-ordinator was supported by a co-ordinating group, which met monthly. As different schemes were planned a person in the group was identified as taking the lead and a planning sub-group was set up.

When the co-ordinator retired from her post as Secretary at the Community Health Council in 1988, she continued to act as co-ordinator on the Community Initiatives Project on a volunary basis. The Health Education Unit provided a base and secretarial assistance.

# Resources

The first award of £5000 was made for the work on community initiatives in 1987. The money was placed in a building society account with the co-ordinator and the Honorary Chairman of the Community Health Council acting as trustees. When the link with the Community Health Council ceased in 1988, the District Health Education Officer replaced the Honorary Chairman of the Community Health Council as a trustee for the award.

The first award covered the period 1987–88. A second sum of £4500 was awarded in 1989 for further work.

The money was spent on resources, materials, venues, seminars, theatre group and fees for speakers and LAYH/LAY tutors.

Secretarial support was initially provided by the Community Health Council but was taken over by the Health Education Unit in 1988. The participating agencies provided staff time and facilities. The co-ordinator gave her time freely, following her retirement in 1988.

# 11 Project Lionheart –
## East Dorset

## Setting – community

Community prevention programmes have significantly helped to reduce coronary heart disease in other countries, especially in Finland and the USA. Project Lionheart in East Dorset draws from these experiences. It is an innovative and comprehensive community action programme designed to help meet local targets to reduce the number of premature deaths from the disease. Volunteers, professionals and the public collaborate in the promotion of healthier lifestyles and better health. The area chosen for the development of the first stage of the project was the rural community around the village of Wool. The next stage involved a suburban area of Poole.

**Key facts**

| | |
|---|---|
| **Location:** | Rural village of Wool and surrounding area.<br>Population 7000<br>Suburban estate of Canford Heath, Poole.<br>Population 14 000 |
| **Timescale:** | Two years' facilitator intervention period<br>Wool 1987–89<br>Canford Heath 1989–91<br>Thereafter local responsibility |
| **Cost:** | Wool – £24 000<br>Canford Heath – £40 000 |
| **Sources of funding:** | East Dorset Health Authority<br>British Heart Foundation<br>LAYH Community Projects Scheme<br>TV South Trust |
| **Initiator:** | Director of East Dorset Heart Programme |

| | |
|---|---|
| **Implementation led by:** | Project Director acted as facilitator in Wool. Project Officer appointed for Canford Heath |
| **Special features:** | <ul><li>Comprehensive community profile prepared</li><li>Programme developed based on community needs</li><li>Facilitated by professionals</li><li>Supported by volunteers</li><li>Builds on existing community networks</li><li>Development of stand-alone groups</li></ul> |
| **Contact:** | Lesley Shucksmith<br>Project Director<br>East Dorset Heart Programme<br>Victoria House<br>Princes Road<br>Ferndown<br>Wimborne<br>Dorset BH22 9JR |
| **Documentation:** | *Interim report – Project Lionheart, Wool* and *Interim report – Project Lionheart, Canford Heath* available from the above address. The final report will be available from April 1991. |

**Good practices**

- Community participation
- Professionals used as facilitators
- Low cost and long term benefits
- Model designed to be adaptable for use elsewhere
- Multi-sectoral collaboration

# Origins

In their document *Health for East Dorset* published in January 1987, the Department of Public Health Medicine set out target reduction aims for individual risk factors and an overall aim to reduce by 30 per cent premature deaths from heart disease by the year 2000. Project Lionheart is a comprehensive programme designed to help meet those targets. The area chosen for the development of the first stage of the project was a rural community centred around the village of Wool with a target population of about 7000. This was a pilot to investigate the feasibility of neighbourhood prevention schemes in general, as well as providing a community based coronary heart disease prevention programme for Wool. Having ascertained that the model was workable, it was repeated in Canford Heath, a high density, modern suburban area of Poole with a fast-growing catchment population of about 14 000.

# Objectives

- To investigate the feasibility of neighbourhood prevention programmes.

- To involve all sectors of the local community in the promotion of healthier lifestyles and better health.

- To establish an independent steering group.

- To develop an adaptable model which might be useful elsewhere and to others.

# What happened

The East Dorset Heart Programme Project Director devoted approximately half her hours, for a period of two years, to acting as facilitator in the development of Project Lionheart in Wool. The first task was to set up preliminary meetings with local residents and networks. Following this, a neighbourhood committee was formed. This group included a GP, a teacher, and volunteer representatives from Wool and outlying villages. A comprehensive programme was developed, linking existing activities and networks and establishing new projects. These included local resuscitation training sessions, a new school programme, training of professionals and volunteers in screening and prevention work, and the development of risk factor support networks.

As a result of the initiative, there are now established local primary care screening programmes and lifestyle intervention courses.

In Canford Heath, Project Lionheart has been fortunate in having a Project Officer funded by the British Heart Foundation for two years. The project started with the development of a

# PROJECT LIONHEART
## PROGRAMME MODEL

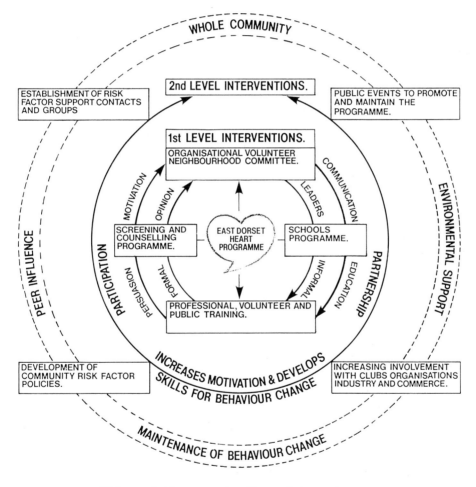

This model incorporates the various programme
initiatives and the processes involved in the development
and diffusion of the project.

Start in the middle and ripple out!

**Fig. 11.1** The Project Lionheart programme model

comprehensive community profile. This showed that there were a number of specific local problems, for example an unacceptable level of teenage smoking, high fat and low fibre food on some pub menus, and the local Leisure Centre facilities were not adequate to meet demand.

Following completion of the profile and the formulation of a needs-related action plan, the Project was launched with a well publicised Healthy Lifestyles Assessment event (offered free to the public) at the local Leisure Centre. Stands included blood pressure checks, fitness testing, diet analysis and individual advice. Over the two evenings 150 people attended the events.

The next step was to set up the volunteer neighbourhood committee to further the aims of the Project and to plan and manage the various events. As a result of the committee's efforts, the local authority has obtained funds to rebuild the dilapidated Trim Trail (an outdoor fitness track). The committee is also organising a campaign for a much needed swimming pool: 'Take your Heart for a Swim' was launched on St Valentine's Day 1990. The authority is also involved in community education activities such as Smokestop and LAYH/ Look After Yourself courses.

# Media coverage

Galvanising the interest of local people was crucial in the effectiveness of the Project, especially in the initial phase. The parish newsletter proved invaluable in Wool. In Canford Heath, the local dairy was involved in the distribution of leaflets advertising the launch. The information thus reached 6000 households. The local press provided regular reports of programme events in both areas.

# Impact

The initial work in Wool generated considerable interest and support. This was mainly due to the skill mix and enthusiasm of the volunteer neighbourhood committee. Each member became a respected opinion leader on coronary heart disease prevention. The success in Wool helped to win funding for the larger Project in Canford Heath. The Healthy Lifestyle Assessment evenings here indicated that there was a need to encourage improvements to people's diet, to provide 'Exercise for Beginners' classes particularly for women, and to run a 'Lose Weight' course. Although the Project in Canford Heath is still at a formative stage, there are indications that the Project Officer is being seen as a facilitator, encouraging different statutory, voluntary and commercial agencies to develop the initiatives themselves. The intention is that when the facilitator input is withdrawn, after two years, an independent coronary heart disease group remains.

# Management

Project Lionheart is a specialist programme linked to the East Dorset Health Authority's Health Promotion Unit and Department of Public Health Medicine. The director of Project Lionheart devoted half her hours for two years of the project and was assisted by part-time secretarial support.

The Project Director is a clinical nurse specialist and programme manager. The Project Officer is a senior health promotion officer. There are two part-time secretaries attached to the Project.

The project is supervised by the Director of Public Health Medicine.

# Resources

The cost of the project was as follows:

(a) Wool

|  | Expenditure (1st year) £ |
|---|---|
| LAYH Community Projects Scheme | 4189 |
| Donations, etc. | 229 |
| Programme development including publicity events, educational resources and committee expenses | 1386 |

(b) Canford Heath

|  | Expenditure (projected; over 2 years) £ |
|---|---|
| Project Officer | 25000 |
| Secretary | 6000 |
| Events | 5000 |
| Administration | 4000 |

# 12 Ramadan stop smoking posters – Tower Hamlets, London

## Setting – community

At the time of Ramadan, the month-long fasting period for Muslims, 20 000 posters with the fasting timetable and messages encouraging people to give up smoking were distributed in Tower Hamlets in London. This project was building on a positive practice in the community where many people give up smoking during Ramadan. The main message was: 'If you can stop smoking for 15 hours a day during Ramadan, you can stop for ever'. Five locally relevant languages were used, including English. The posters (Fig. 12.1) were available at three mosques in Tower Hamlets in the week leading up to Ramadan, and the first Friday of the fasting period.

**Key facts**

| | |
|---|---|
| **Location:** | Tower Hamlets, London Population 160 000 |
| **Timescale:** | Three months to plan |
| **Cost:** | £3335 |
| **Sources of funding:** | LAYH Community Projects Scheme |
| **Initiator:** | Local voluntary health campaign |
| **Implementation led by:** | Health Campaign and District Health Promotion with help from relevant community and religious groups |
| **Special features:** | • Poster campaign<br>• Linked Ramadan with giving up smoking<br>• Used mosques as distribution points<br>• Printed in languages of the community |

|  |  |
|---|---|
| **Contact:** | Myra Garrett<br>Tower Hamlets Health Campaign<br>Oxford House<br>Derbyshire Street<br>London E2 6HG<br><br>and<br><br>Nicky Tewson<br>District Health Promotion Officer<br>Tower Hamlets Health Authority<br>Tredegar House<br>97–99 Bow Road<br>London E3 2AN |
| **Documentation:** | Project report to the Health<br>Education Authority |

**Good practices**

- Clear objectives
- Participation by local people in distribution
- Joint planning with local community representatives
- Project has been repeated
- Use of local cultural/religious tradition

# Origins

Smoking is known as a significant contributory risk factor in coronary heart disease. Tower Hamlets report that over half of all Muslim men smoke, and yet they tend to give up during the month-long fasting period of Ramadan, either entirely, or from sunrise to sunset. Most resume smoking after Ramadan. Some 60 000 Muslims live in Tower Hamlets. As part of a local initiative on smoking, the Tower Hamlets Health campaign and Health Promotion Service decided to print and distribute posters with information about the Ramadan fasting timetable and messages encouraging people to give up smoking permanently. The Bengali-speaking Health Promotion Officer and a number of local Bengali and Somali community workers were very supportive of the idea.

# Objectives

- To target a group of people with a high proportion of smokers.

- To provide useful information about the Ramadan fasting timetable with anti-smoking messages.

- To link abstention during Ramadan with long term cessation of smoking.

# What happened

20000 posters, containing a fasting timetable and the message 'If you can stop smoking for 15 hours a day during Ramadan, you can stop for ever' were produced. Local businesses commonly distribute such posters with a timetable as a way of advertising themselves. The timetable is very important information and would ordinarily be pinned up either at home or at work for easy access.

Other messages on the poster were: 'Giving Up Smoking is Good For You and Your Family' and 'Save Your Life, Save Your Money, Show You Care.' The poster was printed in five languages in a bright purple colour (Fig. 12.1).

Three local mosques agreed to allow distribution to take place outside as people left afternoon prayers during the week preceding Ramadan and on the first Friday of the fasting period.

All 20000 posters were handed out with the assistance of the Young Muslim Organisation; with a few going to community organisations, libraries and advice centres. The local Health Promotion Department and the Family Practitioner Committee also assisted with distribution, but by far the largest number were handed directly to worshippers outside the mosques. This was organised by the Health Promotion Officer with a community group.

# Media coverage

The poster campaign was reported in the local press. In 1990, the same campaign is being repeated, and this time it is also being publicised through the health page in a national Bengali newspaper. (There are estimated to be about 50000 Bengali people living in Tower Hamlets.)

**Fig. 12.1** The Ramadan 'Stop Smoking Now!' poster

# Impact

No formal evaluation of the effectiveness of the posters was carried out. There were some comments received by the Health Campaign office, a number of community workers were interviewed and a report was produced as to how the project had been conducted.

Anecdotal evidence indicated that the poster was well received. People were appreciative that two important messages were given: information about fasting times as well as encouragement to stop smoking permanently. Posters were seen displayed prominently in many homes. Other timetables were printed locally but this one was thought to be particularly attractive and impressive.

Some people thought that there was too much writing on the poster, and the point was also made that, given the high rate of illiteracy in the Bangladeshi community, alternative designs, such as the no smoking symbol, would have been useful.

The Ramadan posters are being printed again this year. This time the project is being organised jointly by the Tower Hamlets Health Promotion Unit and another local voluntary body, the Health Strategy group. For 1990, 25 000 posters will be produced. Formal evaluation of the project is also planned, this time under the aegis of the Health Promotion Service.

# Management

The project was managed by the community based Health Campaign in consultation with the Health Promotion Service.

# Resources

The cost of the project was as follows:

|  | Expenditure £ |
|---|---|
| Project worker for three months | 1600 |
| Printing | 1635 |
| Distribution | 100 |
| Total | 3335 |

These costs were met from the LAYH award and internal funding sources.

# 13 Healthy meat in Hampstead, London

## Setting – activity with commercial sector

As part of the implementation of its District Food and Health Policy, Hampstead Health Authority ran a project to monitor the fat content in meat and meat products sold in the District. During a two-week period in 1988 samples of every type of mince from each retailer in the District were bought and analysed to determine total fat content. The results of the study were fed back to the retailers at a well-attended seminar which began with a 'healthy' supper of lean meat dishes. A month after the seminar, the minces were retested. The results showed a general shift towards a lower fat content. Minces produced by retailers who attended the seminar showed a greater decline in total fat content than those who did not attend.

**Key facts**

| | |
|---|---|
| **Location:** | Hampstead with a population of 110 000 |
| **Timescale:** | November 1987 to May 1988 main study<br>Follow-up in June 1989 and February 1990 |
| **Cost:** | £2500 for analysis and seminar<br>Time of the senior scientific officer |
| **Sources of funding:** | LAYH Community Projects Scheme<br>Public Health Medicine Department, Hampstead |
| **Initiator:** | District Medical Officer |
| **Implementation led by:** | Senior Scientific Officer<br>Hampstead Health Authority |
| **Special features:** | • Samples of mince from each retailer in Hampstead were tested for fat content |

- Analysed results fed back to retailers at a seminar

- All outlets sent a summary of the seminar speeches and discussion notes

- Two months later further samples of mince retested and results compared with first batch

- Testing repeated a year later, results fed back to retailers

- Six months after this, further testing and publicity of results in local newspaper

**Contact:**  Dr Noel Olsen
Director of Public Health Medicine
Department of Community Medicine
21 Pond Street
Hampstead
London NW3
Tel: 071-794 0500

**Documentation:**  DHSS, *Look After Your Heart campaign*
Nicola Dunn, *Improving the nutritional awareness of butchers: a supply-side intervention study*
Both available from Hampstead Health Authority

**Good practices**

- Part of Hampstead Health Authority's activities linked with the promotion of their District Food and Health Policy

- Objectives identified

- Research methodology set out clearly

- Research report provided

- Recommendations for opening a dialogue between health professionals and food suppliers

- Information available for other Districts to replicate

# Origins

Hampstead Health Authority, as part of the activities to promote their Food and Health Policy, wanted to tackle a project aimed at food retailers. As their first target, they decided to identify retailers who sold food high in saturated fats, as coronary heart disease is associated with a customary diet which is high in saturated fats. Meat and meat products were identified as one of the principal sources of saturated fat consumed in British homes, and within this group mince was chosen as the most suitable product for an intervention study.

There were two reasons for choosing mince – firstly, that it was popular with a wide range of customers, because of its cheapness and versatility, and secondly its total fat content can be controlled by the retailer by using leaner cuts and classes of meat.

At about the same time, the Camden Department of Environmental Health identified the sale and production of meat as an area of concern and the Meat and Livestock Commission launched a 'Lean Choice Campaign' designed to encourage the sale of lean meat and meat products.

# Objectives

- To raise the nutritional awareness of food retailers.
- To improve the nutritional behaviour of retailers as food suppliers.
- To increase the supply of healthy foods available in the district.
- To encourage the supply of healthy foods available in the district.
- To develop a research methodology so that other districts can replicate the project.

# What happened

First phase

Camden Environmental Health Department issued a press release outlining their plans to monitor the quality, storage and sale of meat and meat products. They reminded retailers that environmental health officers had the right to take samples of their products to ensure that they complied with certain standards of composition. They highlighted the fact that mince should not contain more than 25 per cent fat, and that retailers could produce lean varieties with a fat content of not more than 10 per cent.

This was followed by a visit from an environmental health officer to each meat retailer in Hampstead when the message in the press release was reinforced and information on the Meat and Livestock Commission's 'Lean Choice Campaign' was distributed.

**Pilot study**

A small pilot study was carried out to test the methodology to be used in the main study.

**Second phase**

During a two-week period in November/December 1989 a member of the Community Medicine Department visited each of the retailers in the District and bought a 500 g sample of every type of mince on sale. These were individually sealed and sent to a public analyst who determined the total fat content of each sample using the Foss-Let method.

Meats with fat content at less than 10 per cent were identified and three weeks later they were sampled again. Those minces that on both occasions had fat content of less than 10 per cent qualified as 'lean' under the terms of the study.

**Third phase**

This stage involved communicating the results of the study to the meat retailers and highlighting the health issues they raised.

Each outlet was sent a brief description of the study, a coded league table of results and an invitation to attend a seminar. They were told that the seminar would consist of speeches from the health professions and the Meat and Livestock Commission and it would include presentation of the Lean Mince Awards.

Each meat retailer was telephoned a week before the seminar to see how many representatives they would be sending and to answer questions about the study.

**Seminar**

The seminar began with a 'healthy supper' of lean meat dishes and during this time the retailers were given their coded number in a sealed envelope. This enabled the representatives to privately compare the fat content of their own mince with the rest of the population. This was followed by the educational section of the seminar with guest speeches followed by a discussion.

The evening ended with six outlets receiving certificates which indicated that on the occasions they were tested they were found to be selling lean mince. Overall one mince was selected as 'best buy' in terms of leanness and price. The awards were valid for two months. The event and prizewinner were featured in the local press.

The seminar was well attended and included local butchers, local retail store managers and senior head office representatives from the larger retail chains. In addition each outlet was sent a summary of seminar speeches and discussion notes.

After two months the Department retested all the minces to enable them to evaluate whether the intervention had had any effect on the retailers' behaviour, by assessing the change in fat content.

Follow-up a year later

A year later fresh mince from all the retail outlets was retested. Letters were sent to the retailers: those with a low fat content were congratulated; those in the middle bracket were encouraged to improve; those with a high fat content were told this was unacceptable on coronary heart disease and public health grounds and were informed that the results could be published. Six months later those with a consistently low and high fat content were retested. This time a journalist from the local paper was involved. The journalist reported the results in the paper giving the names of the retailers.

# Impact

The results showed a general shift towards lower fat contents in the mince although overall the average fat content was not lowered significantly. However, minces produced by retailers who attended the seminar showed a significantly greater decline in the total fat content than those who did not attend.

On retesting a year later, it was found that the improved results reported after the seminar were maintained.

The study showed that the gathering of scientific data which is of interest to the retailer is an effective way of opening a dialogue between health professionals and food suppliers.

The District feel that the method that they have developed could be successfully used by other health authorities and they are going to produce a step by step guide to help others.

# Management

The project was devised by Hampstead's Director of Public Health. The study was carried out by the senior scientific officer. She ran the pilot, collected the samples, found the public analyst; organised the seminar; did the follow-up testing and wrote the reports. The senior scientific officer searched for a suitable independent analyst – prices ranged from £30 to £7 per sample tested. The public analyst charged £7 per test. At today's prices (1990), the cost would be £10 per test.

# Resources

The LAYH Community Projects Scheme awarded Hampstead £2000. This went mainly towards paying for the samples to be analysed and the seminar. The Public Health Department covered the cost of the salary of the senior scientific officer who carried out the work. Any shortfall was met from the Public Health Department budget.

# 14 Heartbeat Award – North Kesteven District Council and the Boundary Cafe

### Setting – public places

The Heartbeat Award is one of the initiatives of the LAYH programme. It aims to encourage caterers to take an active role in helping to reduce coronary heart disease by promoting healthy food choices on menus, providing non-smoking areas and having good standards of hygiene. Catering establishments meeting defined requirements receive a certificate and the right to display the Award and use it in any promotion for one year (Fig. 14.1). The scheme is run by environmental health officers (EHO), who visit local eating places to decide whether they meet the criteria laid down by the Award. In 1989 over 890 Certificates were awarded nationally. North Kesteven District Council has been running the scheme for about 18 months and the Boundary Cafe, 10 miles outside Lincoln, illustrates how the scheme works in a simple transport cafe providing food for working people and passing trade (Fig. 14.2).

**HEARTBEAT AWARD**

**PRESENTED BY NORTH KESTEVEN DISTRICT COUNCIL**

*Department of Environmental Services*

**Fig. 14.1** A Heartbeat Award, for display on approved premises

**Key facts**

| | |
|---|---|
| **Location:** | North Kesteven District Council in Lincolnshire. Population 85 000 |
| **Timescale:** | Award scheme started in 1988 |
| **Cost:** | No specific budget allocated Environmental Health Officers assess establishments as part of their role Fee charged for hygiene courses – this covers their costs |
| **Sources of funding:** | North Kesteven District Council Heartbeat Award materials and video supplied free of charge by the LAYH programme of the HEA |
| **Initiator:** | Environmental Services Department |
| **Implementation led by:** | Senior Environmental Health Officer |
| **Special features:** | <ul><li>Commitment from Authority members to support the Heartbeat Award scheme</li><li>Environmental Services Department targeted 24 eating establishments which were given information packs about the Heartbeat Award</li><li>Six were eligible for the Heartbeat Award – one third of tables non-smoking, one third of menu healthy, one third of staff trained in basic food hygiene</li><li>Environmental Services Department runs basic food handlers course. Most establishments want all staff to receive this training</li><li>Close liaison with dietitian from Health Authority who accompanied the environmental health officer on visits to advise on menus</li></ul> |

- Boundary Cafe fulfils Heartbeat Award criteria and provides 'healthy food for working people and the travelling public'

- Many pensioners come to the cafe as the food is nutritious and cheap

**Contact:**
John Gibson
Senior Environmental Health Officer
North Kesteven District Council
Offices
The Hoplands
Boston Road
Sleaford
Lincs NG34 7EF
Tel: 0529 414166

**Documentation:**
Heartbeat Award information pack available from the Health Education Authority

**Good practices**

- Clear objectives

- Collaboration between local authority and health authority

- Managed within existing budgets

- Reaching establishments catering for those most at risk from coronary heart disease

# Origins

In 1988, South Lincolnshire Health Authority called a meeting of the environmental health officers from the five District Councils covered by the Health Authority, to discuss the Heartbeat Award. North Kesteven District Council expressed an interest in adopting the scheme and the Health Authority's dietician offered to help them in assessing healthy food choices.

Information packs for caterers and for environmental health officers, plus a video, were available, free of charge, from the Health Education Authority's Look After Your Heart programme. Support for the work of the environmental health officers on this award was obtained from the Council.

# Objectives

- To involve those premises who might be eligible for the Heartbeat Award.
- To provide a Heartbeat Award information pack to these premises.
- To run basic training courses for food handlers.
- To enlist the help of the Community Dietitian employed by the Health Authority to vet menus and provide advice on healthy food.
- To promote the Award in the District and raise the awareness of the public about the Award.

# What happened

The Environmental Health Officer with responsibility for implementing the Heartbeat Award selected a range of smaller eating establishments most frequently visited by the local population. Twenty-four establishments were identified and visited by the officer and provided with information about the Award. Six expressed interest and, with some additional help from the Environmental Services Department, it was thought they would be eligible.

The Environmental Services Department put on a basic training course for food handlers. Most of these organisations wanted all their staff to receive the training, not merely the 30 per cent which the scheme required as a minimum standard. Three of the six establishments had at least 30 per cent of their tables as no smoking and the remainder decided to go completely no smoking.

The Community Dietitian subsequently visited the establishments with the Environmental Health Officer to vet menus and provide advice on 'healthy' ways of preparing food.

In 1989, these six establishments were presented with the Heartbeat Award, receiving substantial coverage in the local media.

Boundary Cafe – a prefabricated transport cafe located on an old airfield on the A15 trunk road between Sleaford and Lincoln – was one of the establishments receiving the Award. The proprietors, Mr and Mrs Penfold, aim to provide healthy food for working people and travellers at a reasonable price.

# Menu

### Boundary Cafe
Sleaford Road
Nocton Heath
Lincoln
Lincs. LN4 2AW
Tel: (0522) 810404
*Proprietors: Ray & Ann Penfold*

October 1989

## BREAKFAST TIME

| | |
|---|---|
| Traditional Breakfast | £2.00 |
| Bacon, Egg, Sausage, Fried Bread, Beans/Tomatoes & BB. | |
| Simple Breakfast | £1.30 |
| Bacon, Egg, Beans/Tomatoes & BB. | |
| Double Breakfast | £3.50 |
| 2 Bacon, 2 Eggs, 1 Sausage, Fried Bread, Beans, Tomatoes, Potatoes & BB. | |

### Healthy Choice Breakfasts
Fresh Orange/Grapefruit with either:

| | | |
|---|---|---|
| a. | 2 Poached Eggs on Wholemeal Toast & low fat Spread | £1.45 |
| b. | Beans on Wholemeal Toast & Spread. Griddled Bacon slice. | £1.85 |
| c. | Griddled Bacon, Beans/Tomato, Poached Egg with Wholemeal Bread and Spread. | £1.74 |

Extras may be added to the above at an additional charge e.g. Mushrooms 35p, Potatoes 25p, Black Pudding 30p, Cereals 50p, Grapefruit 70p.

## SANDWICHES
These are made to order with white or Wholemeal bread with butter or low-fat spread.

| | |
|---|---|
| Sausage (2) | £1.00 |
| Bacon | £1.00 |

## SANDWICHES (Cont.)

| | |
|---|---|
| Egg (griddled if liked) | £0.70 |
| Ham (Home boiled) | £1.00 |
| Cheese | £0.80 |
| Corned Beef | £1.00 |
| Roast Meat (if available) | £1.00 |
| Chip Butty | £0.80 |
| Salad (Subject to available ingredients) | £0.80 |

Extras may be added subject to availability e.g. Pickle 5p, Onion 5p, Salad 20p, Tomato 5p

## CONFECTIONERY
A selection of homemade Cakes and Pastries are shown in the cabinet. Sausage Rolls and Scones are made fresh daily. — £0.40

## SNACKS
Wholemeal or white bread can be used as prefered.

| | |
|---|---|
| Toast (white) | £0.22 |
| Toast (Wholemeal) | £0.23 |
| 2 Eggs on 2 pieces of Toast (poached or fried) | £1.00 |
| 2 Scrambled Eggs on 2 pieces of Toast | £1.45 |
| Beans on 2 pieces of Toast | £1.15 |
| Tomatoes on 2 pieces of Toast | £1.15 |
| Cheese on 2 pieces of Toast | £1.15 |
| Cheese and Side Salad, 2 pieces of Bread and Butter | £1.45 |
| Jacket Potato and Coleslaw with Butter or low fat Spread | £1.20 |
| Beefburgers (2) 4oz | £1.15 |
| Toasted Teacakes | £0.40 |
| Sausage Roll | £0.40 |
| Cakes (see in Cabinet) | £0.40 |

## CHIP MEALS

| | |
|---|---|
| 2 Eggs, Chips & BB | £1.45 |
| 2 Sausages, Chips & BB | £1.62 |
| 1 Sausage, 1 Egg, Chips & BB | £1.45 |
| 2 Sausage, 1 Egg, Chips & BB | £1.92 |
| 2 Sausage, 1 Egg, Chips, Beans & BB | £2.28 |
| Chicken Portion, Chips, Beans & BB | £2.64 |
| Battered Fish, Chips, Peas & BB | £2.64 |
| Shepherds Pie, Chips, Peas & BB | £2.22 |
| Gammon, Pineapple or Egg, Chips, Garnish & BB | £3.12 |
| Meat Pie (Homemade when available) Chips, Peas | £2.22 |
| Fish Fingers, Chips & BB | £1.74 |
| Fish Cakes, Chips & BB | £1.74 |
| Corned Beef, Chips, Beans & BB | £1.74 |
| Cooked Ham, Egg, Chips, Beans & BB | £1.85 |

## DRINKS

| | | | |
|---|---|---|---|
| Tea (various available) | 20p | 22p | 38p |
| Coffee | 25p | 30p | 40p |
| (Instant, Filtered or de-Caffeinated) | | | |
| Chocolate | | | 45p |
| Bovril | | | 40p |
| Milk | | | 35p |
| Bottled Spring Water | | | 30p |
| Fresh Orange/Grapefruit Juice | | | 40p |
| Squash - (Orange/Blackcurrant) | | 25p | 35p |
| Cola and Fizzy Drinks | | 32p | 40p |
| Low Cal Cans | | | 35p |

*Cold Drinks are usually kept in the Fridge*

*Lunches Changed Daily see Board Behind Counter*

*Meals marked with Heart are suitable for Healthy Choice Foods.*

**Fig. 14.2** The Boundary Cafe's menu, with healthy eating choices clearly marked

They are particularly noted for their healthy breakfast of griddled bacon, poached egg, wholemeal bread, baked beans, preceded by half a fresh grapefruit or fruit juice – price £1.74.

The cafe has become popular with pensioners who appreciate the fresh food and healthy choices at a price they can afford.

The cafe seats 40 people at one time with a third of the tables for non-smokers. These tables are well used.

All the staff, including the part-time staff, have received the basic food handlers training.

# Impact

Although the proprietors of the Boundary Cafe are proud to display their Award, they do not think that the public know what it means.

The Environmental Services Department promote the scheme because they think it is a worthwhile project, but they feel that more national public awareness about the Award would encourage other establishments to join.

The Heartbeat Award was launched nationally on 26 April 1990 with the aim to promote it to local authorities and the catering industry. At present over 40 per cent of local authorities participate in the Award and major catering companies have demonstrated their commitment to achieving the Award in their premises across the country.

The need to promote the Award to the public is recognised, and promotional activity is being planned by the HEA.

# Management

The implementation of the Heartbeat Award in North Kesteven is managed, as part of his work, by a senior environmental health officer with a special interest in health promotion. He is supported by his chief officer and the District Council.

The District Council cuts across two health authorities. The community dietitians from both authorities have provided much helpful advice and guidance.

# Resources

The Health Education Authority's LAYH programme provides information packs and resources free of charge to environmental health departments wishing to implement the Award.

The environmental health officers visit the establishments as part of their normal duties and no special budget has been allocated.

They charge a fee of £14 for the basic training course for food handlers, of which £7 goes to the Institution of Environmental Health Officers and £7 goes towards covering the rest of the training.

# 15 Birmingham Look After Your Heart campaign

## Setting – city-wide

Following the national launch of the Look After Your Heart campaign in April 1987, a Look After Your Heart committee chaired by the Assistant Director of Environment Services (Public Health) was set up and all departments of the City Council were requested to identify how their departments could contribute to the campaign. The committee comprised senior officers of the Council and district health promotion officers from the five Birmingham Health Authorities, the Regional Health Authority and voluntary organisations.

The LAYH campaign acts as an umbrella for bringing together those involved in health promotion throughout the city. It provides a forum for pooling ideas and resources and it acts as a stimulus to action. The main departments contributing to funding and organising activities are environmental services, the education service and the libraries department. The health authorities and other City Council departments provide expertise and human resources. The Regional LAYH/Look After Yourself officer is based in the Recreation and Community Services Department in the Council. She has organised tutor training for key staff in the organisation, who now run classes in all the City Council departments. No formal evaluation has been carried out. The campaign has 'grown' rather haphazardly but it has the backing of the Council and has proved an excellent tool in exerting pressure for change.

**Key facts**

| | |
|---|---|
| **Location:** | Birmingham. Population one million, including 180 000 schoolchildren |
| **Timescale:** | Built on publicity arising from the launch of the national campaign in April 1987. Ongoing |
| **Cost:** | In 1989–90 – promotion/activities costs £15 000 shared between Education and Environmental Services. Several aspects of the Schools and Young Peoples Health Education Programme (£400 000) and other programmes undertaken by supporting organisations have been co-ordinated with the support of the LAYH 'umbrella' |
| **Sources of funding:** | Since 1987 – Education Department Joint financing Environmental Health LAYH Community Projects Scheme Commercial sponsors |
| **Initiator:** | Director of Public Health Division of Environmental Services in City Council |
| **Implementation led by:** | Jointly by: Sarah Eden District Health Promotion Officer Shama Sharif District Health Promotion Officer Pat Taylor District Dietitian |
| **Special features:** | • Involves every department in the City Council identifying funds and action • Led to close collaboration and planning between the City Council and the five Birmingham Health Authorities and Regional Authority • Provides an umbrella for a continuous programme of activities • Much media coverage obtained |

- Many of the activities have involved children and young people

- LAYH/Look After Yourself an important aspect

- Smoke-free Birmingham by the year 2000 initiative launched in March 1990

- Learning from developments within the European Community and Australia

**Contact:**

Jo Harvey
Health Promotion Unit
Environmental Services Department
67 Curzon Street
Birmingham B4 7XQ
Tel: 021-235 3884

**Documentation:**

Evaluation report on the 1989 Junior School Super Quiz

**Good practices**

- Strong support from members and senior officers

- Implementation led by enthusiastic managers

- Led to joint planning of health promotion throughout the City. Establishing priorities and pooling resources

- Stimulated all departments of City Council to take action

- Funding and activities increased as programme developed

# Origins

Following the launch of the national LAYH programme in April 1987, a LAYH campaign committee chaired by the Assistant Director of Environmental Services (Public Health) was established. Members included representatives from City Council Departments, District and Regional Health Authorities and voluntary organisations.

As a major contribution a Healthy Heart Day was held in October 1987, at the Council House, to which leading figures from the world of politics, commerce, the trades unions, the health professions and management were invited. This was followed by a Healthy Heart Day for members of the committee in December and in May the following year a Healthy Heart Day for Headteachers. These activities raised the awareness of key people in the community about the need to take action on heart disease prevention, and they provided a springboard to develop further activities.

# Objectives

- To target health promotion activity and service provision to reduce the incidence of coronary heart disease in the following groups:

    - young people
    - inner-city groups (including ethnic minority groups)
    - unemployed

- To highlight the following issues in relation to coronary heart disease (targeted reductions currently under consideration):

    - smoking
    - diet
    - alcohol
    - exercise/stress

# What happened

In July 1988, all departments in the City Council were requested to identify funding for the next three years for those areas of work highlighted by the LAYH campaign.

The main departments that have provided funding have been Education and Environmental Health. The Libraries have allocated an information officer. The appointment of a health education adviser for schools by the Local Education Authority was an important move. He convened the Schools Health Education Group which involved representatives from a number of City departments (e.g. Recreation and Community Services and Environmental Health) and representatives from the five District Health Promotion Units. This group provided a basis for joint planning of activities and pooling resources, talents and training. The group also has links with the LAYH 'Smoking' subgroup for planning specific activities with schoolchildren, such as the junior school super quizzes, National No Smoking Day activities in schools, and Smokebusters and Youth against Tobacco initiatives.

The area senior officer from the Environmental Health Department is secretary to the main LAYH campaign committee which meets every six weeks, and is responsible for ensuring that the activities identified by the committee actually take place. This committee has a variety of subgroups, such as the healthy eating group, problems in inner cities group, women's group, food for health group and smoking groups.

**HEALTH·FOR·ALL**

**Fig. 15.1** A leaflet on the overall 'Healthy Birmingham 2000' campaign

The Regional LAYH officer is based in the Recreation and Community Services Department and she has run tutor training courses for officers in a variety of different departments. LAYH/ Look After Yourself classes are now being run by these trained tutors in every department of the City Council.

The City has just launched its new initiative Smoke-free Birmingham by the year 2000, and in March declared itself a WHO Healthy City. Under the Healthy City banner, LAYH will become a task group.

## Impact

No formal systematic evaluation has taken place. Records have been kept about the main events. The campaign has grown and blossomed in a way that was not envisaged originally. It has proved an extremely useful means of getting change in City departments and in providing a format for joint planning on health initiatives throughout the region.

## Management

The LAYH campaign committee consisting of senior officers from the City departments, the Health Authority and voluntary organisations meets once every six weeks. The meeting is now chaired by the Director of Environmental Services and serviced by a Senior Environmental Health Officer. The initiatives in schools and with young people are led by the Schools Adviser on Health Education.

## Resources

The main budget for LAYH activities comes from the Education Department. In 1988/89, the budget was £400000. This includes the salary of all the staff employed by the City working on health topics with young people. Approximately £200000 goes on salary and £200000 on resources and training.

The Environmental Health Department spent about £10000 in 1988–89 on promotional activities linked to LAYH.

# 16

## Yorkshire Heartbeat –
## primary health care team
## workshop programme

### Setting – primary health care

Tackling the problem of heart disease has been given high priority by Yorkshire Regional Health Authority (RHA) who have funded a five year (1988–92) heart disease prevention programme – Yorkshire Heartbeat (Fig. 16.1). The programme has a full-time co-ordinator and one of the main activities has been to assist in the development of a series of workshops for those working in primary health care. This is being done in collaboration with the Health Education Authority (HEA), the Regional Adviser in General Practice, Health Authorities and Family Practitioner Committees (FPC) in the Region. The programme of Primary Health Care Team workshops in Yorkshire form part of a national initiative – with an increasing number of events being organised throughout the country. This national initiative is being co-ordinated by the HEA National Unit for Health Promotion in Primary Health Care.

The Primary Health Care Team workshops are aimed to

PARK PARADE · HARROGATE HG1 5AH · TEL: 0423 500066

**Fig. 16.1** Yorkshire Heartbeat

encourage and stimulate the participation of primary health care teams in health promotion and preventive activities that can readily be undertaken within or alongside the everyday work of the general practice. The workshops provide an important learning opportunity for the teams involved.

They follow a problem solving model and thereby aim to encourage the development of teamwork, organisational and planning skills, and improve understanding and communication between those working together in the general practice and primary health care arena.

The main function of each workshop is for the primary health care teams to produce a practice plan for promoting health and preventing disease in their practice population.

**Key facts**

| | |
|---|---|
| **Location:** | Yorkshire Region which comprises 17 Health Authorities and 7 Family Practitioner Committees. Population: 3.8 million. |
| **Timescale:** | Pilot Workshop June 1987. Yorkshire Heartbeat's co-ordination began September 1988. |
| **Sources of funding:** | Yorkshire Heartbeat HEA FPC reimbursement, Section 63 (up to April 1990) |
| **Initiator:** | Health Education Authority – Dr Deryck Lambert Primary Health Care Consultant Advisor and Co-ordinator of the PHC Training Programme. |
| **Implementation led by:** | Yorkshire Heartbeat Co-ordinator Caroline Hawkridge (until July 1990). |
| **Special features:** | • Programme involves close collaboration between HEA Primary Health Care Adviser, Yorkshire Heartbeat Co-ordinator and the Regional Adviser in General Practice. |
| | • A regional (Yorkshire Heartbeat) co-ordinator identified to co-ordinate the local dissemination of the workshop programme by providing support for the activities of district organising teams. |

- Such district organising teams participated in their own workshops in order to prepare for the task of developing workshop events for primary health care teams.

- Multi-disciplinary organising teams were established in 15 out of the 17 Health Authorities to run workshops for primary health care teams in their District.

- The Primary Health Care Team workshop programme and strategy have been evaluated by the HEA and a report is available from the HEA National Unit for Health Promotion in Primary Health Care.

- Outcomes from the evaluation programme demonstrate that the Primary Health Care Team workshops improve communication and team working, and promote a multi-professional/multi-disciplinary planned approach to health promotion.

**Contact:**

Yorkshire Heartbeat
Yorkshire Health
Park Parade
Harrogate HG1 5AH
Tel: 0423 500066

HEA National Unit for Health Promotion in Primary Health Care
Old Road Headington
Oxford OX3 7LJ
Tel: 0865 63371

**Documentation:**

Jill Spratley. *Disease Prevention and Health Promotion in Primary Health Care. Team workshops organised by the HEA. Evaluation Report.* HEA September 1989.

**Good practices**

- Appropriate objectives clearly identified.
- Carefully planned dissemination strategy for the workshop programme.
- Multi-disciplinary approach to primary health care team development.
- Resources identified.
- Evaluation built into the process.
- Plan for the workshop programme to become established as part of continuing education initiatives in primary health care.
- Potential for other regional health authorities to develop a dissemination strategy.

# Origins

The HEA has developed a programme of workshops for primary health care teams in order to help them develop their plans and strategies for health promotion and prevention activities.

In Yorkshire 50 000 people visit their local GP's surgery every day and around 90 per cent of the population will visit their GP every five years. Primary health care teams recognise that they have an important role to play in the prevention of heart disease, for example, and engage in a range of activities designed to encourage people to develop a healthier lifestyle.

Following meetings in Yorkshire between representatives from the Yorkshire RHA, the Regional Adviser in General Practice and officers of the Health Education Centre, a pilot workshop was run for seven primary health care teams. When Yorkshire Heartbeat was launched in September 1988 one of its main objectives was to develop initiatives in primary health care, and it has subsequently played an important part in co-ordinating the local dissemination of the workshop strategy.

It was always envisaged that the workshop strategy should be disseminated at a local level and as a result, a series of four $2\frac{1}{2}$-day residential workshops were run for district organising teams in the Region in order to provide participants with the opportunity to experience a workshop format similar to that which they might subsequently go on to plan for primary health care teams.

# Objectives

- To develop a dissemination strategy for running Primary Health Care Team workshops in each district.

- To set up multi-disciplinary local organising teams in each district.

- To enable each district organising team to run at least one residential workshop a year for primary health care teams in their district.

- To support district organising teams in their activities.

# What happened

Discussions between the HEA, Yorkshire Heartbeat, and the Postgraduate Regional Advisor in General Practice resulted in the establishment of a programme of workshops with participants attending as District Organising Teams.

Participants in the District Organising Teams included, for example, senior officers from FPC, managers of nursing services, health promotion/education officers, primary health care facilitators, consultants in public health, and a variety of other individuals including community dietitians, practice managers and practice nurses.

By the end of June 1990, fifteen Primary Health Care Team workshops had been organised and run by District Organising Teams in the Yorkshire Region with some districts having run two workshops. These 15 workshops have involved a total of 77 primary health care teams with 380 primary health care professionals involved.

Support for the primary health care teams attending the workshop is provided by the District Organising Team in a variety of ways both before and after the workshop. Primary health care teams are generally offered the opportunity to meet together after a number of months in order to review progress with their plans.

## Impact

The development of the Primary Health Care Team workshop programme is a national initiative of the HEA, and other regions, apart from Yorkshire, are now developing local organising teams to disseminate the workshop programme. Valuable experience has been gained from the developments in the Yorkshire Region which have informed the organisation of such developments elsewhere. Yorkshire Heartbeat still offer support for the workshop programme as appropriate.

Following on from the existing evaluation report relating to the Primary Health Care Team workshop programme, further evaluation work is currently being undertaken, which is examining the dissemination of the workshop strategy.

## Management

The day-to-day liaison work concerning the development of the Primary Health Care Team workshop strategy locally in the Yorkshire Region has been carried out by the Yorkshire Heartbeat Co-ordinator in collaboration with the HEA Primary Health Care Consultant Advisor.

# Medical Knowledge: Doubt and Certainty

Edited by Clive Seale, Stephen Pattison and Basiro Davey

Published by Open University Press

Written and produced by The Open University

Health and Disease Series, Book 1

**OPEN UNIVERSITY PRESS**

Buckingham  •  Philadelphia

## The U205 Health and Disease Course Team

The following members of The Open University teaching staff and external colleagues have collaborated with the authors in writing this book, or have commented extensively on it during its production. We accept collective responsibility for its overall academic and teaching content.

Basiro Davey (Course Team Chair, Senior Lecturer in Health Studies, Department of Biological Sciences)

Kevin McConway (Senior Lecturer in Statistics)

Stephen Pattison (Reader, The Department of Religious and Theological Studies at Cardiff University)

Clive Seale (Reader in Medical Sociology, Department of Sociology, Goldsmiths' College, University of London)

The following people have contributed to the development of particular parts or aspects of this book.

Steve Best (graphic artist)

Teresa Dowsing (course manager)

Sheila Dunleavy (editor)

Rebecca Graham (editor)

Celia Hart (picture researcher)

Pam Higgins (designer)

Jeanne Samson Katz (critical reader), Lecturer, School of Health and Social Welfare

Mike Levers (photographer)

Jean Macqueen (indexer)

Jennifer Nockles (designer)

Rissa de la Paz (BBC producer)

John Taylor (graphic artist)

Joy Wilson (course manager)

## Authors

The following people have acted as principal authors for the chapters listed below.

### Chapter 1
Stephen Pattison, Reader, The Department of Religious and Theological Studies at Cardiff University.

### Chapters 2, 7, 8 and 9
Clive Seale, Reader in Medical Sociology, Department of Sociology, Goldsmiths' College, University of London.

### Chapter 3
Basiro Davey, Senior Lecturer in Health Studies, Department of Biological Sciences, The Open University; and Clive Seale, Reader in Medical Sociology, Department of Sociology, Goldsmiths' College, University of London.

### Chapter 4
Charles Webster, Fellow of All Souls College, Oxford.

### Chapter 5
Andrew Cunningham, Wellcome Trust Senior Research Fellow in History of Medicine, Department of History and Philosophy of Science, Cambridge University.

### Chapter 6
Mary James, formerly a Lecturer in the Department of History, University of Essex.

## External assessors

### Course assessor for second editions
Professor James McEwen, Henry Mechan Chair of Public Health and Head of Department of Public Health, University of Glasgow.

### Book 1 assessors
Professor Michael Bury, Professor of Sociology, Department of Social Policy and Social Science, Royal Holloway, University of London.

Professor Ludmilla Jordanova, Professor of History, Department of History, University of East Anglia.

Professor Roy Porter, Reader in the Social History of Medicine, The Wellcome Institute for the History of Medicine, London.

## Acknowledgements

The Course Team and the authors wish to thank the following people who, as contributors to previous editions of this book, made a lasting impact on the structure and philosophy of the present volume.

Nick Black, David Boswell, Gerald Elliott, Alastair Gray, John Greenwood, Richard Holmes, Perry Morley, Jennie Popay, Steven Rose, Phil Strong.

The editors and authors would like to thank Charles Webster for his advice in preparing the present volume.

## Cover images

Background: Nebulae in the Rho Ophiuchi region (Source: David Malin/Anglo Australian Observatory). Middleground: Globe (Source: Mountain High Map™, Digital Wisdom, Inc). Foreground: Anatomical illustration of the head and neck, dissected to show major blood vessels, nerves and muscles (Source: adapted from Gray's Anatomy, 35th edn, by permission of the publisher Churchill Livingstone).

Open University Press, Celtic Court, 22 Ballmoor,
Buckingham, MK18 1XW.

e-mail: enquiries@openup.co.uk

website: www.openup.co.uk

and

325 Chestnut Street, Philadelphia, PA 19106, USA.

First published 1985. Completely revised second edition
published 1994.
Full-colour second edition published with amendments 2001.
Reprinted 2003.

A catalogue record of this book is available from the
British Library.

Library of Congress Cataloging-in-Publication Data is
available.


Edited, designed and typeset by The Open University.


Printed and bound in the United Kingdom by the
Alden Group, Oxford

ISBN 0335 20834 7

This publication forms part of an Open University level 2
course, U205 *Health and Disease*. The complete list of
texts which make up this course can be found on the
back cover. Details of this and other Open University
courses can be obtained from the Call Centre,
PO Box 724, The Open University, Milton Keynes
MK7 6ZS, United Kingdom: tel. +44 (0)1908 653231,
e-mail ces-gen@open.ac.uk

Alternatively, you may visit the Open University website
at http://www.open.ac.uk where you can learn more
about the wide range of courses and packs offered at all
levels by the Open University.

3.2

# CONTENTS

# A note for the general reader

*Medical Knowledge: Doubt and Certainty* provides a critical introduction to the nature, status and practice of medical knowledge. The book draws principally on the insights and resources of the social sciences and the social history of medicine to develop a critical perspective on this subject.

There are nine chapters in the book. After a brief introductory chapter, Chapter 2 looks at different healing methods and belief systems in contemporary Western society, including lay beliefs about health and disease, and at alternative or complementary therapies. This chapter makes it clear that the medical knowledge which forms the basis of most Western doctors' practice is only one way of approaching health and disease. That perception is amplified in the next four chapters which selectively look at some case studies in the history of medical theory and practice. Chapter 3 gives a general overview of some major trends in the history of medicine as a background to the case studies in Chapters 4 to 6. These chapters focus on (respectively) tuberculosis, blood and hysteria. It will be demonstrated that beliefs, perceptions and approaches to health and disease have changed radically over time and that social and cultural factors have exercised considerable influence on the evolution and form of medical knowledge.

The last three chapters of the book return to present times. In Chapters 7 to 9 various aspects of the use and context of medical knowledge in contemporary society are considered. Social and cultural influences on the construction and use of medical knowledge in modern medical practice are highlighted in Chapter 7. Chapter 8 focuses on the role of doctors within the social order and the way in which social problems and situations can come to be seen as medical problems. Finally, Chapter 9 explores the ways in which doctors and patients interact at the point where medical knowledge is applied in the doctor–patient relationship.

The book is fully indexed and referenced and contains a list of abbreviations and an annotated guide to further reading and to selected websites on the Internet. You will also find details of how to access a regularly updated collection of Internet resources relevant to the *Health and Disease* series on a searchable database called ROUTES, which is maintained by the Open University. This resource is open to all readers of this book.

*Medical Knowledge: Doubt and Certainty* is the first in a series of eight books on the subject of health and disease. The book is designed so that it can be read on its own, like any other textbook, or studied as part of U205 *Health and Disease*, a level 2 course for Open University students. General readers do not need to make use of the study comments, learning objectives and other material inserted for OU students, although they may find these helpful. The text also contains references to a collection of readings (*Health and Disease: A Reader*, Open University Press, second edition 1995; third edition 2001) prepared for the OU course: it is quite possible to follow the text without reading the articles referred to, although doing so should enhance your understanding of the contents of *Medical Knowledge: Doubt and Certainty*.

## Abbreviations used in this book

| | |
|---|---|
| AIDS | acquired immune deficiency syndrome |
| BCG | bacille Calmette Guérin |
| BHMA | British Holistic Medical Association |
| BMA | British Medical Association |
| CFS | chronic fatigue syndrome |
| GMC | General Medical Council |
| GP | general practitioner |
| HIV | human immunodeficiency virus |
| ME | myalgic encephalomyelitis |
| MOH | Medical Officers of Health |
| MRC | Medical Research Council |
| NHS | National Health Service |
| RHA | Regional Health Authority |
| TB | tuberculosis |

# Study guide for OU students

*(total around 48 hours, including time for the TMA, spread over 3 weeks)*

Chapter 1 is very short while Chapters 2 and 4 are substantially longer than other chapters. There are also a large number of Reader articles associated with this book, though some of them are very short. Optional Reader articles for this book will be set reading for later books, so you could usefully study them now and revise them later in the course. You should pace your study accordingly.

## 1st week

| | |
|---|---|
| Chapter 1 | **A journey through medical knowledge** |
| Chapter 2 | **Health and healing in an age of science**<br>TV programme 'Why me? Why now?';<br>Reader articles by Helman (1978) and Sharma (1990) |
| Chapter 3 | **An historical approach to medical knowledge** |
| Chapter 4 (start) | **Tuberculosis**<br>Reader article by Sontag (1978); the Reader articles by McKeown (1976) and Szreter (1988) are also relevant, but optional |

## 2nd week

| | |
|---|---|
| Chapter 4 (complete) | **Tuberculosis** |
| Chapter 5 | **Blood** |
| Chapter 6 | **Hysteria**<br>Reader article by James (1994) |
| Chapter 7 | **Medical knowledge and medical practice**<br>Reader article by Nettleton (1988) |

## 3rd week

| | |
|---|---|
| Chapter 8 | **Medicalisation and surveillance**<br>Reader articles by Asher (1972) and Illich (1976);<br>the Reader article by Navarro (1976) is also relevant, but optional |
| Chapter 9 | **Doctor–patient interaction**<br>TV programme 'Brief encounter';<br>audiotape 'The consultation'<br>Reader article by Brewin (1985) |
| TMA completion | |

*Medical Knowledge: Doubt and Certainty* emphasises that various kinds of social scientific and historical study can contribute to a critical account of medical knowledge. It provides a basis for subsequent interdisciplinary study in later books where other methods and perspectives, drawn from a wide range of disciplines, will be introduced and explained. The structure of the book is outlined in 'A note for the general reader' (p. 6), and is described further in Chapter 1.

Study notes, where appropriate, are given at the start of chapters. These primarily direct you to important links to other components of the course, such as the other books in the course series, the Reader, and audiovisual components. Major learning objectives are listed at the end of each chapter, along with questions that will enable you to check that you have achieved these objectives. The index includes key words in orange type (also printed in bold in the text) which can be looked up easily as an aid to revision as the course proceeds. There is also a list of further sources for those who wish to pursue certain aspects of study beyond the scope of this book, either by consulting other books and articles or by logging on to specialist websites on the Internet.

The time allowed for studying *Medical Knowledge: Doubt and Certainty* is around 48 hours spread over 3 weeks. The schedule (left) gives a more detailed breakdown to help you to pace your study. You need not follow it rigidly, but try not to let yourself fall behind. If you find a section of the work difficult, do what you can at this stage, and then return to reconsider the material when you reach the end of the book.

There is a tutor-marked assignment (TMA) associated with this book; about 5 hours have been allowed for writing it up, *in addition to* the time spent studying the material it assesses.

(a)

(b)

(c)

(d)

**Figure 1.1** *There are many different methods of treating illness in the modern world, even when the site in the body is the same. (a) A Hopi ear candle, derived from North American Indian treatment methods, is used for many disorders. (b) A general practitioner inspecting a patient's ear with an auroscope. (c) A traditional African healer or 'witchdoctor' (from the Runenzari region of Uganda) curing dizziness. (d) Stimulating acupuncture points in the ear.*
*(Sources: (a) photo: Mike Levers; (b) photo: Mike Levers; (c) Jim Holmes/Panos Pictures; (d) photo: Mike Levers)*

# CHAPTER 1

## A journey through medical knowledge

## 1.1   Going on a journey

It may be helpful if, as you read this book, you think of it as travelling to another country. Travellers are often struck by two things. First, there are some continuities and similarities with life back home, but at the same time many things are different.

Often there is an experience of excitement and misgiving, or of surprise and sometimes shock at what is seen. People's lifestyles may be unlike those you are used to. The indigenous people of some lands may appear to have a completely different way of approaching life and, indeed, of understanding it. You may see the physical remains of ancient civilisations and a guide may tell you something of the beliefs and faith systems that went along with particular religious buildings. It is all very curious and challenging, unsettling even. You may wonder that people can live in such conditions, hold such opinions and views of life and engage in such strange practices even though a number of them may seem quite attractive and more sensible than some of the things that happen back home. They certainly seem to work quite well in their present context. Sometimes you come to feel that some of the wisdom and practices you see and hear about could be universally valuable and useful; why haven't people in our own countries adopted them?

The time comes to re-board the plane and go home to familiar surroundings and customs. Yet, having seen how differently people can live, the traveller is a changed person. Life at home is now less obviously straightforward; a lot of practices now seem strange. The questioning of 'taken for granted' reality has been encouraged by an encounter with people with different lifestyles, practices, languages, beliefs and knowledge. Things are less clear and certain than they were before.

## 1.2   The nature and purpose of this book

This description of travellers' experience may help you to understand the nature and purpose of this book, which is to enrich, question and complicate your view of medical knowledge.

It may be that you already know quite a lot about medical science; perhaps you put a lot of faith in it, or perhaps you feel critical about some aspects. As children, many people are told of scientists such as Louis Pasteur, who made significant discoveries about the nature and existence of bacteria, and Alexander Fleming, who pioneered the development of antibiotic drugs. Such people are often presented as heroes of the human race who added solid and beneficial information to science which can now be applied to disease and illness. This helps encourage a view of the doctor as an authoritative and skilled interpreter of this kind of knowledge who treats illness in a scientifically informed way. On the other hand, discussions of the limitations and sometimes harmful consequences of medical endeavours are increasingly presented in the television and newspaper media.

The point of this book is neither to promote the uncritical admiration of medicine, nor to undermine anyone's faith in doctors' knowledge of disease and its treatment. It will, however, place medical knowledge in its social, historical and cultural context and show its relation to other ways of looking at illness. The book aims to take you on a journey around some different kinds of medical knowledge, familiar and not so familiar, past and present, so you can understand something of their origins, nature, practice, assumptions, strengths, limitations and implications for yourself in a fuller way. You may find yourself becoming increasingly doubtful about previously held certainties, or becoming certain in areas where you previously doubted.

## 1.3   The itinerary

We start in the United Kingdom of the late twentieth century. Chapter 2 begins by considering different kinds of contemporary knowledge and beliefs about illness and health. Although many people would be reluctant to claim that they have much medical knowledge of the kind that doctors possess, everyone has a set of working understandings and explanations for illness which they use in everyday life (for example, many people have theories of what causes diseases like cancers or colds which can sometimes differ from explanations offered by medical practitioners). Most of the healing and caring that goes on anywhere in the developed and developing countries is performed by *lay* people without the involvement of health-care professionals. Furthermore, we are becoming more and more aware of so-called *alternative* or *complementary* therapies. The knowledge based on biomedical principles used by *orthodox* practitioners of medicine is only one kind of knowledge about illness in our society, albeit a dominant and very important kind. The sometimes uneasy relationship between orthodox and alternative practitioners is explored towards the end of the chapter.

There then follow four chapters giving an account of the historical antecedents of present-day orthodox medical knowledge. Chapter 3 presents a brief overview of the historical development of medical knowledge as a whole. This is designed to provide a framework to which the more detailed historical case studies presented in Chapters 4, 5 and 6 can be related. By examining the development of knowledge on the important medical topics of tuberculosis (Chapter 4), blood (Chapter 5) and hysteria (Chapter 6), you will gain a sense of its complexity. Furthermore, you will see how social factors have influenced the evolution of medical knowledge and the use to which it has been put. Although scientific knowledge about disease has led to substantial and beneficial advances in the treatment of illnesses, these case studies show that the course of medical discovery has often not run true. Indeed, in the case of hysteria a real question arises as to whether a disease condition actually exists in the way that tuberculosis is thought to exist. This raises questions about what should count as fact and what should be regarded more as social prejudice or custom.

In the final part of the book (Chapters 7, 8 and 9) we move back again to examine medical knowledge in contemporary practice. Here you will be introduced to critical perspectives on modern medical practice drawn from the social sciences. The view that medicine may not be a wholly rational process devoted to the sole benefit of patients is discussed. The ritual and political functions of medical practice are highlighted here, and you will also be introduced to a radical school of thought which questions the very basis of a rational science of the body, and be invited to consider the strengths and weaknesses of this way of thinking. Chapter 9, at the end of the book, focuses on the modern medical consultation as the place of interaction for medical knowledge, practice and the person, and the role of trust in relations between doctors and patients.

## 1.4  The guides

This book has been compiled by a number of authors and uses several perspectives. In broad terms, the main academic disciplines that have been drawn on are **sociology** (the study of how societies develop and work) with a certain amount of **social anthropology** (the study of human beings in cultures), and the **history of medicine**. However, as you will see, even within one discipline such as sociology or history, scholars take different approaches. We hope you will find your understanding enriched by considering different, sometimes discordant or opposing viewpoints; no doubt you will find some approaches more useful than others. Sometimes a good deal of time will be spent looking at a particular feature, such as a disease or medical practice, in order to understand what can be learned from it. Occasionally, the main feature will be found in the Reader[1] to which you will be asked to turn as this book progresses. In addition, each chapter except this one has a list of objectives with associated questions and answers which you can use to test your understanding of the main points made by the chapter.

## 1.5  The destination

We hope that when you have completed your study of this book you will have done a number of things. First, your own way of thinking about medical knowledge should have been broadened. You should be able to see that there are many ways of looking at and understanding this topic through your study of different kinds of medical knowledge, lay and professional, orthodox and alternative. Second, particularly through your study of the historical case studies, you should understand something of the nature of scientifically based medical knowledge, how it has developed and how it has been related to social and cultural factors as well as to the natural world. You should also have gained understanding of how medical knowledge is used by doctors in practice today, of how it relates to other knowledge systems, and of its relationship with cultural attitudes or social structures, such as beliefs about the proper roles of men and women, and the way in which the medical profession is organised.

---

[1] *Health and Disease: A Reader* (Open University Press, 2nd edn 1995; 3rd edn 2001).

# CHAPTER 2

## Health and healing in an age of science

**Study notes for OU students**

This chapter considers a wide range of issues and practices in contemporary medical knowledge. Associated with it are a television programme and an audiotape sequence, each entitled 'Why me? Why now?' Details of these can be found in the Broadcast and Audiocassette Notes. Ideally, you should watch the programme before reading the chapter, but this is not essential.

During Section 2.2.1 you will be asked to read an article contained in *Health and Disease: A Reader* (Open University Press, second edition 1995; third edition 2001): 'Feed a cold, starve a fever' by Cecil Helman. Section 2.4.3 includes study of another Reader article: 'Using alternative therapies' by Ursula Sharma.

## 2.1  Introduction: the sectors of health care

The work and approach of the medical profession are based on scientific method, defining 'science' in the strictest sense of the word, namely the systematic observation of natural phenomena for the purpose of discovering laws governing those phenomena.... As an integral part of the society in which we live, scientific methodology is generally held to be an acceptable basis on which to set reliable judgements, free from overriding social values and political bias...

Inasmuch as scientific medicine lays such firm emphasis on observation, measurement, and reproducibility, historically it has become inevitably and increasingly separated from doctrines embracing superstition, magic, and the supernatural... (BMA, 1986, p. 61)

As this quotation from the British Medical Association (BMA) suggests, medicine is commonly presented as a body of knowledge based on objective scientific principles. The practice of medicine is often seen straightforwardly as the application of that knowledge by doctors. These are dominant ideas in Western society; we are introduced to them as children. When we are sick — and sickness may sometimes involve a regression to a childlike state of vulnerability and dependence — these ideas can be very comforting.

In this chapter, however, it is argued that this view of medical knowledge and practice is too simple. Medical knowledge is not the exclusive preserve of doctors. We all have medical knowledge and we all practice health care. The *professional* medical knowledge, in which doctors and other formal health-care workers are trained, will be contrasted with the *lay* knowledge of illness and of the workings of the body which we all possess to a greater or lesser extent. Both types of knowledge are associated with particular forms of health care, and the boundaries between the two are not as clear-cut as is often supposed.

*We all have medical knowledge and are involved in health care, most of which is carried out by lay people. (Photo: Mike Levers)*

● How might the boundaries between lay and professional medical knowledge be blurred in developed industrial societies?

■ Professional medical knowledge is presented in 'popular' form in various media: magazines, books and television. Lay ideas about health and illness are often, therefore, similar to those of doctors.

This chapter will also show that although scientific medical practice is now the dominant 'professional' form of health care in Western societies, this has not always been so. Study of the history of medicine shows that the dominance of the present-day medical profession has had to be fought for.[1] Rival groups of healers often based their practice on systems of knowledge that were fundamentally at odds with those of the emerging scientific orthodoxy. The threat to professional power from such *alternative* practitioners remains a concern for some in the modern medical establishment. At the same time, many orthodox medical practitioners are concerned to use therapies that are effective, whatever their knowledge-base may be.

Using this distinction between professional, lay and alternative medical knowledge, Arthur Kleinman, an anthropologist, has observed that health care in most societies occurs in three broad sectors, which sometimes overlap. These are shown in Figure 2.1.

The **professional health-care sector** in Western societies consists of the activities of people in officially recognised occupations such as doctors and nurses. These practitioners are trained to base their practice on principles derived from Western **biomedicine**. The modern sciences of biology and biochemistry[2] are the basis of this form of medical knowledge.

*A Chinese acupuncturist treating a patient. Therapies that may be seen as 'alternative' in Europe are regarded as traditional in China. (Photo: Mike Levers)*

The **alternative health-care sector** consists of the activities of specialist healers working outside the main stream of Western biomedical practice. Sometimes these practitioners derive their practice from biomedical principles and are often referred to as *complementary* to orthodox medicine. But more often some alternative knowledge-base is involved. Thus, for example, *acupuncture* is based on Chinese ideas about the interaction of *yin* and *yang,* complementary 'active' and 'passive' forces that operate within the body but that are also reflected in the outside world. This system of thought is not recognised as valid by many British professional practitioners, although in the last twenty years there has been increasing acceptance of acupuncture therapy by some doctors and nurses, due to its evident effectiveness for some conditions. The fact that there is some use of alternative therapies by practitioners in the professional sector is one reason for the overlap between the sectors in Figure 2.1. There will be a more extensive discussion of the relationship between professional and alternative practitioners later in this chapter.

In the **lay health-care sector**, illness is often treated without any consultation of practitioners in other sectors since, for a variety of reasons, certain illnesses may be judged not suitable for specialist help. Self-medication, often in consultation with family or friends, is the norm. Think of taking a headache pill, or putting a plaster on a child's grazed knee. It has been

[1] This is discussed extensively in another book in this series, *Caring for Health: History and Diversity* (Open University Press, 2nd edn 1993; 3rd edn 2001).

[2] Biomedical methods of scientific research are described in another book in this series, *Studying Health and Disease* (Open University Press, 2nd edn 1994; colour-enhanced 2nd edn 2001).

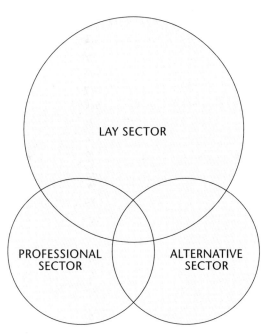

**Figure 2.1**  *Health-care systems.*
*(Adapted from Kleinman, 1980, p. 50)*

estimated that between 70–90 per cent of health care takes place in the lay sector; most is done by women (Kleinman *et al.*, 1978).

All three of these sectors sometimes go under names other than the ones we have chosen to use here (see Box 2.1). It may seem strange to you that the same thing can be described as both 'non-orthodox' and 'traditional'. This reflects the relative position of the alternative sector in different countries. In China, practices such as acupuncture and herbalism have a much longer tradition than does Western biomedicine. The co-existence of the two traditions is such that there are really two parallel 'orthodoxies' in that country, and two types of 'professional' that the Chinese patient may consult. Our choice of terms reflects the fact that this book is largely intended for use in the Western context.

Initially, the focus of this chapter will be on the *lay* sector, where ill-health is first experienced. Lay care, however, is sometimes judged by those who are ill to be inappropriate. The variety of means that people use in order to decide to consult either professional or alternative healers is also described later in this chapter. Figure 2.1 shows overlap between the lay sector and the other two sectors. Some lay knowledge is influenced by biomedical principles and some derives from family traditions and 'folklore'. Some lay knowledge is influenced by the principles of alternative medicine, especially where lay care is practised by people from countries that have their own medical traditions, such as India or China. The boundaries between all three sectors are flexible and negotiated.

**Box 2.1   Terms used to describe the three sectors of health care**

| *Professional* | *Alternative* | *Lay* |
| --- | --- | --- |
| Orthodox | Non-orthodox | Popular |
| Formal | Traditional | Common-sense |
| Biomedical | Complementary | Informal |
| Scientific | Folk | |
| Western | | |

The negotiation of boundaries between professional and alternative practitioners is the focus of the final section of this chapter.

## 2.2   Health beliefs

Within the lay sector, **health beliefs** often inform treatment. These consist of views about what causes, prevents and cures illness, which are held by people who may have no formal training in health care. Anthropologists have long studied belief systems in **traditional societies**, that is, where the customs and way of life have remained virtually unchanged for thousands of years. (Early anthropologists used terms such as 'primitive' or 'savage', to describe such societies. Modern terms might be 'pre-industrial' or 'non-Western'. The term 'traditional' is an attempt to use a word that is reasonably value-neutral.) It is only more recently that they, together with sociologists, have turned to the study of lay beliefs in societies like that of the modern United Kingdom.

To begin our account of health beliefs then, let us consider an example, from a study of a group of people called the *Shribit*, by the African anthropologist Utu Ofiy.

> To the Shribits with whom I lived all sorts of malign influences were thought to undermine bodily and spiritual health. Elders would hold forth in long discourses on the evils of eating animal flesh, which many saw as containing a magical substance, *loretseloch*, blocking the movement of vital forces around the body. A type of dance, known as *goj,* was indulged in, sometimes to excess by the younger members of the group. This *goj* was an unusual type of ritual, in that its purpose was entirely protective against future misfortune. It was also unusual in that it was often done early in the morning, by individuals or in pairs — I never observed more than three people together in this dance. *Goj* is not done in a fixed location, but done, as it were, on the run, sometimes over extremely long distances. I never observed any one episode of this dance from start to finish, as my several attempts to accompany an individual taken by the spirit of *goj* ended in personal exhaustion long before the performer had finished. Humiliating indeed is the memory of those occasions where I have been forced to walk back to the living place, sometimes from miles away, only to be greeted by chuckles from the dancer, long since returned and by now free of the possession that had impelled him to the dance.

> In fact moral connotations and personal failings are never far away when a Shribit discusses his bodily ailments. Young (1976) has distinguished between cultures that believe in external causes of illness, such as sorcery, or the influence of the planets, and cultures that have an internalised view, where imbalance within the body leads to it falling sick. Much of Shribit belief lies firmly within the internalising camp. As a result, Shribits seem to possess an insatiable capacity for self-blame once ill and for moralising about the illnesses of others. There is great concern to distinguish between genuine sufferers and those who simply mimic suffering in order to absolve themselves from their social duties — for work is very onerous in

the complex Shribit society, with its detailed division of labour. Once illness is identified, the cause is almost always located as having its origin in some action of the sufferer. An explanation may be sought in the immediate past behaviour of the sick person: a failure to perform sufficient *goj*, or an excessive intake of *loretseloch*, for example. If the sufferer himself cannot be blamed, the parents of the sufferer may be implicated, through a magical influence that is said to pass between men and women at the moment of conception, described by a term that has no parallel in any other culture with which I am familiar: *ytidereh*. This substance is said to influence all manner of characteristics in the offspring of parents, including appearance, character and even minor mannerisms that may be shared between parents and their children. (Ofiy, 1993)

●   Who are the Shribit?

■   They are the British. Utu Ofiy is U205, the Open University code for the course associated with this book. Horace Miner (1956) originally wrote a 'spoof' piece satirising the health beliefs of Americans (the Nacirema). (Try to unravel the other words that are in italics, and see if you agree with this description of British health beliefs.)

It is a little unfair to spring an anthropological joke like this on you so early in the course. (All of the other examples in this book are genuine.) It was done to make a point that our own health beliefs are not always so far from those that we may regard as less advanced. It also illustrates the difficulties that we normally have in making our own society appear **anthropologically strange**, as though we are anthropologists stumbling across our own culture for the first time. It is easy to see the beliefs of other cultures, or of people in past times in this way. It is harder to do this with the culture we live in.

*The thought and practices of people in other cultures can seem irrational or bizarre, but they help us to see our own actions as anthropologically strange. (Left) The 'Jura' treatment: two men preparing a steam bath to drive out sickness; Orokaiva in Papua New Guinea, from Williams, F. E., 1930,* Orokaiva Society, *Oxford University Press, Oxford, Plate XXXLI. (Source: The Wellcome Library, London) (Right) Keeping fit, or a ritual dance to prevent misfortune? (Photo: Mike Levers)*

## 2.2.1 Modern health beliefs in the United Kingdom

One study that is particularly effective in subverting our common sense ideas was conducted by Cecil Helman, an anthropologist who was working as a general practitioner (GP) in North London in the 1970s. Turn now to the Reader and study his article 'Feed a cold, starve a fever' which was written in 1978.[3] When you have finished, answer the following questions, which are the first of a series on Helman's article occurring at other points later in the chapter.

● For which type of illness do people blame themselves?

■ Colds and chills. They are seen to result from carelessness or lack of foresight, by going outside with wet hair, excessive exposure to night air, or returning from a holiday in a hot place.

● For which type of illness do people blame forces outside their control?

■ Fevers. They are thought to be due to invisible germs, bugs or viruses. These are malevolent entities with personalities, their influence arising from social contact.

● How have these health beliefs changed over time?

■ Younger people, brought up as the first 'antibiotic generation' are more likely to ascribe both hot and cold types of illness to germs or viruses, resulting in a weaker sense of personal responsibility for becoming ill.

Certain features of lay health beliefs are common across cultures. They may also persist from past times, long after official medical ideas have rejected them. An example is humoral theory. This theory probably has its origins in ancient folklore, but it was developed by the Greek and Arabic medical traditions, particularly in the work of Hippocrates (born in 460 BC) and later Galen (AD 129–216?), who lived in Rome and whose work influenced Arabian physicians. The human body was seen as a microcosm of the world, its inner workings a parallel to those of the universe, or macrocosm (see Figure 2.2). Nature, whose elements were earth, fire, air and

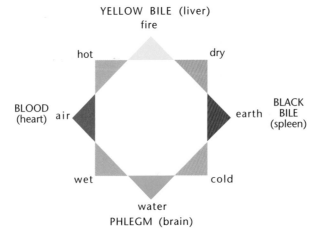

**Figure 2.2** *This diagram shows the relationship between the four qualities, the four humours and the four elements. The humours need to be kept in balance if illness is to be avoided.*

[3] *Health and Disease: A Reader* (Open University Press, 2nd edn 1995; 3rd edn 2001).

water, corresponded to the bodily *humours*, which survive in the English language as descriptions of temperament or character: melancholic (black bile), phlegmatic (phlegm), choleric (yellow bile) and sanguine (blood). Associated with these elements and humours in a complex theory were the four *qualities*, wet, dry, hot and cold.

Humoral theory, via the Moorish occupation of the Iberian peninsula, influenced Spanish and Portuguese physicians, who in turn took these ideas to South America. Latin American folk medicine still shows this influence, explaining bodily and mental disorder by the effect of heat or cold. These words do not refer to *actual* temperature, but to a symbolic power contained in substances such as food. Thus menstruation is considered to be a hot state; menstruating women must avoid certain foods classified as 'cold' lest they clot the hot menstrual blood. In humoral theory, illness is caused by an imbalance of humours or qualities, so treatment consists of altering the balance. The practices of bleeding, purging and vomiting were used by European physicians up until the nineteenth century. Later in this book (Chapter 5) these practices will be described in more detail.

● Helman's description of English lay health beliefs shows the persistence of humoral theory. What treatments designed to redress imbalance does he describe?

■ Coughing up the muck, sweating, washing out germs with fluids such as tea, salt water or cough mixture.

In fact, many of the remedies that are bought over the counter in chemists' shops are designed to appeal to the persistence of humoral theory in lay beliefs. Sweet lemon-flavoured drinks for colds and cough mixture are examples. Helman suggests that doctors sometimes go along with these beliefs, accommodating their patients by prescribing cough mixture even when it has no effect.

Sometimes lay health care is based on theories derived from traditional practices in other countries. In the 1980s, Nikki Thorogood, a British sociologist, interviewed 32 Afro-Caribbean women in Hackney, asking them what measures they took to maintain their health and cure illness. She found a considerable residue of belief and practice derived from folk traditions in the Caribbean, particularly among the older women. A very common medicine was the *washout*, this often being some combination of senna, castor oil, salts and 'physic'. This might be added to a 'tonic' or vitamin supplement such as 'Seven Seas' or cod liver oil. Washouts were taken either regularly, or on special occasions such as bank holidays. Their general purpose was as a type of purgative or laxative, to keep your 'insides clear' or, as Thorogood puts it, 'something like Dyno-rod for humans'. Two of the people interviewed described the purpose of the washout:

> Liquid of Life…you can buy it in the chemist. It kind of purifies the body or something, it wash all the rubbish away, cleans out the body.

> Cerasee — that's a form of washout. That cleans not only your digestive system but it cleanses your womb and everything. (Quoted in Thorogood, 1990, p. 148)

Sheila Kitzinger, who studied health practices in the Caribbean, describes the origins of these ideas.

> Jamaican concepts of sickness are composed of two in some ways disparate body cosmologies, one derived from the medieval European 'humours' and the other from West African concepts of blockage by objects which, whether by sorcery or other means, have obstructed passages so that body substances can no longer flow…. This is related to the bodily concept in which there is one passage leading between the mouth and the lower orifices, passing through the uterus and the stomach on the way. (Kitzinger, 1982, pp. 198–9)

Cecil Helman's study reminds us that such practices are not only to be found in immigrant groups in Britain. A study that ran in parallel to Thorogood's, found widespread use of laxatives among white women of British origin. Many of the washouts and tonics described by the people Thorogood interviewed were available in high street shops — camomile tea, Epsom salts, vitamin preparations, Complan (a 'build-up' drink) — marketed to and used by the population as a whole.

## 2.2.2  The moral dimension: why me, why now?

Peoples' ideas about the causes of ill-health can be thought of as attempts to answer two questions: why have I become ill, and why has it happened now? The television programme and audiotape associated with this chapter[4] show that moral considerations can influence peoples' attempts to answer these two questions. People are often concerned about the extent to which they should shoulder the responsibility for their illness. Iris, interviewed by Jocelyn Cornwell in the television programme, is a good example. As long as she believed she had depression, she did not consider herself to be suffering from an illness that she could legitimately take to a doctor. In her eyes, depression is something to hide, something she should be able to get over on her own. When at last she did consult a doctor, Iris's diagnosis, of an underactive thyroid gland, freed her from the discrediting or stigmatising effects of mental illness because it removed responsibility for the illness from her.

The moral evaluations that pervade our beliefs about illness are deep-seated. Among the first categories of disease that emerge in some societies with elementary systems of health belief are those that serve as a warning against violating moral codes. The *Hadza* of East Africa, for example, do not have terms in their language that describe specific disease entities (Fabrega, 1979). They refer to symptoms, such as a pain in the chest, or coughing, but do not put together groups of symptoms and give them a name. The one exception to this is a condition suffered from by men, called *lingedako*. Symptoms involve an appearance of burning skin which peels, the vomiting of pus and eventual death. It is said to be caused by frequent adultery, or intercourse with one's sister. The disease operates as a partial myth in *Hadza* society, whose complex symbolic meaning represents the dire consequences of transgressing *Hadza* moral codes.

● What diseases can you think of that some people in the United Kingdom use as moral warnings?

---

[4] Both are entitled 'Why me? Why now?' and have been prepared for Open University students. Listen to the audiotape *after* watching the television programme.

■  The most obvious are those associated with sexual activity disapproved of by some people. Sexually transmitted diseases, AIDS and even cervical cancer have been seen in this way. Lung cancer in relation to smoking, and cirrhosis in relation to alcoholism are other examples.

Mildred Blaxter[5] found in her study of British lay health beliefs that a common view of what makes a person healthy emphasised virtuous behaviour. Here are some examples of people describing others whom they considered to be healthy.

> I call her healthy because she goes jogging and she doesn't eat fried food. She walks a lot and she doesn't drink alcohol. She takes care of herself. She was the sickly one as a baby, but she's the healthier one now. She does all the right things. She eats plenty of fruit. Why do I call her healthy? She leads a proper respectable life so she's never ill. (Quoted in Blaxter, 1990, pp. 23–4)

Ill-health is often equated with general misfortune. Here is another of Blaxter's respondents saying why he considered a friend to be healthy.

> Although he has TB he's been aware of his problems and has got over them. Though he was made redundant, since then he's done his own thing, just worked the way and when he wanted to. He didn't worry about being redundant, and he hasn't taken on too much in the size of house and garden. He enjoys life. (Quoted in Blaxter, 1990, p. 22)

Clearly, for this person, remaining healthy is bound up with coping with bad luck or adverse events generally. In fact these two categories are not distinguished in a number of societies. The *Gnau* people of New Guinea, for example, have no word that differentiates illness from other types of misfortune. *Wola* means 'ill', 'bad', 'wretched', 'evil', 'harmful', 'forbidden' and 'potentially dangerous'. *Neyigeg* is a word used by the *Gnau* to describe an impaired sense of wellbeing as a whole, but this does not include illnesses affecting specific parts of the body. *Neyigeg* is caused by evil beings, magic or sorcery.

●  What modern parallels to magical beliefs about the causes of illness does Helman identify?

■  Germs are like invisible, malign spirits. Pollution and radiation are also regarded as evil substances that cause illness.

To Helman's list might be added the idea of 'stress'. This is a common explanation for illness, used in all three of the sectors of health care. Stress may be seen as weakening defences against infectious and other illnesses, or as reducing vital energies in a less specific way. It is sometimes seen as arising from strains in personal relationships, the difficulties of living in crowded, polluted, urban environments, and of competing with others in modern society. Accusations of sorcery in some societies have their origins in stress in personal relationships. Thus witchcraft is a metaphor for the destructive hatred and envy that people from time to time feel for each other, and our own ideas about stress and illness run in close parallel.

---

[5] Mildred Blaxter is one of the sociologists whose work is shown in the television programme 'Why me? Why now?' associated with this chapter.

### 2.2.3  Public and private accounts

Mildred Blaxter found that, when talking about the causes of their *own* ill-health, people were most likely to blame their own behaviour, stress and family relationships. However, when talking about the causes of ill-health in society *as a whole*, other factors also became important. Particularly among more educated people, poor material circumstances, poor housing and standards of living were said to be important; ironically, working-class people attached less importance to these factors. Thus people in different contexts gave different accounts of the causes of illness. Blaxter says that peoples' replies may have been influenced by a desire to give the officially 'correct' or 'expected' answers. Jocelyn Cornwell has taken this idea further in her distinction between 'public' and 'private' accounts of health and illness.

> ...public accounts in general draw attention to aspects of peoples' experience and to ideas and values that they believe are likely to win 'public' approval...they draw attention to aspects of experience, ideas, and values that people believe are acceptable to doctors and compatible with a medical point of view.... The place where medically unacceptable and incompatible opinions and values are stated is in private accounts. (Cornwell, 1984, pp. 204–5)

Accounts of health and illness can be seen as attempts to make sense of events that are otherwise mysterious and threatening. In constructing them people can draw upon a number of sources, including residual beliefs from past times, current popular theories in magazines and newspapers, or indeed the pronouncements of doctors. Increasingly, these days, lay accounts incorporate ideas and expertise from the professional sector of health care. Even our most private accounts, whose audience may be ourselves alone, may fluctuate depending on our current needs. We should therefore be careful about assuming that health beliefs are in some way fixed entities, either in our own or in other cultures.

To summarise this section on health beliefs, we can conclude that the lay sector of health care is influenced by a variety of health beliefs, some of which are derived from past medical theories, such as humoral theory, others of which are influenced by the medical traditions of other countries, as in the case of the washouts used by some Afro-Caribbeans. Moral connotations are never far away in lay attempts to explain illness causation, and accounts are likely to vary according to the audience.

## 2.3  From lay to professional health care

### 2.3.1  The illness iceberg

Doctors only treat a small proportion of illness. The majority of symptoms that trouble people, if treated at all, are dealt with in the lay sector of health care. If you walk into any high street pharmacist you will see a vast array of pills, potions and preparations. Temperatures, headaches, indigestion and sore throats are the most common causes for self-medication. The extent of the lay sector of health care has led some to describe the symptoms that doctors see as the tip of a **clinical iceberg**, the majority of symptoms remaining hidden from their view because they are not brought to the surgery. Table 2.1 shows the results of a study of 79 women aged 16–44 on a housing estate in London. They were asked to keep a diary for six weeks, recording any symptoms they suffered from, and consultations they had with doctors.

- Which are the three symptoms most likely to lead to a consultation with a doctor?

- 'Others', where for every eight episodes of symptoms there was on average one trip to the doctor (one consultation per eight episodes, 1 : 8); sore throat (1 : 9); women's complaints like period pain (1 : 10).

- Which are the least likely to be a cause for consultation?

- Changes in energy and tiredness caused no consultations despite 109 episodes; nerves, depression or irritability (in 74 episodes the doctor was only consulted once); headache (1 : 60); backache (1 : 38).

It might be thought that only less serious conditions are kept from the doctor, but some evidence suggests that this is not the case. In 1978 the staff of a mobile health clinic investigated 3 160 people. Of these, 1 800 (57 per cent) were referred to their GP. Three hundred and ninety-six (12.5 per cent of the total) were considered by the GPs to need a hospital admission (Epsom, 1978).

**Table 2.1**  Symptom episodes and medical consultations recorded in health diaries.

| Main types of symptoms recorded | No. of symptom episodes | No. of occasions on which symptom episode precipitated medical consultation | Ratio of medical consultation to symptom episodes |
| --- | --- | --- | --- |
| headache | 180 | 3 | 1 : 60 |
| changes in energy, tiredness | 109 | 0 | – |
| nerves, depression or irritability | 74 | 1 | 1 : 74 |
| aches or pains in joints, muscles, legs or arms | 71 | 4 | 1 : 18 |
| women's complaints like period pain[1] | 69 | 7 | 1 : 10 |
| stomach aches or pains | 45 | 4 | 1 : 11 |
| backache | 38 | 1 | 1 : 38 |
| cold, flu or runny nose | 37 | 3 | 1 : 12 |
| sore throat | 36 | 4 | 1 : 9 |
| sleeplessness | 31 | 1 | 1 : 31 |
| others | 173 | 21 | 1 : 8 |
| **Totals** | 863 | 49 | 1:18 |

[1] Stomach aches and pains and backache were classified as period pains if so defined by the women themselves.
(Source: Scambler et al., 1981, p. 748, Table 1)

## 2.3.2  Deciding to seek medical help

### Triggers

How then are illnesses defined as worthy of medical attention? The answer to this question varies across different cultures. A classic study in America was carried out in 1973 by Irving Kenneth Zola, a sociologist. He interviewed people in hospital clinics in Boston and found that there were five identifiable **triggers for seeking medical help**. These were as follows:

1    The occurrence of an interpersonal crisis (e.g. a death in the family);

2    Perceived interference with social or personal relations;

3    'Sanctioning' (pressure from others to consult);

4    Perceived interference with vocational or physical activity (e.g. paid work);

5    A kind of 'temporalising of symptomatology' (the setting of a deadline, for example, 'If I feel the same way on Monday…', or 'If I have another turn…'). (Adapted from Zola, 1973)

Zola found that Italian-Americans tended to report the first two triggers the most frequently. Irish-Americans were more likely to report the third and fourth triggers. People of Anglo-Saxon origin also preferred the fourth. Complaints of pain and generalised malaise were more common amongst the Italians. Zola suggests the difference between ethnic groups reflects differences in the cultures of the groups. The Anglo-Saxon preference for the fourth trigger, for example, he feels is related to the pervasiveness of the 'Protestant work ethic', which impels Anglo-Saxons to make work a high priority.

The third trigger, 'sanctioning', shows that other peoples' views may be important in the decision to consult. Here is a case from Zola's research that illustrates this.

> Mr and Mrs O'Brien were both suffering from myopia (short-sight), both claimed difficulty seeing, both had had their trouble for some period of time. The wife described her visit as follows: 'Oh, as far as the symptoms were concerned, I'd be apt to let it go, but not my husband. He worries a lot, he wants things to be just so….he said to me "Your worries about your brother are over now so why can't you take care of your eyes now?"' And so she did. Her husband, coming in several months later, followed the same pattern. He also considered himself somewhat resistant to being doctored. 'I'm not in the habit of talking about aches and pains. My wife perhaps would say "Go to the doctor", but me I'd like to see if things will work themselves out.' How did he get here? It turns out that he was on vacation and he'd been meaning to take care of it,'Well, I tend to let things go but not my wife, so on the first day of my vacation my wife said, "Why don't you come, why don't you take care of it now?" So I did.' (Zola, 1973, pp. 684–5)

### Lay referral

The process by which people talk about their illnesses to networks of friends and relatives in order to decide what to do has been called **lay referral** by sociologists. This parallels the medical referral system operated between doctors in the professional sector. Lay referral may vary according to the nature of the illness, the extent of peoples' social networks, proximity to health-care facilities and a host of other factors.

● An interview with Wendy, describing the events that led to her hysterectomy, is provided in the audiotape associated with this chapter. Was lay referral involved in her decision to consult?

■ No, she says she discussed her problem with no one. She says it is not the sort of topic she would discuss with friends, although she said she could have talked about her symptoms with her mother if she had wanted to.

Different types of social network can influence the decision to consult a doctor. The sociologists who did the study that led to the results in Table 2.1 found that women who talked with relatives were *more* likely to consult their GPs, whereas women with large friendship networks were *less* likely to consult. The researchers suggest that discussions with relatives tend to be more intense and sympathetic, reinforcing the importance of symptoms, whereas talk with friends is more superficial and results in a redefinition of problems as less serious.

### 2.3.3  Illness versus disease

Eventually, however, many people take their illnesses to the doctor. In this context, **illness** can be thought of as a collection of symptoms that trouble the patient. The complex processes occurring in the lay sector ensure that professional practitioners see not just the tip of the clinical iceberg, but a sample of illnesses that has been filtered by cultural factors before it reaches them. Stepping into the doctor's surgery, the person with an illness is transformed into a patient:

> A general practitioner, say, makes a routine measurement of a man's blood pressure and finds it raised. Thereafter both the man and his doctor will say that he 'suffers' from high blood pressure. He walks in a healthy man, but he walks out a patient, and his new-found status is confirmed by the giving and receiving of tablets. (Rose, 1981, p. 1 848)

The patient's view of *illness* can be contrasted with the doctor's view of **disease**. Broadly speaking, modern scientifically based medical thought defines disease in terms of the following characteristics:

1 There is an underlying physical *cause*. This has an effect on the body at the cellular or even biochemical level and sometimes involves another biological organism such as a bacterium or a virus.

2 There is a disturbance to a part or parts of the body's physical structure that causes the manifestations of the disease such as pain or a raised temperature. This physical disturbance is know as a **pathological lesion**.

3 There is a recognisable *course* which may be a sequence of stages marked by characteristic symptoms. This course is not necessarily exhibited by all people who have a disease, but all cases can be theoretically related to a definite stage.

4 Disease, or pathology, is identified and defined by the fact that it represents a deviation from what is **normal**. Taking a person's temperature or pulse, or listening to their chest, establishes whether some aspect of their bodily functioning deviates from what is normal.

The anthropologist Leon Eisenberg draws out the contrast between the patient's 'subjective' concern with the experience of illness and the doctor's preoccupation with 'objective' pathology and disease thus:

> To state it flatly, patients suffer 'illnesses', physicians diagnose and treat 'diseases'...illnesses are *experiences* of disvalued changes in states of being and in social function; diseases, in the scientific paradigm of modern medicine, are *abnormalities* in the *structure* and *function* of body organs and systems. (Eisenberg, 1977, p. 11)

As in the case of the man with high blood pressure, it is possible to have disease, but not illness. People can have high blood pressure, raised blood cholesterol or HIV infection, and feel perfectly well; yet to the doctor they are not. Conversely, it is possible to have illness and yet not be classified as diseased; people may feel they have something wrong with them, experiencing distressing feelings of an emotional or physical nature, and yet be told by their doctor that nothing is wrong. They may be classified as suffering from psychosomatic disorders, hypochondria or even malingering. More usually, patients who experience illness are offered a **disease label** by doctors, that is the professional name, or a lay version of it, by which the disease is known.

### 2.3.4  Non-compliance

A great irritation for many doctors is the patient who does not follow their advice about treatment. The medical term for this phenomenon is **non-compliance**, and it is very extensive. Studies in the United States have estimated that about a third of all patients do not follow medical advice. Here are two examples of non-compliance.

> P.K. is a person whose understanding of her diagnosis is good, but whose compliance is poor. She consulted with the doctor because of headache, double vision, stomach ache, lethargy and tiredness. She thought her symptoms might be related to hypoglycaemia (low blood sugar) and stress. The doctor confirmed her suspicions and recommended a change in diet and increased exercise. For about a month she followed the diet fairly well and said she felt much better. Two weeks after the diagnosis she said 'Food has become the answer for everything'. However, at 17 weeks post-diagnosis, while her conception of her hypoglycaemia and its treatment remained essentially unchanged and quite similar to that of the physician, she rarely adhered to the diet. She said she felt worse, but she was unable to stay on the diet because of the demands of her life as a graduate student and teacher. She found the treatment useful in dealing with specific instances of symptom onset, but too cumbersome to employ on a day-to-day basis. (Hunt *et al.*, 1989, p. 323)

> When I was young I would try not to take it.... I'd take it for a while and think, "Well, I don't need it any more", so I would not take it, deliberately, just to see if I could do without. And then (in a few days) I'd start takin' it again, because I'd start passin' out.... I will still try that now, when my husband is out of town.... I just think, maybe I'm still gonna grow out of it or something. (Woman explaining her non-compliance with anti-epilepsy drugs, quoted in Conrad, 1985, p. 34)

Various attempts have been made to explain non-compliance. First, it might be due to a lack of education about medical matters in patients. Second, it could be due to the lay beliefs of patients being in conflict with the medical view of the cause of the disease. Third, it could be due to a desire to assert control over illness, and adjust medical regimes to the demands of everyday life.

● Which of these three theories best explains the behaviour of the two people above?

■ P.K. is a teacher and graduate, so the first theory *might* not fit her. The second theory *certainly* would not, since her view of the cause of her illness does not conflict with that of her doctor. Either of the first two theories *might*, however, fit the second woman — we can't tell without knowing more about her beliefs and level of education. The third theory *certainly* fits both the women.

In fact, sociologists who have studied non-compliance have found that it often makes sense when seen from a patient's point of view. People have been found to experiment with medical regimes, or pursue alternative treatments in order to cope with their particular illness in their specific circumstances. Broadly speaking, medical practitioners in the professional sector tend to be trained to see the patient as the 'carrier' of a disease. This means that some doctors can have difficulty in recognising the uniqueness of each episode of illness in an individual's life. This difference between the doctor's and the patient's view can be summarised by saying that doctors try to *cure disease*, whereas patients may be more concerned with *healing illness*. This distinction may help to explain why some people consult alternative practitioners when ill; one of the claims of many such practitioners is that they address the patient as a unique individual whose illness is but one aspect of their life.

## 2.4   Choosing a healer

When they judge themselves ill enough with a non-urgent condition to need medical help, most people in the United Kingdom go first to their GP. In the National Health Service (NHS), the GP is the gatekeeper to a range of other services. Normally, we think of professional referral as being from GP to specialist, perhaps in the hospital. In recent years, however, GPs have become more willing to refer patients to practitioners in the alternative sector. They may even themselves be qualified in the practice of some alternative therapy, such as acupuncture or osteopathy, and see these methods as complementing orthodox medicine. A survey in 1986 of GPs in Oxfordshire showed that 12 per cent had received training in one or more forms of alternative therapy, and 42 per cent said they would like such training, particularly in the areas of manipulation (osteopathy and chiropractic), acupuncture, homeopathy and hypnotherapy (Anderson and Anderson, 1987). 59 per cent had referred one or more patients to an alternative practitioner — usually in one of the above disciplines — in the past year.

How large is the alternative health-care sector in the United Kingdom and how does this compare with the situation in other countries? Why do people consult alternative practitioners in preference to orthodox professionals? We turn to these questions next.

*Practitioners of alternative or complementary therapies claim to treat the patient as a whole and unique individual. (Photo: Mike Levers)*

### 2.4.1   The size of the alternative sector

Within alternative medicine there is great variety. Some therapies — acupuncture, for example — arise from traditions whose historical origins lie further back than those of Western medicine. Others are more recent creations. Some require lengthy periods of training resulting in formal registration as a practitioner — osteopathy and chiropractic, for example — others do not. Consultation of practitioners in this sector has risen sharply in recent years, although in practice it is quite difficult to estimate the size of the alternative sector.

The first systematic attempt at doing so was in 1981 when Stephen Fulder and Robin Munro made strenuous efforts to count all alternative practitioners in seven areas of Britain (Fulder and Munro, 1985). In these areas they estimated there were 12 such practitioners per 100 000 population. There were about four times this number of GPs. However, alternative practitioners on average saw fewer patients than did GPs and most worked part-time.

By 1997, the number of registered practitioners in the alternative or complementary sector in the UK had risen to 40 000, with many more thousands in a wide range of specialities working outside any registration system. A fifth of UK general practices provided some alternative or complementary services by a member of the primary health-care team, and around 4 000 orthodox health-care professionals also practised as alternative or complementary therapists, (Zollman and Vickers, 1999). Almost half the GPs in the UK referred patients to alternative practitioners on occasions, and around 70 per cent of these referrals were paid for by the NHS.

### 2.4.2   Traditional medicine

In spite of signs of increased interest in recent years, it remains the case that the professional sector based on biomedical science dominates in the United Kingdom and other Western or developed countries. This is not the situation in many other countries, where *traditional* forms of medicine are more important. In many rural areas of Africa, for example, access to Western medicine is poor, and traditional practice both fills the gap and is sometimes preferred by patients. Thus in Sokoto, Northern Nigeria, it was estimated in 1986 that there was one Western trained doctor for every 100 000 people. 85–90 per cent of people consulted traditional practitioners for advice (Tahzib and Daniel, 1986).

The attraction of traditional medicine in Africa may be partly due to its effectiveness in satisfying patients' needs to *explain* their illness. The therapeutic benefits of some forms of traditional medicine may rest entirely in giving the illness a meaning and assigning it a name or cause that make sense to the sufferer — in much the same way as receiving a diagnosis may bring relief in an orthodox medical consultation.

In India there exist traditions of medical practice that have developed separately from Western medicine, whose practitioners are widely respected and used. The *Ayurvedic* (Hindu) and *Unani-Tibb* (Islamic) traditions are based on humoral ideas, including the 'hot/cold' concept. Government support is given to practitioners of these systems in India.

Sometimes these traditions influence immigrant groups in the United Kingdom. This has been shown by medical doctor Rajinder Singh Bhopal, who investigated the use of traditional medicine amongst the Asian community in Glasgow. He found widespread use of remedies (such as ginger or garlic for arthritis or asthma) based on Asian medical concepts. People using these remedies did not usually see them as being in conflict with the advice of biomedically trained doctors, whom they visited and whose advice was respected. Yet most were reluctant to discuss these practices with doctors because they feared disapproval and believed doctors lacked knowledge or interest in traditional medicine (Bhopal, 1986).

Some European countries contain more established traditions of alternative practice than the United Kingdom. This is particularly the case in Germany where, for example, *homeopathy* was developed in the nineteenth century. Homeopathy is based on the principle of treating like with like; practitioners treat patients with very small quantities of the substance that they believe is making the person ill, on the grounds that this will stimulate the body to heal itself. This contradicts the principles of Western bio-medicine, in which drug treatments are based on the principle of *allopathy*, or treatment by opposites, and drugs are used to oppose the action of disease.

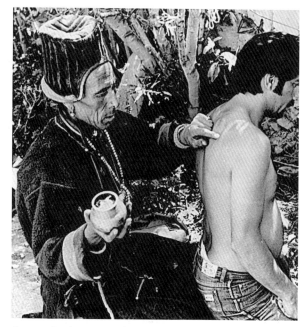

*Sonam Gyelson, a traditional doctor practising Tibetan medicine in Ladakh. Elements of humoral medicine survive and flourish on the Indian sub-continent. (Source: Rex Features)*

Co-existence between biomedicine and traditional medicine has not always been easy, especially when practitioners' livelihoods have been at stake. Oscar Lewis, an anthropologist, describes how, in Tepoztlan, Mexico, a Western-style medical cooperative was set up in the early 1950s (Lewis, 1955). Already in the area existed three types of healer, *curanderos, magicos* and 'el doctor' who, in spite of his title, was not qualified in biomedicine.

> There was continuing faith in the practices of the *curanderos*.... Local interest groups, headed by the leading *curandero*, Don Rosa, [saw] the medical co-operative as a threat. He killed the clinic by discrediting it. The researchers were administering a Rorschach test[6] to all the schoolchildren. Don Rosa persuaded the parents that this was an immoral activity by distributing pornographic pictures which he had acquired in a neighbouring town, saying that these were the tests that were being given to the children. (Stacey, 1988, p. 22)

The mayor, schoolmaster and local fascist leader were also threatened by the clinic, and so opposed it. This resulted in its eventual closure.

## 2.4.3  The users of alternative medicine

Unlike those in Mexico in the 1950s, in the United Kingdom the treatments that we are calling alternative are not most people's first resort. It used to be fashionable to speak of 'fringe' culture and 'fringe' medicine. Subsequently the term 'alternative' became popular in the early 1970s, when a variety of 'alternative' lifestyles were gaining much media exposure. A more recent designation for these therapies is

---

[6] A type of psychological test involving the interpretation of random ink blots.

'complementary'. This usage represents a political statement about the positive value of these therapies and their relationship with the professional sector. It is debatable whether it accurately describes some therapies, such as homeopathy, whose principles are decidedly opposed to the biomedical principles of professional medicine.

Alternative therapies are sometimes characterised as a part of an alternative culture, part of a comprehensive rejection of mainstream values by certain groups of people. Some studies, however, throw doubt on the idea that users of alternative medicine are on the margins of society, although they are in some respects different from the rest of the population. In 1989, MORI, an opinion polling agency, was commissioned to survey a representative sample of the general population, asking people whether they had used various alternative therapies. The results for different age groups, social classes and sexes are given in Table 2.2.

●   What does the table show about users of alternative medicine? Look at which groups have the highest proportion of users.

**Table 2.2**   Percentages of various sex, social class and age groups in the United Kingdom who had used alternative therapy, September 1989 figures. (The figures are the percentage of the people in each group who had used at least one therapy, in a random sample of 1 826 adults.)

|  | Sex | | Social class[1] | | | |
|---|---|---|---|---|---|---|
|  | Men | Women | AB | C1 | C2 | DE |
|  | 20% | 22% | 26% | 22% | 21% | 17% |
| Sample size (N) (= 100%) | 869 | 957 | 312 | 409 | 562 | 543 |
|  | Age (years) | | | | | |
|  | 18–24 | 25–34 | 35–44 | 45–54 | 55–64 | 65+ |
|  | 14% | 20% | 23% | 26% | 29% | 18% |
| Sample size (N) (= 100%) | 279 | 321 | 276 | 261 | 257 | 349 |

[1] Social class is measured here using category A to mean 'professional/senior managerial' and E to mean 'unskilled manual labourer', with other letters referring to grades in between. (Source: MORI (1989) *Alternative medicine,* 21–25 September, MORI, London)

■   There is not a large gender difference, but the users are more likely to be in the middle age groups, and in higher social classes. (20 per cent of the 869 men questioned had used at least one therapy; 22 per cent of the 957 women had done so, and so on.)

Ursula Sharma, a sociologist then at Keele University, interviewed thirty people about how they came to use alternative medicine, and in 1990 wrote a report, entitled 'Using alternative therapies: marginal medicine and central concerns.' Please read the extract from this report which is in the Reader[7] now, and then try to answer the following questions.

[7] *Health and Disease: A Reader* (Open University Press, 2nd edn 1995; 3rd edn 2001).

● How representative of users of alternative medicine are the thirty people?

■ The sample was taken from people answering newspaper advertisements in the Stoke-on-Trent area. It could be that the volunteers were not representative. For example, they might have been people who were keen to advertise the benefits of their treatment. Sharma claims, however, that being representative 'was not the purpose of the research.'[8]

● How did the people hear about the practitioners they consulted?

■ Mostly through the recommendations of people in their social networks — lay referral. Only one was referred by a GP.

● Did the users consult as part of a general philosophical commitment to alternative values?

■ On the whole, no. Sharma stresses the practical, experimental approach of most of her respondents. Many were trying out different things, having started with professional medicine, to see what worked.

The reasons that Sharma's respondents gave for consulting fell into five categories:

1  Conventional medicine failed to get at the 'root cause' of chronic illness or to take a preventative approach, treating the symptoms only.

2  The fear of drugs as habit-forming or having side-effects.

3  Fear or dislike of treatments considered too radical or invasive.

4  A perception that conventional medicine failed to cope with social and experiential aspects of illness.

5  Dissatisfaction with the conventional doctor–patient relationship as giving patients little control.

Consultations with alternative therapists are generally longer than consultations with doctors. One study (Fulder and Munro, 1985) estimated, on the basis of replies by practitioners themselves, that an average length was 36 minutes, six times as long as the average for NHS GPs. Many alternative practitioners like to stress that while professional medicine treats the *disease*, alternative medicine treats the *person*. To do this, time needs to be spent getting to know the patient. Indeed, some alternative therapies, such as homeopathy, require that diagnosis is based on extensive enquiry into the patient's social and emotional life, as well as physical examination. The linking of mind and body is a thread running through a number of alternative therapies. Alternative practitioners often claim that this **holistic** approach contrasts with the separation of these elements in professional medicine which adopts a **reductionist** approach in the sense that the body and mind are *reduced* to a collection of component parts.[9]

---

[8] The importance of representative sampling in this sort of research is discussed more fully in *Studying Health and Disease* (Open University Press, 2nd edn 1994; colour-enhanced 2nd edn 2001), Chapter 5.

[9] Holistic and reductionist approaches to biomedicine are also pursued further in *Studying Health and Disease*, Chapter 9.

## 2.5    Boundaries and boundary maintenance

> The boundaries between what is to count as legitimate knowledge
> and what is not are...not given states of affairs. They have to be
> achieved, and conflict takes place on the margins of science as to
> what is to be incorporated and what rejected. (Bury, 1986,
> p. 145)

Science is usually seen as an objective description of a world that exists independently
of people, a body of knowledge with ever-increasing specialisms, dividing into
sub-specialties over time as discovery reveals more of the complexity of the world.
Scientific knowledge, on this view, is determined by the nature of the world that is
actually out there, waiting to be described and understood. The subdivisions of
medical science, and the organisation of professional medical practice into its
specialist disciplines, are thought to follow this logic. According to this view of
science, the history of medicine is simply the accumulation and ordering of a
mountain of facts, chosen for their truthfulness. Medical practice consists of the
application of the more useful facts.

This picture is challenged by studies of how medical knowledge and specialties
actually develop. The message of many sociologists and historians of medicine is
that, as in the quotation above, a substantial proportion of the content of medical
knowledge is determined by conflict between rival groups and the striving for
**professional dominance**. Far from being purely a revelation of natural laws, the
divisions of medical science can also be seen as achievements in setting boundaries,
between science and non-science, and between medical and non-medical
practitioners. These boundaries are institutionalised and then maintained against
threats. Some argue that the driving force in all this is not scientific discovery, but
the achievement of professional dominance and a monopoly of practice.

### 2.5.1    Professions

Underlying this claim is a particular view of the occupational strategy of the medical
profession, which has resulted in a generally high social standing, and a position of
dominance over most other groups involved in health care. Eliot Freidson, a
sociologist who has written extensively on the profession of medicine, has stated
that:

> It is useful to think of a profession as an occupation which has
> ...[gained] control over the determination of the substance of its
> own work...it is autonomous or self-directing...[sustaining] this
> special status by its pervasive profession of the extraordinary
> trustworthiness of its members. (Freidson, 1970a, p. xvii)

An essential part of doctors' occupational strategy to achieve this end is to restrict
entry to the profession by using control over the training and qualifications required
for membership.[10] By limiting the supply of doctors, a high demand for their services
is ensured.

A second strategy is to create and impose a code of professional ethics, whereby
doctors are committed to placing the interests of their patients first. Critics of medical
dominance argue that by maintaining control over the disciplining of members,
professions are able to prevent the sort of public scrutiny of their affairs that could

[10] The evolution of the professional status of doctors from 1500 to the present day is discussed in
*Caring for Health: History and Diversity* (Open University Press, 2nd edn 1993; 3rd edn 2001).

threaten their altruistic image. The medical profession, so the argument goes, does this in the United Kingdom through the General Medical Council (GMC), which is responsible for disciplining doctors.

●   How might members of the General Medical Council counter this argument?

■   Far from being primarily a means of preventing scrutiny by members of the public, the GMC serves the public interest by ensuring that high standards of professional conduct are maintained in medical practice.

A third essential element of the professional strategy is to claim that only doctors are qualified to provide medical services. In the case of doctors this has been recognised by law since the middle of the nineteenth century. It is illegal to impersonate a medical practitioner. This has ensured professional monopoly of practice.

For any occupation, professional status of this sort is desirable, for with it comes high social status, control over one's own work, and substantial material reward. The medical profession has fought long and hard to attain this status and to maintain it in the face of contemporary threats to medical dominance in health care.[11]

Our present concern, however, is the place of medical knowledge in these professional struggles. David Blane, a sociologist who is also a doctor, has claimed that

> ...the acquisition of these professional powers occurred before doctors had the means to alter the course of most diseases to any significant extent.... The development of effective knowledge...was produced by a health care system over which doctors had already achieved considerable professional control. (Blane, 1991, p. 227)

David Blane clearly believes that much medical knowledge *is* effective in curing disease, but that this was not the reason for the granting of professional status to doctors. Study of disputes between professional practitioners and others tends to support the view that medical effectiveness has not been the only issue at stake, although it is an important one.

## 2.5.2  The boundary between alternative and professional sectors

The conflicts between alternative and professional medicine provide many examples of boundary maintenance disputes. The effectiveness of the therapies concerned is often hotly disputed. In 1986 the British Medical Association (BMA) published a report on alternative medicine. Having defined science as objective and value-free (in the words quoted at the beginning of this chapter), the authors went on to say that:

> Herein lies the first and most important difficulty that orthodox medical science has with alternative approaches. So many of them do not base their rationale on any theory which is consistent with natural laws as we now understand them.

[11] Threats to doctors' professional dominance in modern UK health care are discussed in two other books in this series, *Caring for Health: History and Diversity*, 3rd edn 2001, Chapter 7, and *Dilemmas in UK Health Care* (Open University Press, 3rd edn 2001).

The fact is that the steadily developing body of orthodox medical knowledge has led to large, demonstrable, and reproducible benefits for mankind, of a scale which cannot be matched by alternative approaches...

...New and unconventional techniques should be evaluated with the same scientific methods as have been applied to [orthodox] therapeutic methods now known, through the results of careful evaluation, to be effective. In the results of such studies does progress lie. (BMA, 1986, pp. 62, 75)

The report assessed the claims of a number of alternative therapies and concluded that some of them could be effective. Acupuncture for analgesia, hypnotherapy for some conditions (for example, asthma), and manipulation (i.e. osteopathy or chiropractic) for pain arising from spinal disorders were the chief benefits that the BMA recognised. However, concern was expressed about the harmful effects of some therapies — such as herbal remedies — and doubt expressed about the validity of the underlying theories of even those therapies where benefit was recognised. Patients' belief that treatment would make them better[12] was felt to be a powerful factor in the testimony of many users of alternative therapies that the treatment had worked.

At the same time, the report argued that part of the appeal of alternative therapy was the time that practitioners spent with patients, addressing their reactions to their illness, and helping them cope with its consequences. The BMA recognised that this was often not done by busy NHS doctors, and welcomed developments in the NHS that stressed this more holistic view of patient care.

The British Holistic Medical Association (BHMA), founded in 1983 to promote holistic approaches within professional medicine, and containing many medically qualified practitioners of alternative therapies, published a response to the BMA report, an extract of which is given here.

No approach has a monopoly on the truth. Our world views and the meaning we attribute to phenomena more or less fit a negotiated reality. Unfortunately the authors of the BMA document have taken the primitive...stance that 'whoever is not for me is against me'.... It is interesting that Galileo's theories threatened the church to such an extent that Galileo was put on trial for his thinking. It seems quite a comment on the difficulty that small minds have with truth when it brings change or shifts in thought.

...The BMA Report fails to understand medicine both in relationship to society and in a historical context. The concept of disease reflected in the document belongs to a limited scientific model which characterises constellations of physical symptoms and the biological conditions which underlie them, and ignores social factors, psychological correlates, and illness behaviour.

[12] Sometimes called the *placebo effect,* which is discussed in *Studying Health and Disease* (Open University Press, 2nd edn 1994; colour-enhanced 2nd edn 2001).

…The personal implications of illness, how symptoms are perceived and responded to, how they have been handled in the past, and the personality of the patient, all influence illness behaviour. Yet [the Report] fails to include any of these aspects…By neglecting these areas of personal, social, political, and cultural influence the Report fails to grasp the importance of some 'alternative' practices, and why people are turning to those practices.

…[In the Report] scientific methodology is described as 'generally held to be an acceptable basis on which to set reliable judgements, free from overriding social values and political bias'. This is not true…. Science is not an objective reality, it is constructed as a social entity by persons. To say that science is true and value free is rather like saying that Islam is true because everyone subscribes to the faith in Iran. (BHMA, 1986, pp. 9, 22–3, 64, 67, 69)

● How does the BHMA view of science differ from the BMA view?

■ For the BMA, science is the one true way to knowledge; for the BHMA, science is just a belief system, like any religion.

The BHMA view of science is **relativist**. Relativism is a philosophical view based on the idea that there is no single system of ideas that is privileged above others in its access to the truth. Taking a relativist view, science is simply a system that has been more successful than others in gathering allegiance, particularly in modern Western cultures. There is no objective yardstick by which to assess claims to the truth which in practice can only be resolved by power struggles between rival groups. Unfortunately for relativists, however, there is no objective way of deciding whether relativism itself is true or false.

The BMA, however, has no such problem. The way to decide the truth is to subject alternative therapies to scientific procedures designed to test their effectiveness. The BHMA appears to believe that it has a broader conception of illness than the BMA, and that alternative therapies succeed in addressing this. The response of some other alternative therapists to the challenge to prove effectiveness has, however, been equivocal. Some alternative practitioners take the view that their effectiveness *cannot* be evaluated. Fulder, a promoter of alternative medicine, has tried to explain his reasons for this.

The methods of clinical evaluation are designed for modern medical procedures and are completely inappropriate to test complementary medicine. This is because complementary medicine does not offer treatment for a disease, only for a person. Therefore it is impossible to compare treatments between groups. Can one compare one group of 50 patients receiving a drug, with another group receiving 50 different treatments for conditions that are not necessarily the same? In addition complementary treatment must change and develop in response to the changing symptom picture, and the treatment must be monitored over a long period, longer than is usually possible in clinical trials. Furthermore success cannot be judged on the basis of symptoms since complementary and conventional medicine do not define them or remove them in the same way. There are many other problems. (Fulder, 1986, p. 240)

At this stage you may feel unable to judge the wisdom of Fulder's view.[13] Suffice to say that, in spite of Fulder's objections, attempts have been made to evaluate the effectiveness of a number of alternative therapies, though with mixed results.

Focusing on the lack of scientific evaluation of alternative therapies is not altogether fair. You will see later in this book that a great deal of medical practice is based on tradition; the effectiveness of many surgical procedures in particular has not been proven, although the BMA demands such proof for alternative therapies. Further, there is growing documentation of the harmful side effects of many professional treatments, and of the inability of medicine to treat many conditions. These are all points that have been made by alternative practitioners in boundary maintenance disputes. None of them, however, really succeed in assaulting the central tenet of the biomedical view: that scientific methods of evaluation *ought to be* the ultimate arbiter of the worth of therapies. Wherever possible, the medical view requires that the rationale for therapies of proven effectiveness is compatible with scientific views of how the body works.

### 2.5.3   Exclusion and incorporation

The various political strategies used by the medical profession to deal with threats to their professional dominance can be categorised into two broad areas: **exclusion** and **incorporation**. The response to alternative medicine as a whole has largely been one of exclusion. Sometimes this has been because the alternative therapists have refused offers of incorporation. On other occasions, alternative therapists have struggled hard for recognition, but have been brushed aside by doctors in the professional sector.

One of the triumphs for professional medicine was the achievement of a state register of recognised doctors in 1858. By law, only those on the Medical Register, entry to which is controlled by the medical profession, are allowed to practice as doctors. The major employers of doctors — most importantly in the context of the United Kingdom, the NHS — are constrained to employ only registered practitioners. This mechanism ensures virtual professional monopoly. After the 1914–18 war, many groups of healers sought state registration in the hope that similar benefits would become theirs. For the most part their justification for this was the protection of the public against poorly trained practitioners. This, indeed, had been the medical justification for the Medical Register. Charles Newman, Chief Medical Officer, reacted to such aspirations by herbalists in 1923 in these words:

> The object is obviously to secure legal recognition for herbalists, and the next step would be to claim for registered herbalists all the rights of qualified medical practitioners. No doubt the argument of the promoters would be that if people wish to be treated by herbalists, it is better that they would be treated by herbalists who have had some kind of training than by those who have had none. I do not know how herbalists are trained, and it is at least doubtful whether a trained herbalist is any less dangerous than an untrained one, but if any official recognition is to be given to herbalism it cannot be denied to any other type of unqualified medical practice. (Quoted in Larkin, 1992, p. 117)

---

[13] Methods for evaluating the effectiveness of therapies are discussed in *Studying Health and Disease* (Open University Press, 2nd edn 1994; colour-enhanced 2nd edn 2001) and *Dilemmas in UK Health Care* (Open University Press, 2nd edn 1993; 3rd edn 2001).

*Nineteenth-century caricature by George Cruikshank of doctors as quacks.*
*The 1858 legislative triumph allowed doctors to exclude other practitioners*
*and 'quacks' from medical practice. (Source: Hulton Getty Picture Collection)*

● Is there an appeal to scientific criteria in Newman's judgement?

■ No. He proudly displays his ignorance of anything to do with herbalism,
including its effects which he characterises as more or less dangerous. His main
concern is to avoid opening a door through which other rivals might then
pass.

Herbalism was thus *excluded* from medicine, rather than *incorporated*. The strategy
of incorporation has been used in the case of a number of occupational groups. At
various points in history, groups such as nurses, pharmacists and radiographers,
have desired greater independence and higher status. The medical profession has
generally tried to bring such groups under its wing, and to define their skills and
knowledge as subordinate parts of a greater medical enterprise.

Gerald Larkin, a sociologist, describes how this was done with radiographers. The
discovery of X-rays in 1895 led to a proliferation of radiographic technicians who,
for a fee, would provide X-ray pictures for the purpose of diagnosis. The private
practices of these technicians were sometimes very lucrative. At the same time the
medical specialty of *radiology* began to develop.[14] In 1921, the Society of
Radiographers was formed to enhance the status and training of technicians.

> The first president, Sir Archibald Reid, was a former chairman of
> the electrotherapeutic section of the Royal Society of Medicine,
> and was chairman of the British Association of Radiology, which
> indicates the extent of medical involvement in technician

[14] The suffix *-graphy* here indicates a science of description only; the suffix *-ology* indicates that
scientific reasoning is involved.

organisation. Very quickly disputes developed, between the sections of the membership, over the critically sensitive issue of 'reporting' on X-ray plates or, increasingly, films. Boundary disputes developed which, if settled in the technicians' favour, could mean a loss of control by doctors over information often vital for accurate diagnosis. Clearly any encroachment upon what the doctor regarded as his function, 'interpretation' as opposed to 'production', would be resisted. Both radiologists, and other (medical) practitioners, could only be alarmed by the prospect of technicians controlling a new and strikingly successful diagnostic technique.... In the medical professional view, the interpretation of all X-ray plates necessitated a full medical training.... Radiographers could not possibly develop such skills of judgement, and more significantly should not be trained in them. (Larkin, 1978, pp. 847–8)

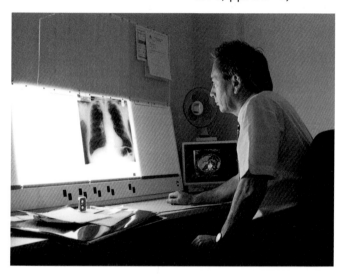

*Consultant radiologist examining an X-ray. The medical specialty of radiology took over the function of reporting on X-rays, which had originally been carried out by non-medical radiographers. (Photo: Mike Levers)*

In order to gain legal recognition from the Board of Trade, the technicians' society was forced to agree to medical demands to supervise all cases taken on by them, on pain of exclusion from the society. The doctor in charge of the case was to remain responsible for diagnosis. After 1925, if a radiographer 'reported' on an X-ray (i.e. gave a diagnosis) they were to be struck off the register. The medical specialty of radiology became the preserve of more theoretical knowledge, and doctors' monopoly over diagnosis was maintained. The non-medical radiographers found themselves defined as possessing craft-skills, rather than medical knowledge, and were subordinated to doctors.

The professional position of doctors, and with it the boundaries of medical knowledge, has been fought for on numerous fronts, and is still subject to challenges which are vigorously resisted. The role of medical knowledge in these disputes is complex. The appeal to science, or to proof of therapeutic effectiveness, is the focus for many of these disputes, although we have seen examples of both sides being influenced by other considerations. Incorporation of rival systems of thought necessitates their re-interpretation by medical theory. This may raise doubts about the objectivity of medical science, but science nevertheless retains its appeal for many people.

## 2.6   Conclusion

This chapter has taken you on a rapid tour of the three main sectors of health care. In the lay sector, you saw something of the variety of sources on which people draw in order to understand and treat themselves when ill. The idea that illness and health are invested with moral connotations was stressed. The complex factors that lead people to decide to seek medical help, and which type of medical help to seek (professional or alternative) were explored. This was followed by a discussion of boundary maintenance disputes between professional medical practitioners and others, and the role of different conceptions of medical knowledge in these was emphasised. By now, you should be aware that arguments about methods of gaining true knowledge are not merely arid disputes between philosophers of science. They are intricately bound up with claims to professional authority, in ways that are not always easy to disentangle.

You will have seen that this discussion of present-day medical practice has frequently referred to historical studies. In attempting to understand the present, it is often helpful to look into the past in order to see the origins of the ideas and institutions with which we are so familiar. What is familiar may then be seen in a new light. The next four chapters will explore the history of medical knowledge.

## OBJECTIVES FOR CHAPTER 2

When you have studied this chapter, you should be able to:

**2.1** Define and use, or recognise definitions and applications of, each of the terms printed in **bold** in the text.

**2.2** View the health beliefs of your own culture as anthropologically strange.

**2.3** Describe the extent and overlaps between the three sectors of health care: lay, alternative and professional.

**2.4** Describe how people decide to consult healers, choose between types of therapy and decide whether or not to comply with the treatment prescribed.

**2.5** Recognise the strategic importance of the appeal to science in struggles to assert professional dominance.

## QUESTIONS FOR CHAPTER 2

**1**   (*Objective 2.2*)

The 'messages' on the Andrews tins (Figure 2.3) read:

> (1911 tin) This preparation acts especially on the liver and kidneys. It cleanses and imparts a vigour to the whole system, and takes away that heavy and depressed feeling so common to people with a sluggish liver. For heaviness, headache, sickness, giddiness, and all forms of indigestion it is invaluable.

**Figure 2.3**    *(left) A 1911 tin of Andrews salts, and (right) a 1984 tin of Andrews salts. (Photos: Mike Levers)*

(1984 tin) Andrews wakes up your natural sparkle. Sparkling effervescent Andrews freshens the mouth, settles the stomach and quickly revives the system. When your natural sparkle has been over-run by the effects of modern living, wake it up with a glass of sparkling Andrews. Thousands of tiny bursting bubbles give you an instant and refreshing lift. Andrews will help if you've over-indulged the night before and your stomach's feeling queasy. The antacid in Andrews gives you the soothing relief you need without irritating an already upset stomach. The dose may be increased, as directed, to make a pleasant laxative.

The humoral medical theory of classical and medieval times emphasised the importance of the liver, which was thought to secrete two of the four humours — yellow and black bile. Can you spot other references to humoral theory?

**2**  (*Objective 2.3*)

Look again at Figure 2.1. Does the size of the circles represent the size of the sectors in the United Kingdom? Why do they overlap?

### Questions 3 and 4

First, look again at the photograph of the person using Hopi ear candles (Figure 1.1a; the frontispiece to this book). The makers of these candles, which are hollow and are placed in the ear before burning, claim the following:

It was through the Hopi Indians, a people characterised by their extensive knowledge of healing techniques and their great spirituality, that the practice of ear treatment candles reached Europe...During the burning phase, the silver-foil lining reflects a gentle, soothing flow of heat inwards. Locally applied heat always has the effect of stimulating peripheral blood circulation which, in turn, strengthens the immunological defence system and enhances lymph circulation. The heat phase likewise stimulates the reflex zones and the energy points within the area of application. The whole process is pleasant and non-invasive. Recipients of the treatment regularly describe feeling an intensive yet harmonious relaxing and calming effect over the whole system.

Now answer Questions 3 and 4 below.

**3**  (*Objective 2.4*)

Which aspects of the general attractions of alternative medicine does this text invoke?

**4**  (*Objective 2.5*)

Which aspects of this text appeal to science for legitimation?

# CHAPTER 3

## An historical approach to medical knowledge

**Study notes for OU students**

This chapter forms an introduction to Chapters 4 to 6, in which three historians of medicine each present a different case study chosen to illustrate important aspects of the development of medical knowledge. These are the stories of tuberculosis (Chapter 4), blood (Chapter 5) and hysteria (Chapter 6). The present chapter sets out the rationale for selecting the history of these three topics for detailed inspection and for presenting them in the order given above. By presenting three contrasting case studies, we can more easily show how medical ideas and techniques of investigation and treatment have been applied to specific topics of medical interest. These accounts therefore contain considerably more depth and detail than might have been given in a broad overview of the historical development of medical knowledge as a whole. However, you will find it helpful to know something of general developments in medical knowledge over time, in order to place the case studies in context, and to see how they interrelate. This is the prime function of this chapter.

## 3.1    Why take an historical approach?

In the previous chapter you encountered a broad spectrum of different models of disease co-existing today, many of them detectable within a single society. The range included divine retribution, spirit possession, social deviance, disequilibrium between qualities such as 'hot' and 'cold', and disordered biology. We attempted in Chapter 2 to make contemporary models of disease and medical knowledge and practice appear *anthropologically strange,* so that you can more easily stand back and see the strangeness usually obscured by familiarity. This is not always easy when the subject is one that involves us personally. Each of us tends to believe that 'our' models are somehow natural and real, others are odd or simply wrong.

An historical approach to medical knowledge enables us to set aside personal involvement in current issues and, by looking at the past, observe the rich mixture of beliefs, observations and rituals that interact in every situation in which medical knowledge plays a part.

> The apparent strangeness and distance of the past enable one to discern features there that are camouflaged in the present by the very taken-for-grantedness of every experience. We use the past to shake confidence in the obvious appearance of medicine today.
> (Wright and Treacher, 1982, p. 2)

But in looking back, we must avoid the pitfall of seeing the past in much the same way as early explorers once inspected 'savages' in far-off lands, viewing them solely as repositories of false beliefs. Bear this in mind as you read the case studies in Chapters 4 to 6.

### 3.1.1    Why tuberculosis, blood and hysteria?

We selected tuberculosis, blood and hysteria as the focus for detailed consideration in this book partly because they represent three contrasting areas of medical interest: a major infectious disease, an aspect of human physiology, and a mental disorder. But a more important reason is that they demonstrate clear variations in the extent to which modern medical knowledge based on scientific research is accepted as the dominant **paradigm** in explaining human health and disease. 'Paradigm' is a useful term, which occurs frequently in this and other books in this series. It means an influential set of ideas about the way the world (or an aspect of the world) is — a 'world view' if you like — which tends to exclude or discredit alternative views, at least for a time.[1]

In the late twentieth century, in Western industrialised countries, **scientific medical knowledge** became the most influential set of ideas (i.e. the *dominant* paradigm), shaping our beliefs about the functioning of the human body in sickness and in health. It is based on systematic investigation of all aspects of human biology, from the largest anatomical feature of the body to the smallest biochemical substance, and includes experimental manipulation of body functions and testing of treatments under scientifically controlled conditions.[2] It is a synthesis of knowledge gained

---

[1] The theory of 'paradigm shifts' formulated by the philosopher Thomas Kuhn is discussed in *Studying Health and Disease* (Open University Press, 2nd edn 1994; colour-enhanced 2nd edn 2001), Chapter 2, and again in *World Health and Disease* (Open University Press, 2nd edn 1993; 3rd edn 2001), Chapter 11.

[2] A review of methods of scientific investigation of human biology is given in *Studying Health and Disease* (Open University Press, 2nd edn 1994; colour-enhanced 2nd edn 2001), Chapter 9.

from research in laboratories, clinical trials conducted on large numbers of patients and volunteers, and the everyday observations of doctors and other health-care professionals at the 'bedside'.

Other paradigms co-exist with it — for example, as Chapter 2 described, the *humoral* paradigm persists from antiquity and has been joined by several paradigms of *alternative* medicine, which are often based in the traditional knowledge of other cultures — but these are subordinate to the scientific medical paradigm in most sections of Western populations. Disease is *primarily* (though not exclusively) conceptualised — even by lay people — in general accordance with the definitions used in scientific medicine, rather than as (say) demon possession or a lack of inner harmony with nature.

- Within the paradigm of modern scientific medicine, how is a 'disease' defined? (think back to Chapter 2).

- A disease is considered to be a significant disturbance of the normal function of a specific part of the body, detectable by instruments or by chemical analysis in specific organs, cells or body fluids and thus objectively 'real'. It produces characteristic signs and symptoms which can often be attributed to a specific underlying cause (e.g. an infection, a blockage in a blood vessel, excessive production of a certain hormone, etc.).

The three historical case studies in the chapters that follow demonstrate how the power of scientific medical knowledge to describe and explain the workings of the human body in health and disease displays **cultural relativism**, that is, it has varied across time and from place to place. It has not always been the dominant paradigm.

We begin with tuberculosis (TB) which, at the present time, has largely shed the spiritual, romantic or polluting connotations that adhered to it in the past, when the disease was variously seen as an expression of delicacy and artistic temperament or a blameworthy consequence of filth and vice. Today TB is viewed as a scientifically detectable disturbance of normal bodily function, most commonly found in individuals made vulnerable to the action of a specific bacterium by the debilitating effects of poverty, poor nutrition and overcrowding. Hardly anyone in Western societies would dispute that TB *is* a 'real' disease or that medical knowledge can be appropriately applied to its prevention and treatment.

But even here, in this apparently undisputed territory, there is a question mark over the extent to which the paradigm of scientific medicine deserves its dominant place. TB is a disease of poverty — a subject barely addressed by medical knowledge. The history of TB reveals relentless progress towards defining the disease in strictly medical terms, with the centre stage in the last 150 years taken by researchers and practitioners of scientific medicine disputing rival theories and treatments. So successful were they at promoting medical knowledge as holding the answer to TB that it may come as a shock when you discover in Chapter 4 that medical intervention can be credited with only a small fraction of the massive decline in TB as a major cause of death.[3] And when TB re-emerged in the 1990s, medical knowledge was again at a loss to contain it.

The paradigm of scientific medicine also predominates in the contemporary Western view of blood but, in contrast with TB, other more ancient paradigms persist in

[3] The reasons underlying the decline in TB in Europe are discussed in detail in *World Health and Disease* (Open University Press, 2nd edn 1993; 3rd edn 2001), Chapter 6.

having widespread significance today. The reliance of many branches of medical practice on the doctor's ability to sample or manipulate the patient's blood has not erased its power as a symbolic or spiritual substance. For example, blood figures prominently in the English language as a rich source of imagery and metaphor.

● Can you suggest some examples?

■ 'She wept blood', 'your blood's worth bottling' (a compliment!), 'you can't squeeze blood out of a stone', 'he made my blood boil!', 'blood is thicker than water', 'he's a red-blooded male', 'she's got blue blood in her veins'. There are many more.

As you will see in Chapter 5, the scientific investigation of blood and the incorporation of that knowledge into the medical paradigm has not wholly displaced such 'non-scientific' thinking.

The study of hysteria takes us even further outside the scientific medical paradigm into territory where the relevance of medical knowledge is more hotly disputed in the twenty-first century than it has been for several centuries past. An unresolved but passionate debate continues as to whether hysteria can be defined as a disease at all, using the criteria currently favoured in modern medicine. Some medical experts assert that it can, but they face strong opposition (most but not all from outside medicine), arguing that hysteria is a *socially constructed* affliction — either a reaction to intolerable pressures in the social world, or a product of the cultural stereotypes about female behaviour contained in medical knowledge. Yet until the last half of the twentieth century there was little disagreement with the view that hysteria existed as a discrete medically defined disease with characteristic signs and symptoms and identifiable underlying causes.

It is tempting to ask what went wrong. As you will see in Chapter 6, the story of hysteria may in part be a case study of the medical profession's tendency to view all human distress as explainable in medical terms and treatable by medical means, and the willingness of the laity to believe that this is so.

## 3.2   The development of medical knowledge

Before you begin the detailed analysis of the three topics, we must point to a potential danger in the historical case-study approach. A reader who does not already have a broad knowledge of medical history in which to locate the case study, may assume incorrectly that the events and ideas current in that time and place had an immediate influence on medical knowledge 'across the board'. In reality, 'progress' towards the views held by practitioners of scientific medicine today did not advance on a broad front, but in a piecemeal and erratic manner. An historical approach to the development of medical knowledge shows that it was often diverted into blind alleys, that there were protracted disputes and disagreements, earlier beliefs were renounced and later resurrected, only to be modified and perhaps discarded again. 'Pockets' of medical knowledge that we might now consider to be modern can be detected centuries before the weight of medical opinion accepted that view, and in other times and places practitioners clung on to beliefs and practices that the majority of their colleagues had long since rejected.

Thus, the 'state of the art' of medicine was highly variable from place to place, and across time, even within a single country. For example, the dominant explanation for hysteria as taught by specialists in the Paris medical schools in the last quarter of the nineteenth century (see Chapter 6) was fundamentally different from that used by general physicians in the towns and villages of France. There are parallels in the present day: medical practice in specialist teaching hospitals may differ in key respects from the clinical management of a disease by a general practitioner, and there are variations between medical 'experts' and between common practice in different countries, even where scientific medicine is the dominant paradigm.

Moreover, a history of medical knowledge focuses on the thoughts and actions of a relatively restricted section of society, whose present 'high profile' may deceive us into imagining that important medical discoveries in the past had an immediate impact on society as a whole. For example, in Chapter 4 you will learn about the 'bacteriological revolution' which took place primarily as a result of research in European laboratories in the second half of the nineteenth century. But for decades after those vital early experiments had demonstrated that many diseases were caused by infectious micro-organisms, the relationship of lay people to their environment was little changed. The discoveries had a 'revolutionary' impact on a relatively restricted section of the population, that is the scientific and medical community, while the mass of population remained oblivious to the presence or significance of 'germs'. There are parallels in the 'genetic revolution' in progress since the 1990s, when the prospect of being able to replace a faulty gene with a normal gene and so 'cure' selected diseases is causing great excitement among medical scientists, but has as yet had little impact on lay people's lives.

Keeping in mind these caveats against assuming a linear progression in the development of medical knowledge over time, it is possible to distinguish several shifts in the *dominant* paradigm within medicine. In the twenty-first century, *scientific medicine* is the dominant paradigm. The historical case studies in Chapters 4 to 6 contain many insights into the manner in which it gained ascendancy. In each case study, three highly-overlapping earlier paradigms can be distinguished, which have made a fundamental contribution to the scientific medicine practised today. They can be described as *bedside medicine*, *clinical medicine* (sometimes called *hospital medicine*) and *laboratory medicine*. These paradigms consist of three interacting systems of medical concepts, each with some characteristic techniques of medical practice, which determined the sort of questions that were asked about human health and disease, as well as the sorts of answers that were constructed.

Although it is broadly true that bedside medicine is the oldest of the three paradigms, and laboratory medicine is the most recent, it is a mistake to think of a linear progression from one to another. Medical knowledge accumulates rather like barnacles on a ship's hull — some bits are scraped away or lose the competition for space as time passes, but some of the most ancient remain to the present day.

## 3.2.1  Bedside medicine

Until roughly the middle of the eighteenth century, disease was conceptualised and treated very differently from the way we see it today. The great majority of illness was treated at home (i.e. at the bedside), primarily with lay remedies and only sporadic recourse to a variety of mainly part-time practitioners in various healing arts.[4] Medical knowledge was not yet the 'property' of doctors, but was shared

[4] See *Caring for Health: History and Diversity* (Open University Press, 2nd edn 1993; 3rd edn 2001), Chapter 2.

**Figure 3.1** *Drawing from Heymandus de Veteri Busco's Ars Computistica, published in 1488, showing the figure of an 'Astrological Man' in which the body is surrounded by zodiacal signs, related to their appropriate parts by a cord. (Source: The Wellcome Library, London)*

among the whole population. The term **bedside medicine** encompasses the dominant concepts of disease and the rationale underlying popular techniques for restoring health in an age before the hospital clinic and the laboratory came to dominate medicine.

In bedside medicine, all aspects of what we would now call the patients' emotional and spiritual life, as well as physical experience, were potentially important in understanding their illness. Cosmic influences were given great importance, although their nature was hotly debated (see Figure 3.1), but so too was the local environment and the habits and 'constitution' of the patient. Although much of ancient and medieval medical knowledge took no account of astrology, an emphasis on the relationship between the person and the natural and supernatural environment is a characteristic of bedside medicine which has retained some of its power even in the twenty-first century. The emphasis on a *holistic* view of the patient, in which disease was an expression of disharmony between multiple interacting forces, meant there was an acceptance of a 'common nature' to all diseases and the body was seen as a microcosm of the universe.

However, the holistic view that all illnesses had an underlying commonality was combined with a detailed medical knowledge of the particular characteristics of each disease, which required the practitioner to make the most detailed bedside observation of the patient in order to reach a diagnosis.

> Speech, behaviour, silence, thoughts, sleep, absence of sleep, dreams — of what kind and when, plucking, itching, tears upon exacerbation, bowel movements, urine, sputum, vomiting, how many transitions of disease from one kind to another, as well as abscessions toward a fatal or a critical issue, sweat, chill, frigidity, coughing, sneezing, hiccupping, breathing, belching, flatulence silent or noisy, hemorrhages, and hemorrhoids. These things and what they bring must be considered. (Hippocrates, *Epidemics*, I.23; I: 180)

There were many rival theories among medical practitioners about the causes of and remedies for particular diseases, arising partly from the great variety of writings attributed to Hippocrates and Galen, and from rival traditions, which allowed enormous scope for different (but not always mutually exclusive) interpretations of medical knowledge. For example, bedside medicine is commonly associated with the Hippocratic theory that epidemics of disease were spread by **miasmas**, a term derived from the Greek word for a stain. The theory of miasmas identified the cause of disease as pollution of the air by rotting organic matter or stagnant water. It remained influential until well into the nineteenth century, but for most of its history co-existed with the less influential theory of **contagion**, derived from the Old Testament, which held that tiny seeds acted as infective agents and could be

**Figure 3.2**  *This dissection scene, from Johannes de Ketham's* Fasciculus Medicinae, *published in Venice in 1495, represents an early anatomical lesson at Padua. While a senior student reads from Mundinus' text, and an assistant performs the dissection, the professor attempts to relate book to body. (Source: The Wellcome Library, London)*

passed from person to person causing specific diseases. Contagion clearly prefigures 'germ' theory which developed in the nineteenth century. There were no universally accepted ideas about which diseases were caused by miasmas and which by contagion, and it was possible to believe in both and in humoral theory simultaneously.

Medical knowledge about the human body as we currently understand it developed slowly, in part because of the reverence for ancient texts and because of the stigma attached to opening corpses to reveal their anatomy by **dissection**. The emphasis in some of the earliest dissections was on demonstrating that human anatomy conformed to the predictions of classical writers, rather than being used as a source of new knowledge that might challenge the dominant paradigm. However, an increasing interest in dissection (see Figure 3.2) came to be associated with a highly experimental investigation of nature from about 1500 onwards, which was *empirical* in orientation, that is, based on observations of the real world rather than on speculation.

### 3.2.2  Clinical medicine

In the later eighteenth and early nineteenth centuries, the 'centre of gravity' for the generation of new medical knowledge moved from the bedside to the recently founded hospitals.[5] This should not be taken to imply that bedside medicine suddenly came to an end, or that the concepts associated with this paradigm were

---

[5] See *Caring for Health: History and Diversity* (Open University Press, 2nd edn 1993; 3rd edn 2001), Chapter 3.

rejected. Rather they came to be challenged by a new paradigm — **clinical medicine** — which gradually came to predominate without ever wholly submerging the bedside tradition. Clinical medicine was really the culmination of a way of thinking about the human body in health and disease that had been developing for some time, and on many fronts. The hospital — an institution that afforded doctors the opportunity to examine large numbers of patients, who were for the most part poor and whose bodies could often be dissected at death — became the crucial site for the development of this form of medical knowledge.

**Figure 3.3** *Plate from John Bell's* Engravings Explaining the Anatomy of the Bones, Muscles and Joints, *published in Edinburgh in 1794. An accepted description of the normal body was constructed in the words and pictures of medical texts. (Source: The Wellcome Library, London)*

The formalisation of medicine as a profession, with an accepted programme of clinical training and education, enhanced the power and prestige of the teaching hospital and led to the proliferation of medical textbooks. As an accepted description of the normal body was constructed in the words and pictures of medical texts (see Figure 3.3), doctors became interested in relating the abnormalities that they found in the bodies of their hospitalised patients after death to the bodily appearance and abnormal sensations experienced by those patients when alive. Practitioners of clinical medicine developed ways of investigating the living body, for example, the stethoscope and the thermometer.

The success of clinical medicine depended on the specialised investigation of particular diseases. Distinctions between clusters of signs and symptoms gradually became accepted as the basis for categorising different sorts of disease, for distinguishing separate diseases that had previously been believed to be the same, or (as in the case of TB) unifying as a single disease category a disparate collection of manifestations previously thought to be separate diseases. These systems for classifying diseases (or *nosologies*) were gradually related to underlying pathological lesions within the body, so that 'families' of diseases were identified, whose common site (for example, the chest, the heart, the brain) formed the chapter headings of medical textbooks, and were the basis for medical specialisation.

Increasingly, the patient came to be seen as a *carrier* of a disease. This is not to imply that a theory of the passing on of germs had developed, but that the patient's body was a vessel containing the thing that was of true interest to the doctor — the disease itself.

- ● In what way is this a departure from the conceptualisation of disease associated with the paradigm of bedside medicine?

- ■ The older tradition was holistic in its approach to disease, which was considered to be the result of disharmony or lack of balance in the 'cosmos' of the patient's physical, emotional and spiritual world. In bedside medicine the whole patient is an *expression* of the disease. In clinical medicine the patient is seen as *distinct from* the disease.

**Figure 3.4** *Orthopaedic mannikin, from Hieronymus Fabricius ab Aquapendente,* Opera Chirurgica, *published in Padua in 1647. A contrivance like this one, used for correcting dislocations, lent support to the notion that the human body might also perform like a machine. (Source: The Wellcome Library, London)*

As the paradigm of clinical medicine gained ascendancy over bedside medicine, the classification of diseases as distinct entities came to require a description of not only their characteristic signs and symptoms, but also their underlying pathology. A view of the body as a *machine* became widely accepted, building on a much earlier tradition (see Figure 3.4). The mechanics of muscle movement, the hydraulics of the blood system and many other physiological systems were increasingly investigated and interpreted in this functional manner. Disease came to be seen in terms of the body as a broken mechanism.

### 3.2.3 Laboratory medicine

The third medical paradigm emerged from and remains hand-in-hand with clinical medicine. The hospital ward, operating theatre and dissecting room are limited arenas in which to investigate the workings of the human body, and in the second half of the nineteenth century the focus of medical research gradually swung towards the laboratory and the use of other animal species as substitutes for humans in experiments.[6] However, although the paradigm of **laboratory medicine** came to *dominate* medical knowledge in this period, it can be detected first in ancient traditions, which were resurrected in the seventeenth century by William Harvey, who used laboratory science to discover the circulation of the blood (Chapter 5). Laboratory medicine was given new impetus in the nineteenth century by progress in understanding the nature of chemical elements and the availability of improved

---

[6] The use of animals as 'models' for human biology in laboratory research is discussed in *Studying Health and Disease* (Open University Press, 2nd edn 1994; colour-enhanced 2nd edn 2001), Chapter 9.

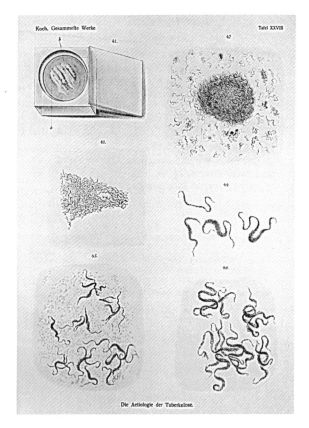

**Figure 3.5** *Tubercle bacilli (Koch's term for the bacteria that cause TB) from Robert Koch, Gesammelte Werke, published in Leipzig in 1912 (originally published 1882). Laboratory medicine was associated with a knowledge of the cell, and a theory of the role of 'germs' in causing disease. (Source: The Wellcome Library, London)*

instruments such as the microscope and thermometer. This re-emergence and revitalisation of a much older tradition warns against thinking of a simple chronological progression in the source of medical knowledge from bedside, to hospital, to laboratory.

Laboratory medicine is characterised by the further reduction of the body into its constituent parts, this time with the aid of a technology of enlargement, in which the microscope played an important role. In the laboratory, the study of disease was subsumed in a wider enterprise of biological and biochemical enquiry into nature, focusing in particular on the workings of the cell. Among other things, laboratory medicine is associated with the ideas of **germ theory**, which identified the underlying cause of some diseases as the entry of micro-organisms into the body, from which a causal chain develops that disrupts normal bodily function (see Figure 3.5).

Germ theory was made possible by laboratory medicine, which both extended the sight of the research worker to ever smaller things, and developed a logic of experimentation which inferred the existence of organisms too small to be seen, even with the aid of a microscope.

### 3.2.4  The case studies

As you read the following chapters on tuberculosis, blood and hysteria you will see that in their various ways they illustrate the medical paradigms just outlined. You will also realise that the account here has been extremely condensed, merely sketching some of the outlines of a much more detailed story. As you read the case studies, think back to this chapter and try to assess how far each of them illustrates the paradigms identified here. Questions at the end of each case study are designed to help you do this.

When you have studied this chapter, you should be able to:

**3.1** Define and use, or recognise definitions and applications of, each of the terms printed in **bold** in the text.

**3.2** Justify the use of an historical approach to studying medical knowledge and identify some of its potential pitfalls.

**3.3** Explain what is meant by a dominant paradigm within medical knowledge and distinguish between the paradigms of bedside medicine, clinical medicine, laboratory medicine and modern scientific medicine.

**1**    (*Objective 3.2*)

How might an historical approach to medical knowledge enable you to counter the claim that it has advanced steadily and on a broad front from the ignorance of antiquity to the certainty of present-day medicine?

**2**    (*Objective 3.3*)

The sociologist Mildred Blaxter analysed the responses of 46 middle-aged, working-class women interviewed in Scotland about their health beliefs in the early 1980s. Which of the paradigms discussed in this chapter is most consistent with the women's views about the causes of disease?

> There appeared to be a positive strain towards accounting for their present bodily state, or describing their accumulated experience, by connecting together the relevant health events. It did not seem reasonable to them to suppose that one part of their body had gone wrong at one stage, and another part at some other time, in a totally random fashion…they believed that their childhood experiences, their pregnancies and deliveries, their work and environment and other major illnesses they had suffered must all be connected. (Blaxter, 1983, p. 67)

# C H A P T E R  4

## Tuberculosis

### Study notes for OU students

In Section 4.3 of this chapter you will be asked to read an extract from Susan Sontag's book, *Illness as Metaphor*, contained in *Health and Disease: A Reader* (Open University Press, second edition 1995; third edition 2001). You may also wish to read there the articles by Thomas McKeown and Simon Szreter, which are concerned with the role of medical and non-medical factors in the decline of tuberculosis (TB) towards the end of the nineteenth century. These articles are set reading for *World Health and Disease*, but you could usefully read them now if you have time. TB is discussed in *World Health and Disease* (Open University Press, second edition 1993; third edition 2001) and in *Caring for Health: History and Diversity* (Open University Press, second edition 1993; third edition 2001) where you will notice that TB remained important enough to become one of the main preoccupations of the expanding health services after the Second World War.

The biological details of infectious diseases caused by bacteria, and the immune response to infection, are given in another book in this series, *Human Biology and Health: an Evolutionary Approach* (Open University Press, second edition 1994; third edition 2001); we do not assume any prior biological knowledge as you study the present chapter.

# 4.1  Introduction

Tuberculosis (TB) is an infectious disease caused by the bacterium given the Latin name *Mycobacterium tuberculosis*, which is transmitted by the coughing and sneezing of persons in whom the disease has reached the infectious stage. It is also possible to contract another strain of TB from the milk of infected cows (known as *bovine* TB). Given these two ready means of transmission, TB bacteria are extremely widespread. Until recent decades the TB bacterium was harboured by the great majority of the population in the industrialised economies, and this remains the case in developing countries today. The retreat of TB in the developed nations for most of the twentieth century and its re-emergence in the 1990s, illustrates the importance of this disease, which has probably been responsible for more destruction of life and debilitation than any other infectious disease.

Because TB has exerted great impact over a long period of time, this disease has occupied high priority in the field of medical research. Investigations into the disease and its treatment have involved centuries of effort, attracting the attention of many of the best-known names in medical science. This disease is therefore an ideal case study to demonstrate the character of medical knowledge in the field of infectious disease.

It is tempting to reduce the account of TB into a story of 'discovery' and 'conquest'. TB offers much to attract this triumphalist view of the history of medicine, and it would be perverse to deny the achievement of individual researchers or the effectiveness of major therapeutic innovations. Yet it is also important to obtain a balanced view of the process of innovation. A more qualified review of the long-term pattern of enquiry enables us to appreciate the erratic nature of the growth of medical knowledge, and the many factors that have stood in the way of balanced understanding, or in applying this knowledge to optimum practical effect. Therefore, as in the cases of blood and hysteria, considered in Chapters 5 and 6, analysis of the generation of knowledge in the case of TB illustrates the themes of doubt and certainty which constitute the main theme of this book. A more critical account of medical discovery enables us among other things to understand why TB has proved such an elusive target and cannot be regarded as a problem of the past.

The present chapter concentrates primarily on the West and on the nineteenth and twentieth centuries, which constitute the zenith of research in this field, and when TB assumed the highest priority as a medical problem. You will find out how, during the nineteenth century, TB became recognised as a *unified* disease caused by a bacterial agent. You will then investigate the course of a series of much-heralded discoveries in the field of prevention and treatment in the twentieth century. You will observe that the most humane, effective and economic therapies were not necessarily the alternatives most actively pursued. Indeed, you will notice that the devising of comprehensive and appropriate programmes of prevention and treatment was delayed until the later-twentieth century. Even then, the absence of the means to apply these programmes effectively has created a situation in which TB has never come under control in developing countries, and has now re-emerged as a dangerous threat to health in the West. Thus, contrary to the impression conveyed by triumphalist accounts, the twentieth century emerges as a series of false dawns in the field of TB research. Once again the disease seems poised to outrun the resources of medical knowledge in the new millennium.

## 4.2   The biology of TB

TB attracts less immediate attention than its main rivals among the epidemic infectious diseases because it is generally slow-acting, sometimes exerting its effect over many years. The bacteria are capable of remaining quiescent in the body for long periods, but the infection can become active again in appropriate circumstances, for example when the immune system is deficient. This contributes to the association of TB with poverty, malnutrition, and now with human immunodeficiency virus (HIV) infection as it progresses to acquired immune deficiency syndrome (AIDS). Thus, although less dramatic in its action than such epidemic diseases as plague or cholera, TB has constituted a more constant threat to human life. Once entrenched, the infection is difficult to treat because the waxy protective coating of the bacteria makes them extremely resistant to chemical attack, with the result that even the most active drugs need to be applied over a long period (typically 6–8 months). The TB bacterium also has the ability to evolve drug-resistant strains, which contribute to its resistance even in Western populations.

The TB bacterium can circulate throughout the body and may settle in many different sites, giving rise to a wide range of symptoms. The bovine strain of TB is apt to infect the bones and joints of children and cause *osteomyelitis* (inflammation commencing in the bone marrow), deformity and crippling. Alternatively the bacterium can infect the skin and give rise to *lupus vulgaris* (ulceration starting in the area of the nose or ear, resulting in facial disfigurement). When it causes swelling of the lymph nodes (part of the immune system), especially in the neck, it is called *scrofula*.

The most common site of infection is the lungs, where it is called **pulmonary TB**. The **tubercles** from which the disease takes its name are most easily detected in the lungs. These begin as pockets of infection which develop into ulcers, expanding until they completely erode the lung substance. As the tubercles increase in number and size, gradual impairment of lung function occurs, starting with the breathing irregularities for which the disease is best known and which often provide the first symptoms. However, the manifestations are by no means confined to the lungs. There also occurs a slow-acting disruption of the gastro-intestinal system, with attendant weight loss and general physical deterioration, with the result that this form of disease is called by the Greek name *phthisis* or by its Latinised equivalent **consumption**. Although TB is generally slow-acting, if it strikes at the central nervous system and the brain the effects are more dramatic, and in these locations *tuberculous meningitis* results in rapid death.

It is now understood that the above diversity of conditions originate from a single bacterial agent, and are accompanied by similar cellular responses throughout the body, but this *integrated* conception of the disease took centuries to build up. For most of its history, what is now known as 'tuberculosis' was thought of as a variety of separate diseases each affecting a specific site and disconnected with one another.

●   What does it mean to say that the present-day view of TB is 'integrated' or 'unified'?

■   Scrofula, consumption, pulmonary TB and tubercular meningitis are now seen as manifestations of a single disease. With knowledge of their causative agent (*Mycobacterium tuberculosis*), conditions previously thought to be diverse diseases have now been classified together.

## 4.3 The impact of TB

In the seventeenth century, John Bunyan (the author of *The Pilgrim's Progress*) called consumption 'the Captain of all these men of death'. This was a shrewd and probably accurate observation and was confirmed by the **Bills of Mortality**, which since the early seventeenth century recorded deaths in London by their cause. This source suggests that up to 25 per cent of deaths in the capital were attributable to consumption. The Bills of Mortality represent the most complete record of deaths by cause, but there is no comparable source of data from outside London. For the most part, before the nineteenth century, we are reliant on small samples, the estimates of doctors specialising in this field, or the impressionistic experience of social commentators.

Popular myths about the consumptive 'character' arose, and were perpetuated in literature and the arts. In the first part of the nineteenth century Emily Brontë, John Keats and Frédéric Chopin died of TB at the ages of 30, 25 and 39 respectively. The American writer Susan Sontag has described the myths that have arisen concerning particular diseases, such as AIDS or cancer, as *metaphors*. You should now read the extract in *Health and Disease: A Reader*[1] from her book *Illness as Metaphor* in which she discusses romantic images of TB.

*The death of Chopin, from a painting by F. J. Barrias. Chopin asked the Countess Potocka, draped in white, to sing to him. (Source: Mary Evans Picture Library)*

● According to Sontag, what qualities were thought to be conveyed by those suffering from TB?

■ Gentility, delicacy, sensitivity, refinement, creativity, together with an air of languor and a thin appearance thought becoming in aristocratic and literary circles. (Sontag suggests that mental illness ('insanity') nowadays attracts similar sentiments.)

The great French investigators of TB, Gaspard Laurent Bayle and René-Théophile-Hyacinthe Laënnec, whose work will be discussed below, died from the disease at the age of 42 and 45 respectively. Unlike many infectious diseases which affect childhood, TB is predominantly a disease of late adolescence and maturity. It was therefore much feared by the poor because in the short term it was likely to cause loss of employment, robbing the poor of their income and orphaning countless children. In the longer term it resulted in total destitution.

Taking all the evidence into account it is likely that in the early nineteenth century one in four deaths in the cities of Europe was attributable to consumption. To this must be added the deaths due to other 'diseases' of the period which we now recognise as forms of TB. Given the generally high levels of mortality at the time, it is clear that TB was devastating urban populations. This impression was confirmed when city authorities, partly under pressure from doctors and other pioneers of public health, began assembling more adequate **epidemiological data** (i.e. data

[1] *Health and Disease: A Reader* (Open University Press, 2nd edn 1995; 3rd edn 2001).

on the distribution of deaths in different sections of the population).[2] Early records on the role of pulmonary TB were collated by the pioneer American epidemiologist Lemuel Shattuck in 1850 (see Table 4.1).

These early data confirmed the importance of TB as the most *consistently* serious threat to health among urban populations. Although the three main cholera epidemics of 1831, 1848–9 and 1853–4, resulted in about 100 000 deaths in England and Wales, and occasioned more immediate panic, they were limited in their effect on the population compared with TB. The scale of the TB problem can be deduced from Figure 4.1, which suggests that in the British Isles about 100 000 deaths from TB occurred *annually* in the mid-nineteenth century.

**Table 4.1**  Mortality from pulmonary tuberculosis in certain American and European cities early in the nineteenth century.

| City | Period | Number of deaths from all causes | Number of deaths from pulmonary TB | Deaths from pulmonary TB as a percentage of all deaths |
|---|---|---|---|---|
| Portsmouth (USA) | 1800–11 to 1818–25 | 2 367 | 471 | 19.9 |
| Providence (USA) | 1841–5 | 3 032 | 718 | 23.7 |
| New York (USA) | 1811–20 | 25 896 | 6 061 | 23.4 |
| Philadelphia (USA) | 1811–20 | 23 582 | 3 629 | 15.4 |
| London (UK) | 1840–7 | 397 871 | 57 047 | 14.3 |
| Paris (France) | 1816–19 | 85 339 | 15 375 | 18.0 |

Adapted from Shattuck, L. (1850) *Report of the Sanitary Commission of Massachusetts,* adapted from Waksman, S. A. (1965) *The Conquest of Tuberculosis*, Robert Hale, London, Table 1, p. 20.

The availability of statistics relating to every facet of our daily life is now taken for granted. The gathering of population and medical statistics was one manifestation of a *statistical movement*, which developed in the late eighteenth century, and was concerned with discovering the mathematical basis of the wealth and poverty of nations. Doctors were actively involved in these speculations in the field of political economy and they played a leading part in the embryonic statistical movement. The establishment of the **General Register Office** in Britain in 1837 concerned with all census and registration matters was a typical product of the statistical movement. Significantly the chief official of the General Register Office was the doctor, William Farr (1807–1883), who mobilised this department to gather data relating to disease on an hitherto unprecedented scale. Farr himself was an active theorist of infectious disease. His records provided the first reasonably reliable mortality data on all forms of TB covering all parts of Britain.

It is quite possible that Farr's records marked the end of a long period of high incidence of TB. Even allowing for limitations in accuracy of the data, it is clear that TB entered into a decline in the late-Victorian period (see Figure 4.1). There is currently a debate amongst historians about the extent and rate of this reduction. The registration data suggests an oscillation in levels between 1838 and 1867, the real fall being located in the last 30 years of the century. Those medical officers who believed that deaths from pulmonary TB were often registered as bronchitis

[2] Epidemiology is extensively discussed in *Studying Health and Disease* (Open University Press, 2nd edn 1994; colour-enhanced 2nd edn 2001).

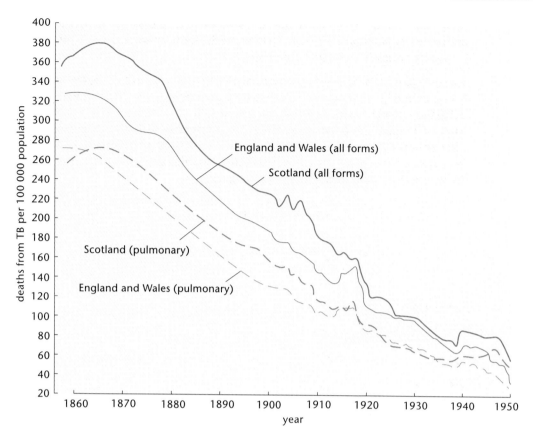

**Figure 4.1** *Standardised death rates from pulmonary tuberculosis and from all forms of tuberculosis combined, per 100 000 population in England and Wales, and Scotland, 1860–1950. For example, in 1860 in England and Wales, approximately 330 people out of every 100 000 died of TB. If you are unsure about 'reading' data from a graph, start by finding the year 1860 on the horizontal axis, then run your eye vertically up the graph until you find the line labelled 'England and Wales (all forms)'. It is level with 330 deaths per 100 000 population on the vertical axis of the graph. Taking the population of the British Isles as about 30 million in 1860, the death rates indicated in Figure 4.1 suggest 100 000 deaths per annum. The death rates in Figure 4.1 have been 'standardised' to make allowances for changes over time in the relative sizes of different age groups in the populations being compared. The calculation of standardised death rates is fully explained in* Studying Health and Disease *(Open University Press, 2nd edn 1994; colour-enhanced 2nd edn 2001), Chapter 7. (Based on Bryder, 1988,* Below the Magic Mountain: A Social History of Tuberculosis in Twentieth-Century Britain, *Oxford University Press, Oxford, Figure 1, p. 7)*

could argue that the decline commenced only in the 1880s. This point warns us of the unreliability of the registration of deaths, especially from diseases such as TB which carried a social stigma.

The role of medical efforts in the decline of TB is somewhat controversial, with Thomas McKeown, for example, arguing that a general increase in resistance brought about by rising living standards and improved nutrition was responsible for driving TB into a decline. Others stress the role of public-health measures in the nineteenth century, such as improved sewage disposal, clean water supplies and better housing conditions.[3] Of course, these explanations for the decline in TB are not mutually exclusive, and both give little credit to medical *treatments*. The

[3] Articles by Thomas McKeown and Simon Szreter addressing these issues are contained in *Health and Disease: A Reader* (Open University Press, 2nd edn 1995; 3rd edn 2001). Public-health reforms in nineteenth-century Britain are discussed in detail in *Caring for Health: History and Diversity* (Open University Press, 2nd edn 1993; 3rd edn 2001).

boundary between medical and non-medical intervention is somewhat arbitrary, and a variety of factors are likely to have been instrumental in strengthening the population's resistance against this disease and reducing exposure.

It is also important not to exaggerate the extent of the retreat of TB. Even in 1900 medical experts regarded TB as the single greatest threat to health. They appreciated that TB maintained its hold among the poor, where the incidence was much greater than indicated by the mortality statistics, because of under-reporting and especially because the majority of cases were not fatal. The adoption of more refined methods of investigation to determine more precise levels of incidence of TB in the twentieth century will be considered later in this chapter.

This section has established the consistent seriousness of the problem of TB, but also the tenuous nature of the statistical evidence, even when official statistics made an appearance. The McKeown debate warns us that modern authorities are apt to make selective use of these data, so compounding the problem of uncertainty over the reliability of our knowledge of the incidence of TB.

## 4.4    Clinical investigation and pathological anatomy

As already mentioned, the major advances in medical knowledge of TB occurred in the nineteenth century. Given the diversity of manifestations of this disease, it is not surprising that its unified character was not appreciated until clinical medicine reached a high degree of sophistication. In the centuries before 1800 little progress towards the understanding of TB may have been made, but as far back as Greek antiquity many shrewd observations were recorded, even on the intractable problem of pulmonary TB. These descriptions were not improved upon until the nineteenth century. Not surprisingly, consumption tended to be conflated with other respiratory problems, such as bronchitis or even lung cancer, rather than being linked with other degenerative changes now recognised as advanced stages of TB.

In the field of **pathology** (the study of the manifestations of disease in the body) the theories of the Greeks were as influential as their observations. Even in the seventeenth century, disease was predominantly explained according to the theories of Claudius Galen (AD 129–216?), whose system of pathology was based on the idea that disease was a manifestation of imbalance between four hypothetical physiological humours (as described in Chapter 2). The intellectual appeal of **Galenic[4] medicine** was increased by its association with physical principles derived from the Greek philosopher Aristotle, particularly the four qualities (hot, cold, moist, and dry) belonging to the four elements (earth, air, fire, and water). (In physical sciences and philosophy, the influence of Aristotle (384–322 BC) was just as enduring as that of Galen.) Explaining disease with reference to degrees of heat or moisture, and humoral fluctuations, became an elaborate computational exercise which required considerable learning for its full expression, and therefore provided a justification for the lengthy classical education of the university-trained elite of the medical profession.

Galenic ideas about pathology were not without their critics. The first major assault in the modern period came from the Swiss doctor and religious thinker, Paracelsus

---

4 The term 'Galenic' refers to medical beliefs and practices based on Galen's medical system of balance between the humours. 'Galenists' are supporters of this medical system in subsequent centuries. Historians are uncertain about the year he died, citing a range 199–216.

(1493–1541), who pronounced the entire Galenic edifice as worthless. Among reformers such as Paracelsus and Thomas Sydenham (1624–1689) an alternative idea of disease developed, which was based on the analogy with biological species. The new theory suggested that, like more visible parasites, diseases were implanted from outside, located at a particular site, and subject to a particular cycle of development. This approach prepared the ground for regarding diseases as distinctive entities rather than stages of physiological disruption.

Sydenham approached pathology in the spirit of a naturalist describing an animal or plant species, placing the emphasis on systematic clinical observation in order to distinguish between the fine gradations of specific diseases. He made important advances in the clinical description of infectious diseases, and he produced some classic descriptions, but he paid little attention to the various conditions we now describe as TB, which is somewhat surprising given the prevalence of pulmonary TB in London at Sydenham's time. However this omission was soon compensated for by Sydenham's follower, the Nonconformist minister and medical practitioner, Richard Morton (1637–1698), whose *Phthisiologia, or Investigations on Tuberculosis* (1689) was predominantly based on Morton's own clinical observations. However, even Sydenham's new methodology was unable to generate a spontaneous transformation in the understanding of consumption. Morton failed to connect consumption with scrofula and lupus vulgaris, but instead followed classical authorities in conflating it with fevers, jaundice and gout.

Further attention to TB was associated with the great revival of anatomy and experimental physiology which took place in the wake of William Harvey's discovery of the circulation of blood (discussed in detail in Chapter 5). François de la Boë (1614–1672) of Leyden and Thomas Willis (1621–1675) in England provided improved anatomical descriptions, each investigator showing evidence of scrupulous investigations of pathology. De la Boë was the first authority to state categorically that the tubercle was an invariable feature of pulmonary consumption and he recognised that tubercles were present at disease sites other than the lungs. He therefore made an important step towards placing the tubercle at the centre of TB, although this particular aspect of his work was not appreciated at the time. More attention was attracted by the explanations of consumption and other diseases based on the profusion of new chemical and physiological theories which emerged in the later seventeenth century.

These theories contributed almost nothing to the advancement of understanding of TB. Although the microscope was invented in the early seventeenth century and became popular in the later part of this period, both the defects of the instrument and the absence of methods of preparing tissue for microscopic examination rendered it virtually useless for pathological investigations.

The study of pathological anatomy within the range of naked-eye observation reached a climax in the general surveys of pathology of Giovanni Battista Morgagni (1682–1771) in the mid-eighteenth century. Morgagni's *On the Seat and Causes of Disease* (1761) not only summed up the work of earlier generations, but advanced knowledge across the entire field of pathology on the basis of vast personal experience with **post-mortem examinations**. In many instances, Morgagni was successful in linking his pathological descriptions with the symptoms of the relevant diseases, thereby providing a more rigorous basis for the localised conception of disease. However, Morgagni was so fearful of consumption that he avoided the corpses of consumptives. Esmond Long, the modern TB pathologist, concluded that 'the discussion of pulmonary TB is accordingly one of the weakest sections of the work' (Long, 1965, p. 71).

*René-Théophile-Hyacinthe Laënnec (1781–1826), a pioneer of clinical investigation into tuberculosis, who died from the disease at the age of 45. (Source: Sigerist, H., 1965,* Grosse Ärzte, *J. F. Lehmanns Verlag, Munich)*

Consequently, despite the considerable advances of clinical investigation and pathological anatomy, the Galenic conception of pulmonary TB as a complication *arising from* inflammatory conditions associated with advanced forms of fever was not actively contested. Discoveries in anatomy and physiology, such as the circulation of blood, were easily adapted to fit this traditional view of diseases such as TB.

### 4.4.1 The clinical revolution: Parisian medicine

A transformation in understanding of TB came about at the beginning of the nineteenth century. It was the immediate consequence of the researches of Gaspard Laurent Bayle (1774–1816) and his successor and friend René-Théophile-Hyacinthe Laënnec (1781–1826). As noted above, both were victims of consumption. The work of Bayle and Laënnec was built on the attainments of the remarkable school of medicine which developed in Paris around the time of the French Revolution (1789), and continued its ascendancy until the widespread European revolutions of 1848. The dominance of Paris as a medical centre was paralleled by its achievement in such fields as philosophy, science and technology. Paris provided in both quantity and quality, career prospects, hospital facilities and a cosmopolitan academic environment that could not be matched elsewhere in France or Europe. Chapters 5 and 6 provide further evidence of the intellectual productivity of Parisian medicine at this period.

TB may well have been at the peak of its impact in Europe at this time. Laënnec estimated that between 20 and 25 per cent of deaths in Paris were caused by TB (18 per cent is given in Table 4.1 for the period 1816–19). It is therefore understandable why this disease attracted the attention of the most able Parisian investigators. Bayle's *Researches on Pulmonary Tuberculosis*, published in 1810, was based on 900 post-mortem examinations, 54 of which were selected for special report in his book.

Bayle's method of exhaustive scientific enquiry, made possible by the facilities and ethos of the Paris medical school, resulted in a transformation of clinical knowledge concerning pulmonary TB and its pathological lesions. Bayle improved on all previous descriptions of the tubercle and its relations to TB cavities developed in the lungs, and he detected the similarity between the ulcerative condition of the lungs, larynx, intestine and lymph glands within the abdomen. He confronted the prevalent theory mentioned above which regarded pulmonary TB as a complication resulting from inflammatory conditions such as fevers or syphilis. He insisted that consumption was an independent, degenerative disease, containing six separate 'species', five of which are now identifiable as stages of pulmonary TB, the sixth now being known as lung cancer. Thus Bayle successfully brought together the major elements needed for the description of TB and eliminated most of the extraneous elements belonging to other diseases.

Bayle's work on TB was extended by Laënnec in *Mediate Auscultation, or a Treatise on the Diagnosis of Disease of the Lungs and Heart* (*De l'auscultation mediate*) (1819). This work introduced his invention of the stethoscope, the importance of which is described in Chapter 5. The central feature of Laënnec's book was its extended discussion of pulmonary TB. He made the revolutionary suggestion that Bayle's 'species' were either stages in a unified disease, or else they were entirely independent diseases such as cancer. Because the development of the tubercle was central to this disease, Laënnec adopted the term *tuberculosis* as the most appropriate term to embrace all the disparate forms. Laënnec's description of the unified phenomenon of TB is given below:

> The tubercles develop in the form of small semitransparent granules, gray in color, though occasionally they are entirely transparent and almost colorless. Their size varies from that of millet seed to that of hemp seed; when in this state, they may be termed *miliary tubercles*. These granules increase in size and become yellowish and opaque, first in the centre and then progressively throughout their substance. Those nearest together unite in the course of growth and then form more or less voluminous masses, pale yellow in color, opaque, and comparable, as regards density, with the most compact kinds of cheese; they are then called crude tubercles...

> In whatever manner these crude tubercles are formed, they finish at the end of a longer or shorter time of very variable duration by becoming softened and liquified. This softening starts near the middle of each mass, which daily becomes softer and moister until the softening has reached the periphery and become complete...

> When the tuberculous matter has completely softened, it breaks its way into the nearest bronchial tube. The resulting aperture being narrower than the cavity with which it communicates, both remain of necessity fistulous even after the complete evacuation of the tuberculous matter. (Laënnec, adapted from Ackerknecht (1967), p. 94)

The above description and Figure 4.2 demonstrate the skilful manner in which Laënnec was able to weave together the disparate findings of anatomy into a dynamic disease process, beginning with minute abnormalities and ending with fatal complications. Laënnec's terminology and descriptions, resting upon apposite analogies drawn from everyday experience, have not been superseded.

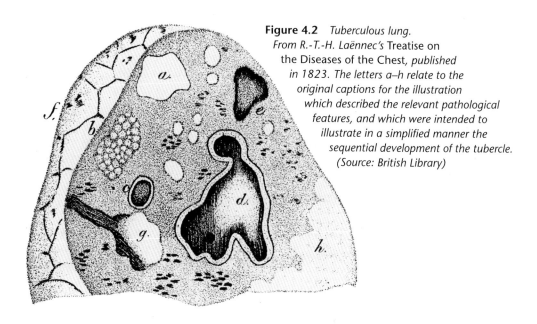

**Figure 4.2** *Tuberculous lung. From R.-T.-H. Laënnec's* Treatise on the Diseases of the Chest, *published in 1823. The letters a–h relate to the original captions for the illustration which described the relevant pathological features, and which were intended to illustrate in a simplified manner the sequential development of the tubercle. (Source: British Library)*

● Identify some everyday analogies contained in the quotation. What do they suggest about Laënnec's background?

■ Laënnec referred to seeds, the smaller millet seed (Latin, *milium,* hence miliary tubercles) and the larger hemp seed, for initial stages, and cheese for the later stages in tubercle development. Laënnec had strong affection for his Breton rural background.

### 4.4.2  Cellular pathology and opposition to cell theory

Further elaboration of the work of Laënnec and his followers was impeded by the limitations of naked-eye observation. However, this situation was soon remedied with the rapid improvements of microscopes and microscopic techniques which took place in the mid-nineteenth century, the further importance of which is discussed in Chapter 5. The immediate effect of microscopy was to give added credibility to **cell theory**: the idea that all living matter was constituted from cells, which possessed the capacity to divide and replicate themselves. In the 1840s this idea became dominant and it was applied to medicine in the theories of 'cellular pathology' of Rudolf Virchow (1821–1902), who argued that all pathological phenomena could be explained in terms of a cellular process.

The stage might have been set for the final consolidation of the findings of Laënnec by explaining the process of TB in cellular terms (i.e. as infectious organisms disrupting the structure and function of body cells). But events proved otherwise. Central to the outlook of Virchow was the concept of *inflammation,* which was correctly understood as a cellular reaction to irritant forces, resulting in an increased blood supply to the affected part. Virchow reverted to the Galenic ideas (which Bayle and Laënnec had contested), by regarding inflammation as the *primary* phenomenon and TB as a *consequence* of inflammation. The authority of Virchow therefore extended the life of the inflammation theory of TB and undermined the idea that it was a discrete disease. Virchow's idea remained current until after the bacteriological discoveries of Robert Koch (discussed below), which were also opposed by Virchow.

## 4.5   Ideas on treatment before the bacteriological revolution

Before the bacteriological findings of Koch in 1882, advancement of knowledge concerning the clinical description and pathology of TB resulted in no immediate insights into improved methods of therapy. TB was subjected to the same regimes as other diseases with which it was associated. It was treated as the by-product of inflammation connected with fevers. In the early nineteenth century the preferred course of treatment was by 'counter-irritation', or 'local depletion', which in practice meant blistering, purging and bleeding. In line with this theory, people with TB were shut away in darkened, airless rooms, and were introduced to a regime of total inactivity. More fortunate patients were introduced to milder hygienic or dietary treatments. The prosperous were dispatched to the Mediterranean. The above regimes were complemented by the almost indiscriminate resort to new lines in medication. Fashionable new drugs like the innocuous cod liver oil, or dangerous substances like creosote or digitalis (derived from the foxglove, a powerful heart stimulant) were tried out on TB patients.

Following Galenist teaching it was generally believed that consumption fell into the incurable class of diseases. This idea was fostered by the growing belief in the nineteenth century that consumption was an hereditary disease. This view seemed to gain support from the prevalence of TB among the poor dwelling in the expanding urban slums. The poor were often regarded as a genetically inferior racial type, prone to fecklessness, intemperance, insanity and diseases such as TB. This generated a somewhat fatalistic approach to TB, but it was believed that the poor could alleviate their condition by moral endeavour and that higher social classes could reduce their proneness to the disease by avoiding the intemperate habits of the lower classes.

● Suggest an alternative explanation for the prevalence of TB among the poor.

■ Overcrowding increased the rate of transmission from person to person of TB, and of course of many other infectious diseases. Poverty increased susceptibility due to poor nutrition, ventilation and exhaustion from heavy work and long hours.

## 4.5.1  Vitiated air

Understanding of the chemistry of air, achieved in the early nineteenth century, provided a new rationale for fevers. It was believed that fevers were induced by a rise in carbon dioxide in air, and by organic impurities emanating from human exhalations, or *miasmas* from rotting organic matter in the environment. This *vitiated* (or corrupted) air was identified as the main enemy of health, and it was held especially responsible for chest and throat diseases such as pulmonary consumption, scrofula, bronchitis, pneumonia and diphtheria. This theory paved the way for a new approach towards TB therapy, based on the doctrine of fresh air and sunlight which occupied a major part in public-health programmes in the later nineteenth century. TB sufferers were now encouraged to take advantage of the open air and exercise, while maximum ventilation and cool temperatures were demanded for the sick-room.

The above theories provided guidelines for the **Medical Officers of Health** (MOH), the public-health professionals, who played an increasingly interventionist role in late-Victorian Britain.[5] The public-health doctors exploited an increasing number of channels to dragoon the poor into habits of cleanliness, but without fundamentally affecting their poverty. Pulmonary consumption was one of the targets for this official public-health action. Despite the claims of public-health officials to success, it is far from certain that the scale of the intervention was sufficient to make a significant indentation on the TB problem. Nevertheless, the seemingly scientific justification and appearance of effectiveness indicated by the declining TB mortality rates, provided a useful means for legitimation and expansion of the public-health profession until the point was reached where public-health measures *were* influential. However, as indicated below, it should not be assumed that the public-health doctors invariably exercised their new powers responsibly or effectively.

In fact, when it was first evolved the new philosophy of treatment was just as arbitrary as the old one, since it was based on a fundamental misunderstanding of the cause of the disease. But the new approach to TB treatment involved adoption

[5] Their work is discussed in *Caring for Health: History and Diversity* (Open University Press, 2nd edn 1993; 3rd edn 2001), Chapter 4.

of practices which were *accidentally* more consistent with the true causes of the disease. The Victorian public-health reformers in this case, as in others, were advocating the right course of action for the wrong reasons.

● Why were fresh air, ventilation and sunlight helpful in the prevention of TB?

■ They reduced the chances of transmission of the infection. (Also the TB bacterium is destroyed by sunlight.)

The fresh-air approach to TB was strengthened by the activities of Hermann Brehmer of Goebersdorf in Silesia. Brehmer was an obscure provincial doctor, but he is an example of the many entrepreneurial figures in the history of TB, who have pursued their patent treatments with fanatical zeal, sometimes with genuine humanitarian motivation, occasionally with the objective of gratuitous fame or financial gain.

*The Schwarzeck sanatorium near Blankenburg-Schwarzatal. The open-air sanatorium became the basis for treating rich and poor during the nineteenth century. (Reproduced courtesy of Professor Paul Weindling)*

Brehmer provides a further example of advocating the correct course of action for the wrong reason. He believed that since TB was a degenerative disease, it could be corrected by building up the metabolism, which required maximising the functioning of the heart and circulatory (cardiovascular) system, physical exercise, and a plentiful diet. He also believed that the cardiovascular system would be assisted by reduced atmospheric pressure, and therefore high altitudes. Brehmer's regime was put into practice at his sanatorium in Goebersdorf. The **sanatorium** idea gained appeal because its institutional setting provided the opportunity for rigorous application of the therapeutic regime — an idea not dissimilar to the modern 'health farm'.

Brehmer's experiment was widely publicised, but even more attention was captured by the rival sanatorium at Nordrach in the Black Forest, founded in 1888, which took into account the new bacteriological approach to TB, but which essentially repeated Brehmer's open-air system. Sanatoria modelled on the Nordrach system were established throughout Europe and the sanatorium became the basis for the treatment of TB for both rich and poor during the bacteriological age. The rationale for treatment was suitably adjusted, but it is important to recognise that the basic regime of open-air treatment in the new sanatoria was taken over virtually unchanged from the pre-bacteriological period.

## 4.6   The bacteriological age

The idea of contagiousness of disease (i.e. that it is spread between persons by some kind of agency) extended back into the pre-scientific age. But the vigorous scientific debate between contagionists and their opponents the miasmatists (see Chapter 3) belongs to the mid-nineteenth century. In the second half of the century conclusive evidence emerged in favour of contagion or infection, and *bacteria* were shown to be the main causal agents for many common diseases. The central figure in establishing new **microbiological principles** (theories relating to microscopic organisms) upon which the above findings were based was Louis Pasteur (1822–1895) who is shown in his laboratory in Figure 4.3. Pasteur carried out fundamental researches demonstrating the connection between fermentation and

**Figure 4.3** *Pasteur in his laboratory. Notice the various flasks on the laboratory bench. The narrow neck of the largest flask, which curves down out of sight, would be sealed after the rich organic broth in the flask had been heated at boiling point for some time. The failure of any organisms to originate in this hermetically sealed container was fundamental to Pasteur's critique of spontaneous generation. (Source: The Wellcome Library, London)*

micro-organisms. In 1860, in beautifully constructed experiments, he demonstrated the fallacy of the widely-held idea of *spontaneous generation* (the theory that organisms can be generated from a suitable medium, rather than being formed by *reproduction* from pre-existing organisms), thereby removing one of the props of miasmatic theories of fevers.

● What was the purpose of the microscope shown in Figure 4.3?

■ To examine the broth for signs of the presence of micro-organisms. This confirmed inferences from experimentation with direct visual inspection.

Pasteur then turned to the problem of protection against contagious disease. Between 1877 and 1884 he established that fowl cholera, anthrax and erysipelas (a disease causing inflammation of the skin), were all caused by bacterial infections. He also investigated the cause of rabies and, although its viral origin was not identified for some years, Pasteur recognised that the infectious agent was *not* bacterial.

However, the first steps towards an understanding of the microbiological basis for TB were made by Pasteur's associate, Jean-Antoine Villermin (1827–1892), whose experiments on rabbits in 1865 demonstrated that TB was a specific infection which could be transmitted by injection. Villermin's *Études sur la Tuberculose* (*Studies of Tuberculosis*) (1868) contained impressive evidence of the infectiousness of TB, which won him influential supporters. He effectively undermined explanations based on miasmatic theory or heredity, but his work left the final identity of the infectious agent of TB unestablished. This last link in the chain was put in place on 24 March 1882 in a lecture to scientific colleagues in Berlin by Robert Koch (1843–1910), who was at that time an unknown Prussian provincial doctor.

As in the case of Pasteur, Koch's ideas were based on elaborate experimental technique. He was dependent on recently developed methods of preparing animal tissue for microscopical examination, and techniques to stain different cells and tissues in different colours using synthetic dyes which had only been recently produced by organic chemists. In evolving these microscopical techniques Koch was assisted by collaboration with his relative Paul Ehrlich (1854–1915), who will be mentioned again in this chapter in the context of chemotherapy (drug treatment). Koch's microscopical studies enabled him to substantiate Laënnec's theory of TB as a unified disease by showing that all stages of pulmonary consumption and all other forms of TB were characterised by the presence of the same bacterium, which we now know as *Mycobacterium tuberculosis*.

Figure 4.4 shows Koch in his laboratory, like Pasteur using his microscope. This was the most sophisticated scientific instrument in the field of medicine. Its prominence in portraits served to enhance the authority of the new speciality of **bacteriology** (the study of bacteria).

● What differences in the glassware are there, in comparison with Pasteur's laboratory (Figure 4.3)?

**Figure 4.4** *Robert Koch, photographed in 1896 or 1897 at work in his laboratory at Kimberley, South Africa. (Source: The Wellcome Library, London)*

■ The round flasks have wide necks which are corked rather than sealed, and the dominant items are circular, flat dishes with lids.

These flat dishes are known as *Petri dishes*, and were important for Koch. They were used to *culture* fluid taken from tuberculous lesions of an infected animal. The fluid was placed on a gelatinous substance, or *culture medium*, prepared in the round flasks and maintained in conditions that allowed the bacteria to multiply. Specimen bacteria from these cultures were stained and identified under the microscope (see Figure 4.5). Koch identified cultures of the TB bacterium and passed samples of bacteria from one Petri dish to another, in each case allowing the culture to multiply before passing a sample to a new Petri dish, over many generations. The bacterial culture surviving to the end of this process proved capable of causing TB in his laboratory animals, proving that the bacteria alone were responsible for causing TB.

On the basis of his investigations into TB, Koch defined conditions of proof for establishing the microbiological source of infectious disease, which became known as Koch's postulates. They can be summarised as:

1   The micro-organism should be found in every type of lesion associated with the disease.

2   It should be capable of cultivation on an artificial medium for several generations.

3   After culture it should be capable of reproducing the original illness in the body of a laboratory animal.

These procedures laid down guidelines which were followed by Koch and have guided other investigators of infectious disease ever since. The stringent requirements of proof evolved by Koch had implications way beyond the field of infectious disease. They pointed to the kind of criteria which would need to be fulfilled in biomedical research more generally.[6]

[6] Scientific methods are discussed further in *Studying Health and Disease* (Open University Press, 2nd edn 1994; colour-enhanced 2nd edn 2001), Chapter 2.

Koch's discovery of the bacterial cause of TB prompted great emotion in those who viewed it as a decisive turning point in an exhausting battle against the disease. Thus in 1908, a TB expert, Leonard Williams, wrote of Koch's achievement:

> ...the riddle of the white plague, which had so long defied solution, had been read at last; the dreary watches of the night were over; and the dawn, with its promise of victory, peace and purity, was really at hand. (Williams, 1908, p. 56)

### 4.6.1 False dawn?

Although Koch's lecture in 1882 is conventionally taken as marking the beginning of active control of TB, we should not exaggerate the immediate impact of his discovery. It is important to appreciate the distinction that exists between the *understanding* of the mechanism of a disease and the *application* of that knowledge for the purposes of prevention and control. There are a number of reasons for this delay in application in the case of TB.

First, theories that TB was hereditary or caused by miasmas were so entrenched that there was a disinclination to regard Koch's findings as more than a partial explanation.

**Figure 4.5** *Tuberculous lesions and cultures of TB bacteria, from Robert Koch's* Gesammelte Werke, *published in Leipzig in 1912 (originally published 1882). (Source: The British Library, London)*

Second, Koch's discovery brought no immediate medical benefits. In 1890 Koch seemed to have arrived at an effective natural form of therapy when he isolated a protein product from TB bacteria cultures which he called *tuberculin*. Great claims were made for a variety of tuberculin preparations over a long period, many of which were supported by Koch's personal authority. The veteran research worker in this field, J. A. Parish, cites a review from 1927 that listed 65 tuberculins and 36 'vaccines', almost all of which were ineffective, positively dangerous, or even fraudulent. Parish concludes that the vogue for tuberculin was 'one of the regrettable episodes in medical history.' (Parish, 1965, p. 94). As noted below, Koch's ideas on chemotherapy (drug treatment) were also unproductive.

Third, the bacteriological camp was also divided over other important issues, especially over the infectiousness of bovine TB (i.e. the strain found in cow's milk). At the important International Conference on Tuberculosis held in London in 1901, Koch declared that the bovine TB bacterium was harmless to humans. It is a reflection of the great authority of Koch that in Britain it required the authority of a Royal Commission, which reported in 1911, to reject his findings. Even then Koch's intervention caused lasting damage, because it hampered the movement for the pasteurisation of milk (whereby milk is heated to destroy the bacteria it contains), and gave greater credibility to the many vested interests resisting health control on cattle, meat and milk. In fact, effective safety of milk was delayed until World War II, with the result that generations of children were unnecessarily exposed to the risks of bovine TB, and resources were absorbed in providing special schools, rehabilitation services and sanatoria for children suffering from this crippling disease.

### 4.6.2  Surgical treatments

The failure to evolve an effective vaccine or chemotherapy to combat the TB bacterium created the opportunity for other forms of treatment to prosper. Surgeons in particular were keen to try their hand at treating the advanced stages of TB. The opportunities for surgical intervention were drastically increased at about the time of Koch's discovery with the development of anaesthesia in the mid-nineteenth century and *aseptic* surgery (i.e. surgery using techniques designed to reduce the risk of wound infection).

The favoured surgical treatment for TB involved inducing the affected lungs to collapse, either by injection of gases into the chest cavity (artificial pneumothorax), or later by more radical operations involving cutting or removing part of the rib cage (thoracoplasty), or paralysing the phrenic nerve which controls movements of the diaphragm and hence lung inflation and collapse. A variety of techniques for such *collapse therapy* were developed in the 1890s. In the absence of effective alternatives, lengthy, hazardous and expensive surgical methods gained the ascendency. As noted by R. Y. Keers, this trend was exacerbated by World War I.

> Collapse therapy had gained a firm foothold on the therapeutic ladder by 1914 when the outbreak of World War I initiated a startling increase in the incidence of tuberculosis in Europe. This increase, which was both an accompaniment and an aftermath of the war, made imperative the mobilization and exploitation of all possible forms of treatment and ushered in an era in which therapy was dominated by the sanatorium, artificial pneumothorax, phrenic paralysis and thoracoplasty. (Keers, 1978, p. 126)

The progress of surgical treatment continued relentlessly during the inter-war period. A survey conducted in 1941 noted that, between 1929 and 1939, 2100 papers were produced on surgical treatment for TB, but only five per cent were concerned with the *effectiveness* of this form of care. In the event *none* of the techniques in use possessed proven validity, a situation which gradually led to a 'morass of doubt and contradiction' (Keers, 1978, p. 162).

This damning conclusion emanating from a leading expert in the field illustrates the gulf between the exacting standards of proof laid down by Koch for the new science of bacteriology and the lack of standards of evaluation in the old art of surgery. The lapses of surgery in the case of TB are by no means an isolated instance, and the pursuit of surgical procedures that are eventually discredited and discarded has remained a problem down to the present day (modern enthusiasm for pursuing surgical treatment for a variety of conditions is discussed in Chapter 7). However, the high status of surgery based on its known successful procedures and high standard of service during emergencies, and especially World War I, provided an elitist image and a defensive mystique which protected the less creditable aspects of its art from critical scrutiny.

Thoracic (chest) surgeons' enthusiasm for making a decisive impact in the area of TB tempted them to make extravagant claims for their methods, which were not based on critical evaluation, but which seemed acceptable in the absence of clearly preferable alternatives. Once the trend to surgical treatment was established, it was maintained by inertia, and surgeons were sufficiently influential to serve as an obstacle to the development of alternative forms of treatment. Their position was further strengthened by the enhanced status given to sanatorium treatment by the presence of patients undergoing advanced surgery. By this means the sanatorium was elevated to the 'premier league' of major hospital specialisms, and there was little inducement for doubt to be cast on the methods which had earned this status.

### 4.6.3  The sanatorium system

The bacteriological revolution failed in the short term to exercise a decisive positive impact on TB treatment. It failed to deliver a cure for the disease, or even an effective new specific treatment. Nevertheless, despite his misjudgements and the disappointing results of his specific therapies, Koch's ideas had some direct positive effects. His bacteriological theory of TB provided a new rationale and increased legitimation for public-health measures. The TB bacterium replaced vitiated air as the justification for the gospel of fresh air, ventilation, sunlight, cleanliness and disinfection.

In Britain, an influential new campaigning organisation, the National Association for the Prevention of Tuberculosis, was established in 1898, and the King Edward VII National Memorial Association, founded in 1910, assumed responsibility for TB services in Wales. An elaborate system of dispensaries, after-care organisations, and sanatoria was built up. Legislation in 1911 and 1921 established the TB service as a high priority among the publicly-funded health services. Parallel developments occurred throughout the industrialised economies. Although, as just noted, thoracic surgery played a significant part in this development, the whole of this enterprise was premised on the bacteriological explanation. Because bacteriological theory established the infectiousness of TB, the isolation of patients assumed paramount importance, especially when they worked in factories or came from overcrowded homes, where they were seen as constituting a hazard to fellow workers, family and neighbours. Thus, even at a time of economic depression, institutional provision for TB assumed high priority and was rapidly expanded. Sanatoria therefore constituted the dominant element in the expanding TB service. An indication of the rapidity of expansion of the sanatorium system is provided by Table 4.2.

**Table 4.2**  Sanatorium beds provided in England 1911–1938.

|      | Local Authorities[7] | Voluntary sector | Total   |
| ---- | -------------------- | ---------------- | ------- |
| 1911 | 1 300                | 4 200            | 5 500   |
| 1921 | 6 531                | 7 015            | 13 546  |
| 1929 | 12 189               | 7 684            | 19 873  |
| 1938 | 15 609               | 7 848            | 23 457  |

Data from Bryder, 1988, *Below the Magic Mountain: A Social History of Tuberculosis in Twentieth-Century Britain*, Oxford University Press, Oxford, Tables 2 and 4, pp. 44, 76.

● What does the table show about the relative contributions of the local authority and voluntary systems?

■ Between 1911 and 1938 local authorities increasingly took over from the voluntary sector in providing the majority of beds for TB patients.

[7] Local authorities of the period provided health and social services funded from local rates and other taxation; the voluntary sector provided services funded by charitable donations. The pattern of expansion of publicly-funded health services is discussed in *Caring for Health: History and Diversity* (Open University Press, 2nd edn 1993; 3rd edn 2001), Chapters 4 and 5.

*The Paimio Sanatorium, Finland, photographed in the 1930s. Sanatoria became the showpieces of the modern hospital system throughout Western Europe. (Source: Reiach, A. and Hurd, R., 1944, Building Scotland, The Saltire Society, Edinburgh)*

The local authority sanatoria provided for the working classes, whereas the voluntary sector dealt also with the middle classes. Sanatoria for the poor contrasted with the luxurious sanatoria for the rich which sprang up in countries such as Switzerland and Finland. TB experts suitably adapted the regime to impose the maximum discipline on poor patients. The publicly provided sanatoria therefore became vehicles for reinforcement of the work ethic. The following statement by Marcus Paterson, one of Britain's leading sanatorium Medical Superintendents in the 1920s, indicates the way in which Koch's ideas were mobilised to justify a harsh regime of physical discipline.

> If we allow our patient to exert himself, we make him liberate a certain amount of tuberculin (the poison) or toxin, to overcome which the body immediately reacts and produces anti-toxin, which at once kills the tuberculosis poison, and we can bring about this happy result simply by means of exercise or graduated work. Exercise or work, in graduated amounts is therefore, in every sense of the term, scientific treatment. (Paterson, 1920, quoted from Bryder (1988), p. 57)

This extract indicates the degree to which the sanatorium took its place alongside the workhouse and other institutions as a vehicle of medical surveillance and social control, a conclusion which is developed in Chapter 8 of this book. The medical profession, in justifying the provision of expensive services such as sanatoria, was anxious to avoid the accusation of extravagance. Accordingly they inclined to over-compensate by surrounding their services with an aura of austerity or even vindictiveness against the classes they were supposed to serve.

The precise benefits deriving from the sanatorium system are difficult to establish, but little was gained by isolation or surgical treatment, and it is doubtful whether

*Male patients doing 'Graduated Labour' c. 1910 with the Royal National Hospital for Consumption, Ventnor, Isle of Wight, in the background. Such an approach at this sanatorium in the voluntary sector provided a model for reinforcing the work ethic in later sanatoria for the working classes. (Source: Bodleian Library, Oxford)*

anything was attained by sanatoria that could not have been achieved by much cheaper non-institutional means. However, the gradual decline in TB mortality (indicated in Figure 4.1 earlier) undoubtedly encouraged the view that the institutional system was contributing to this trend. This may well have been an erroneous impression, but its cultivation was an important element in the legitimation of the substantial vested interests involved in the sanatorium movement.

## 4.7   Screening the population

By 1900, TB accounted for about 12 per cent of all deaths in Britain. This represented a sizeable annual death toll of 75 000. As indicated by Figure 4.1, the improvement was interrupted during World War I and to a much lesser extent during World War II. In 1950 the number of deaths from TB was exceeded by lung cancer, indicating the degree to which in Western nations this once major fatal disease was in rapid retreat.

At the beginning of the twentieth century, biological understanding and medical control of TB were impaired without firmer evidence concerning levels of **morbidity** (a term that refers to sickness or disability, as opposed to **mortality** which refers to deaths). The medical profession was faced with a difficult problem. Clearly, mortality figures in this period gave a completely inadequate impression of the scale of the disease and of its sources of dissemination. In order to establish the population most at risk from TB, it was necessary to introduce a test that would locate non-infectious carriers and potential sufferers of the disease.

**Notification** of some infectious diseases was made compulsory in 1889, involving medical practitioners reporting to a central registration office whenever they encountered a person with a particular *notifiable disease*. TB was not among them because in 1889 there was no direct means of identifying TB infection. However, skin tests were devised, the best-known of which was the test developed by Charles Mantoux in 1910 (based on a skin reaction to tuberculin of those infected with the TB bacterium) and known subsequently as the Mantoux test. Skin tests revealed that a large proportion of the population were non-infectious carriers of the TB bacterium, but most had not developed the disease. Consequently the Mantoux test was of limited value in identifying infectious cases, but they could be identified by a sputum test (in which bacteria were cultivated from sputum). This was useful, but time-consuming to perform. Compulsory notification of TB was introduced in 1913.

The introduction during World War II of mass radiography (chest X-rays, see Figure 4.6) provided an effective mechanism of preliminary surveillance. X-rays provided a reliable method of selecting people for further tests. Thus a method of locating infectious people was devised, but only after TB had ceased to be the highest priority as a medical problem. Although TB accounted for only five per cent of all deaths in Britain by 1940, 66 000 new cases each year were reported at this time, which undoubtedly understated the scale of the problem.

**Figure 4.6**   *Mass radiography, introduced during World War II, provided an effective mechanism of preliminary surveillance. (Source: Macintosh, J. M., 1944,* The Nation's Health, *Pilot Press, London, p. 40)*

Compulsory notification for TB was more unpopular than for any other infectious disease. It was resisted because of the penalties such as loss of employment and social ostracism affecting TB sufferers and their families. Also there was no consistency in practice among doctors responsible for notification. For reasons of clinical judgement, sympathy with patients, or antipathy to 'state medicine', they inclined to neglect the notification procedure (Bryder, 1988, pp. 103–9).

As a consequence of all of the above shortcomings, the attempt to refine information about the distribution of TB in the population was only a partial success.

### 4.7.1  Blaming the poor

As already noted, the association of TB with poverty generated little sympathy for TB sufferers among medical investigators. Victorian TB specialists were apt to regard the poor as victims of their own idleness and degenerative tendencies, and as a reservoir of contamination for their betters. In 1912 Henry de C. Woodcock, a leading TB authority of the time, described TB as a

> …coarse, common disease, bred in foul breath, in dirt, in squalor….
> The beautiful and the rich receive it from the unbeautiful poor.
> (Quoted by Bryder, 1988, p. 20)

This quotation illustrates the continuing moral connotation of disease even after the arrival of a bacteriological explanation.

A more sensitive understanding of poverty and its association with ill-health gradually emerged in the course of the twentieth century through the increasingly comprehensive investigations undertaken by social scientists. Although this scientific investigation of poverty represented a positive advance, it is clear that the perspective of these early social scientists was limited by many of the same social prejudices, moral strictures and hereditarian beliefs which affected the medical profession.

*Woman and children in a 1930s working-class district in London. Organisations like the Eugenics Society kept to the fore the idea that an hereditary underclass constituted a dangerous reservoir of disease. (Source: W. Suschitzky; photo by Edith Tudor Hart)*

Such influential organisations as the Eugenics Society[8] kept to the fore the idea that an hereditary underclass constituted a dangerous reservoir of disease.

Social scientists found it difficult to disentangle the relative importance of such factors as housing standards, overcrowding, nutrition, income, and personal habits. It was not until the 1930s, during the impact of the Depression, that it was established in precise quantitative terms that TB infection was usually an unavoidable consequence of adverse economic circumstances, rather than the effect of moral delinquency. Research into the social aspects of TB underlined the degree to which not all regions, occupations and classes were enjoying the improvements experienced by the better-off. Marked differences in health among people from different social classes persisted, despite the improvement in certain average levels of mortality and an increased degree of welfare provision. An elaborate survey by P. D'Arcy Hart and G. Payling Wright demonstrated the scale of this disadvantage in England and Wales. Some of their findings are indicated in Table 4.3.

**Table 4.3**  Rates of pulmonary TB in the age group 15 to 24, during the periods 1911–13 and 1931–3, for two groups of county boroughs having greater and lesser improvement in housing.[9]

| | | Average TB death rates per 100 000 population aged 15–24 | |
| --- | --- | --- | --- |
| | | 1911–13 | 1931–3 |
| 12 boroughs with greater improvement in housing | males | 129 | 101 |
| | females | 139 | 131 |
| 12 boroughs with lesser improvement in housing | males | 135 | 143 |
| | females | 138 | 160 |

Adapted from Hart, P. D. and Wright, P. G., 1939, *Tuberculosis and Social Conditions in England with Special Reference to Young Adults, a Statistical Study*, National Association for the Prevention of Tuberculosis, London, Table 18, p. 58.

● What does Table 4.3 show about the relationship between housing standards and trends in the incidence of TB over time?

■ Boroughs with improved housing witnessed moderate reductions in TB, particularly for males, where the death rate fell from 129 per 100 000 of the population in that age group in 1911–13 to 101 in 1931–3. However, in those boroughs with worse housing the situation actually deteriorated over time, particularly for females.

● Examine Figure 4.1 (p. 59) again. You will notice substantially higher levels of TB in Scotland before World War I. In the light of Table 4.3 how might the Scottish situation be explained?

[8] Eugenics is the term used to cover the theory and practice of controlling the genetic character of the human race. It is mentioned again in *Caring for Health: History and Diversity* (Open University Press, 2nd edn 1993; 3rd edn 2001), Chapter 4 and in *Human Biology and Health: an Evolutionary Approach* (Open University Press, 2nd edn 1994; 3rd edn 2001), Chapter 9.

[9] The death rates are standardised to allow for differences between boroughs in the proportions of people in different age groups. The process of standardising death rates to allow for age differences is discussed in *Studying Health and Disease* (Open University Press, 2nd edn 1994; colour-enhanced 2nd edn 2001), Chapter 7.

■   Scotland possessed notoriously bad housing in its large areas of heavy industry which provided ideal circumstances for the spread of TB.

The investigation by D'Arcy Hart and Payling Wright conclusively demonstrated that measures to relieve poverty and improve the quality of housing provided the most effective means to contain TB. They also indicated a new level of awareness of gender differences. Their conclusions concerning the adverse position of women were applicable to many other areas of health.[10]

## 4.8   Prevention and its problems

The discoveries of Pasteur and Koch generated the expectation that prevention of TB by **immunisation** was a realistic possibility. Immunisation involves the introduction of *killed* but formerly infectious bacteria, or *attenuated* bacteria (i.e. living, but rendered non-infectious by laboratory treatment), or a harmless but *related* strain of bacteria, into the body. The immune system responds to their presence by mounting a highly specific attack against the micro-organisms. If living infectious bacteria subsequently get into the body, the immune system responds rapidly enough to destroy them before the infection can take hold.[11] This form of protection against TB first became available in 1921, when Léon Charles Albert Calmette (1863–1933) and Camille Guérin (1872–1961) commenced human trials with their vaccine, known subsequently as Bacille Calmette Guérin (**BCG**). This innovation is recognised as one of the great landmarks in the campaign against TB.

Calmette and Guérin worked in Lille and at the Pasteur Institute in Paris. They followed Pasteur's approach by attempting to evolve an attenuated strain of the TB bacterium. Building on the observation that ox bile used as a nutrient had the effect of breaking up colonies of the bacteria into a suspension, they considered that prolonged exposure of the bacteria to ox bile might eventually lead to a stable, attenuated strain. This work began in 1906 and it was patiently continued for 13 years.

The resultant strain of attenuated bacteria proved incapable of producing TB in guinea-pigs, and when injected into laboratory animals it gave complete protection against an infectious strain introduced subsequently.

Following initial, small-scale trials on human subjects which suggested favourable results, BCG was given by oral administration to 50 000 French schoolchildren between 1922 and 1928. An improved method of injecting BCG into the skin was evolved in Sweden and this was used in extensive trials in Scandinavia and Canada. Thus, during the interwar period, BCG passed from the trial stage to mass application in substantial areas of the developed world. However, BCG was not universally accepted. In Britain, Germany and the USA, BCG was not accepted until the 1950s, which represented a delay of 30 years (see Figure 4.7). With hindsight, this delay seems particularly unreasonable because of the undoubted success and safety of BCG, which was not associated with the obvious defects that clouded the path of Koch's tuberculin preparations.

[10] See *Caring for Health: History and Diversity* (Open University Press, 2nd edn 1993; 3rd edn 2001), Chapter 5 for a discussion of the way in which health services also left women at a disadvantage during this period.

[11] The immune response to infection is the subject of *Human Biology and Health: an Evolutionary Approach* (Open University Press, 2nd edn 1994; 3rd edn 2001), Chapter 6.

**Figure 4.7** *British school children in the 1940s waiting to be immunised against diphtheria. Immunisation against diphtheria, like that against TB, was delayed in Britain for 30 years compared with most other Western countries. (Source: Taylor, S., 1944, The Battle for Health: A Primer of Social Medicine, Nicholson and Watson, London, Figure 73, p. 79)*

## 4.8.1 The British opposition to BCG

There were numerous obstacles to the acceptance of BCG, especially in countries like Britain, and these are instructive for revealing general constraints affecting the adoption of medical innovations. First, during the 1920s many rival vaccines made their appearance and most proved to be ineffective or positively dangerous. Consequently public-health agencies tended to react with extreme caution towards even widely-acclaimed vaccines or cures. In 1930 Sir Arthur MacNalty, the official with formal responsibility for TB and the future Chief Medical Officer to the Ministry of Health, encapsulated the establishment's mood of caution:

> While uncertainty still persists as to whether the living vaccine, B.C.G., is free from virulence under all conditions, and doubt is expressed as to its effective immunising properties, its use as an immunising agent, particularly for young children, is unlikely to be advocated in this country on any extensive scale. (MacNalty quoted from Ministry of Health, 1947, p. 60)

Second, statisticians were suspicious of the work of Calmette and Guérin. For instance Professor Major Greenwood of the London School of Hygiene and Tropical Medicine, a respected epidemiologist, claimed to have discovered serious statistical errors in Calmette's work (Greenwood, 1928).

Third, a degree of chauvinism and professional jealousy motivated the adverse response to the French innovation. Rival researchers, annoyed by the failures of their own vaccines, devoted much energy to experiments aimed at demonstrating that BCG (which contained live bacteria) was likely to revert into an infectious form. This work was often backed by powerful funding bodies, who were keen to prove the superiority of their own initiatives. In Britain the antipathy to BCG on the part of the Medical Research Council (MRC) took the form of support for Professor Georges Dreyer of Oxford, inventor of the failed 'Diaplyte Vaccine'. As Linda Bryder, a leading historian of TB, has pointed out, the unjustified bias against BCG, uncritical faith in the judgement of enthusiasts who lacked impartiality, neglect of research into drug treatment, and general lack of commitment to TB research by the MRC, removed Britain from the forefront of advance in this important field of medical endeavour (Bryder, 1988).

Fourth, an outbreak of TB in 1931, known as the 'Lübeck Disaster', provided damaging publicity against BCG, even though subsequent enquiries concluded that the TB contracted by vaccinated schoolchildren had resulted from a serious local error which had allowed BCG to become contaminated by an infectious strain of TB bacteria.

Fifth, in Britain and elsewhere public-health agencies were inhibited by vociferous anti-vaccination organisations motivated by ethical and religious considerations. In a situation where TB was being contained at a reasonably constant level, there was little inducement to introduce a controversial new form of intervention.

Finally, the evident lack of enthusiasm for BCG must also reflect inertia within Britain's 'national TB scheme', which represented the product of many generations of effort. It included its own methods of prevention, entailing campaigns of education and social improvement which were regarded as valuable in themselves, and which would have been undermined by the introduction of a simple method of prevention.

Thus, formidable obstacles stood in the way of general implementation of BCG vaccination in Britain. Expert advocates of BCG eventually went onto the offensive during World War II, but the Ministry of Health, MRC and newly-founded Public Health Laboratory Service were unresponsive. In 1946 the Ministry of Health described its position as one of

> ...interested detachment. Results in other countries have been closely studied and developments awaited which might convince medical men in this country that the time had come for action here. (Ministry of Health, 1947, pp. 59–60)

Eventually, in 1947, preparations were made by the MRC for exhaustive trials of BCG, which were reported between 1956 and 1963. However, the use of BCG was by then so extensive elsewhere that official obstruction collapsed, and BCG vaccination was sanctioned for schoolchildren and other high-risk groups in the course of the 1950s.

## 4.8.2  BCG in the wider world

Before the MRC trials began in Britain, the Danish Red Cross initiated a BCG campaign in Europe and this was soon extended to developing countries, particularly those under European colonial rule. The effectiveness of BCG was improved by the introduction in 1956 of a freeze-dried vaccine. The success of BCG campaigns varied, but under optimal conditions it proved possible to vaccinate virtually all infants, with the result that children were effectively protected. But it soon became evident that vaccination alone would not eliminate TB. The effects of vaccination were not permanent and adults varied in their response to the vaccines. Trials in the 1980s displayed that in some areas BCG gave virtually no protection to adults, with the result that infected adults remained a potent reservoir for the dissemination of the disease to all but the youngest vaccinated members of their communities. As indicated earlier, the rise of AIDS has greatly increased the magnitude of this danger. Consequently the original optimism that the BCG campaign would eliminate TB within a generation proved to be misfounded. Nevertheless, after many false starts, vaccination has been justified as an essential element in the wider programme of TB control.

## 4.9   Zero option?

Vaccination provided the most satisfactory approach to the containment of TB because it seemed to offer the prospects of lifelong protection if administered during childhood. However the limitations of BCG that emerged in recent decades necessitated increasing reliance on other forms of treatment. Drug therapy proved particularly important to the relative success of the anti-TB campaign from the 1950s to the 1970s.

### 4.9.1   Drug treatment: a new dawn?

Effective drug treatment was slow to evolve. Koch's discovery suggested that it might be possible to evolve a drug that would target and destroy the TB bacterium — the idea of the 'magic bullet'. This approach was pursued by Koch's collaborator Paul Ehrlich, who in 1909 synthesised a drug effective in the treatment of syphilis. However, despite advances in many other fields, progress in drug therapy for TB proved elusive. Success was eventually achieved during World War II when attention turned to antibiotics, substances produced naturally by micro-organisms, which were capable of inhibiting the growth of other micro-organisms. *Streptomycin*, manufactured in usable quantities in 1944, was the first effective drug against TB, but its usefulness was limited by adverse side-effects. In the case of TB, antibiotics failed to fulfil early expectations, but progress was soon made with a wide range of synthetic drugs, one of the most successful of which was *isoniazid*, which dates from 1951. It was rapidly discovered that treatment with a single drug was not feasible because the tiny residue of bacteria resistant to any one drug were capable of causing the re-emergence of the disease. This realisation brought an end to the dream of a single 'magic bullet' solution for TB. It was necessary not only to use combinations of drugs (*multiple drug therapy*), but also to take them in a carefully organised pattern every day over a lengthy period (6–8 months).

But advances in drug therapy together with determined commitment to BCG vaccination induced a new spirit of confidence in the treatment of TB from the 1950s onwards. The steady retreat of this disease and availability of cheap and effective drugs convinced expert opinion that TB should be included among the infectious diseases suitable for total elimination. This new mood of optimism was typified by what came to be known as the *approach zero* adopted in the USA in the 1960s. The following extract characterises the mood of that period:

> In the prosperous countries of the world tuberculosis…is well on the way to becoming as unusual as diphtheria or smallpox…. In many of the under-developed countries, however, the disease is still a major scourge. As living standards are raised, the combination of public health measures, new drugs, and our modern knowledge should, with proper organisation, be able to bring the disease under control even more quickly than it has been in our own country. (Office of Health Economics, 1962, pp. 19–20)

The formula for elimination of TB was deceptively simple. Children could be protected by BCG vaccination; infectious adults could be located by X-radiography, followed by sputum tests, and then treated with appropriate drugs. However, even under ideal conditions, TB control could not be achieved by simple intervention. Rather, it necessitated a lengthy and coordinated programme of surveillance and treatment.

In addition, a reservoir of infection was to be found in domestic cattle. A global eradication programme was therefore a considerably more complicated proposition than in the case of smallpox, and it rivalled malaria in its difficulty.[12]

In the 1960s, TB specialists discovered that modern eradication programmes were just as complex and problematic as the national TB schemes evolved by earlier generations. In developed economies, where TB had become a minor problem, rapid strides towards eradication were made, but with regard to the developing world the conditions listed by the Office of Health Economics in the above quotation were extremely difficult to realise in practice. It was rarely possible consistently to raise living standards, evolve systems of public health, afford new drugs, achieve stable organisation of eradication programmes, or even to agree on realistic means of adapting new knowledge to local conditions. It was recognised that, unless TB was eradicated in developing countries, programmes in developed economies would constantly be undermined by infection imported from elsewhere.

Accordingly, the next stage in TB eradication required not further therapeutic discovery, but the evolution of systems for the effective application and diffusion of current knowledge. Progress in this field required the coordination of expertise on an international scale. In practice, this has proved extremely difficult to realise in the case of TB and the many other areas of medical intervention where international coordination is relevant.

An important step in the direction of global collaboration was the establishment in 1964 of the World Health Organisation (WHO) Expert Committee on Tuberculosis. Estimation of the scale of the worldwide TB problem, particularly in developing countries, has always been difficult, but in 1960, on the eve of the WHO's initiative, estimates varied at between 12 million and 25 million seriously infected people worldwide, of which between 4 and 8 million were in India. This situation was described as an 'astronomical computation of distress' (Crofton, 1960, p. 679). From the start, the Committee appreciated the political, economic, social and technical obstacles to the adoption of effective TB policies. They cautioned that, despite all the tools being available to tackle the problem worldwide, progress was being hampered by 'insufficient realism in selecting priorities for application; lack of national planning, co-ordination and evaluation; and failure to re-orient traditional approaches to present knowledge' (WHO, 1964, p. 4). But despite their concern about these obstacles, they cannot have foreseen that the gains made in the battle to control TB in the 1960s and 1970s would be thrown so profoundly into reverse as the new millennium approached.

### 4.9.2  A global emergency

BCG vaccination and more widespread use of the new drugs against TB produced a steady decline in deaths and in incidence (the number of new cases each year) in most countries around the world, until about the mid-1980s. Then a combination of factors overturned the successes of previous decades and TB rates began to climb. By 1993, the situation had deteriorated so rapidly that the WHO declared tuberculosis a 'global emergency', but the spread of TB continued to accelerate. Between 1993 and 1996 there was a 13 per cent increase in TB cases worldwide, prompting Dr Gro Harlem Brundtland, Director-General of the WHO, to address

[12] The broader problems of eradication campaigns are considered in *World Health and Disease* (Open University Press, 2nd edn 1993; 3rd edn 2001), Chapter 8.

the Global Congress on Lung Health held in Bangkok in November 1998 in the following terms:

> We are at a crossroads in TB control. We can allow the global TB epidemic to become more deadly and strengthen its grip on the world. Or we can act now to reduce the suffering and deaths. We can and must strike back with the tools that we have. (Brundtland, quoted in WHO, 1988).

Some key features of the current global TB epidemic are summarised in Box 4.1.

---

**Box 4.1   The current global epidemic of TB**

- Worldwide, TB kills an estimated 2 million people each year, including 100 000 children; more women die of TB than all causes of maternal mortality combined.

- One-third of the world's population is already infected with TB bacteria; by 2020 an estimated 200 million of these people will get sick and 35 million will die unless current trends are halted.

- TB is the leading cause of death among people who are HIV-positive, accounting for 40 per cent of AIDS deaths in Africa and Asia and one-third of AIDS deaths worldwide.

- Throughout the late 1990s and into 2000, around 8 million new cases of TB were occurring each year: 4.5 million in six Asian countries (India, China, Bangladesh, Pakistan, Indonesia and the Philippines), 1.5–2 million in Sub-Saharan Africa, and the rest mainly in countries such as Afghanistan, West African states including Mali, Peru and Bolivia in South America, Thailand, Malaysia and South Vietnam. A quarter of a million new cases per year occur in Eastern Europe, particularly in the countries of the former Soviet Union.

- In the UK and Northern Ireland, 5 658 new cases of TB were officially notified in 1998, but this was estimated as less than a third of the real total.

(Adapted from WHO, 2000a, b)

---

● Several factors underlie the rapid increase in TB in the late 1980s and 1990s. Can you suggest some of them?

■ Poverty — always the friend of TB — increased during this period as the world went into economic recession and countries with already low incomes slid further into debt (Mali, for example, is one of the poorest countries in the world). The inability of poor countries to afford case detection and treatment programmes was compounded by destitution and displacement among large sections of their populations due to wars, food shortages and natural disasters. TB spread rapidly in refugee camps (the number of refugees and displaced people increased ninefold in the 20 years to 1998). The global epidemic of HIV damaged the immune system of HIV-positive people (estimated by the WHO at 31 million in 1997), making them 30 times more susceptible to TB. Drug treatment for TB became less effective as the bacteria evolved resistance to widely used antibiotics.

The relative importance of these factors in enabling the TB epidemic to race out of control varies from place to place. In most of Africa, the spread of HIV infection has had the greatest influence on TB rates: 'It appears HIV infection is pushing the epidemio-logical clock back towards the time of the first encounter of human population with tubercle bacilli.' (Schulzer *et al.*, 1992, p. 58). In war-torn Afghanistan, Kosovo and Chechnya, and in Bangladesh after an unprecedented series of floods in the 1980s and 1990s, the epidemic took hold in the refugee camps and detention centres and spread as people returned to their devastated homes. In industrialised countries, homeless people are most at risk; WHO estimates that around a quarter of London's 'rough sleepers' are infected with TB. And throughout the developing world the cost of curative treatment can be prohibitive — even though it amounts to about US $11 per patient, this exceeds the total annual health budget per capita for the poorest countries. (For example, annual government spending on health care and family planning in Bangladesh is only US $3.50 per head.)

But the cost of *not* treating people with TB effectively has been the evolution of **multi-drug resistant TB (MDR-TB)**. Even where the cost of treatment has been met by aid agencies, it has proved difficult to ensure that drugs are taken consistently over several months by people who are homeless or in refugee camps, or live in remote rural communities or in the shanty towns and tenement buildings of cities around the world. Inefficient methods of 'case finding' and record keeping, and reluctance by some patients to maintain contact with the authorities, have added

*A district nurse observes a young TB patient taking her medication during a home visit as part of the DOTS programme (Directly-Observed Treatment Short-course). Samoa, 1999. (Photo: A. Crump/WHO/TDR)*

to the problem of treatment which is begun but never completed. Incomplete or partial treatment means that a residue of the most drug-resistant bacteria survive and then multiply in the patient, who infects others with this more drug-resistant strain. Every time this cycle of ineffective treatment was repeated, the residual bacteria became even more drug-resistant than their predecessors, until MDR-TB evolved — a strain that is resistant to the two most commonly used anti-TB drugs, isoniazid and rifampicin.[13] The cost of isolating and attempting to treat people who are infected with MDR-TB is 100 times greater than when conventional drugs are used, and there is no guarantee of success even in countries with highly developed health-care systems. The WHO published its first report on the spread of MDR-TB in 1997; the second report, published on World TB Day, 24 March 2000, warned that incidence was rising in many parts of the world, but was particularly worrying in Eastern Europe. In Estonia, for example, the percentage of MDR-TB cases rose from 13.5 per cent in 1997 to 18.1 per cent a year later.

The strategy that holds out the most hope of success in reversing the TB epidemic in the twenty-first century is a worldwide programme known as **DOTS** or **Directly-Observed Treatment Short-course**. In DOTS programmes drug therapy is organised to maximise access for the patient, for example by arranging treatment in homes, rural or urban clinics and workplaces. Patients are directly observed taking their anti-TB medication in the correct combinations every day for at least the first two

[13] The evolution of antibiotic resistance in pathogenic bacteria is further discussed in *Human Biology and Health: An Evolutionary Approach* (Open University Press, 2nd edn 1994; 3rd edn 2001), Chapter 5.

months of their 6–8 month course of drug therapy, and preferably until the course is completed. Accurate records are kept and reported back to a national register. In some parts of the world, if a DOTS patient fails to attend for treatment regularly, a search is initiated and the patient may be held in custody and treated until declared free from TB.

This strategy raises difficult questions about denial of civil liberties for the individual who resists the imposition of such an onerous treatment regime, but in some parts of the world the decision has been taken that denying infected people the freedom to infect others is the lesser of two evils. For example, in 1991, an outbreak of MDR-TB in New York city claimed over 500 lives. Figure 4.8 illustrates why, at the start of the 1990s, newspaper headlines in New York warned of a public-health 'time bomb' and public opinion swung behind campaigns to target the city's homeless, drug addicts and slum-dwellers. Later the city invested in mass screening and enforced treatment in a disused prison of anyone found with infectious TB. Advocates of DOTS point out that 80–95 per cent of patients treated in DOTS programmes worldwide are cured of TB, and countries like China, Peru, Cuba and Nepal, which initiated vigorous DOTS programmes in the mid-1990s, are the only places in the world where MDR-TB is declining. The rapid globalisation of the DOTS strategy is seen by WHO as the best defence against the catastrophic potential of multi-drug resistant strains of TB. But the bacteria that cause TB are not alone in evolving resistance to common antibiotics; the lessons learned from the DOTS programme may have to be applied to the treatment of other infectious diseases.

**Figure 4.8** *TB cases for New York City, 1920–91. (Source: Brown, P., 1992, The return of the big killer, New Scientist, 10 October, p. 32)*

Although it is premature to predict the return of TB to the industrialised Western economies on the scale it achieved in previous centuries, the new alert draws attention to the failure in recent decades to devote adequate resources to comprehensive surveillance, routine collection and reporting of epidemiological data, effective public-health systems and continuing innovation in pharmaceutical research. The development of the first wave of effective drugs against TB quickly led to over-reliance on these 'magic bullets', but lax administration of drug therapy has contributed substantially to a global disease burden which is greater at the start of the new millennium than at any time in the history of TB. Consequently, the rhetoric about the 'conquest of TB' which was dominant since the time of Koch, has been replaced by a greater sense of realism concerning the capacities of modern medicine to vanquish this entrenched 'captain of communicable disease'. Medical certainty has given way to sobering doubts.

When you have studied this chapter, you should be able to:

**4.1** Define and use, or recognise definitions and applications of, each of the terms printed in **bold** in the text.

**4.2** Justify the claim that tuberculosis has a unique history as a disease of global importance.

**4.3** Describe the developments that led to tuberculosis being recognised as a unified and communicable disease caused by a single bacterial agent.

**4.4** Identify the factors that contributed to unsuccessful treatment strategies before new drugs became available in the 1950s, and explain why there was delay in exploitation of BCG vaccination.

**4.5** Discuss the reasons for the limited effectiveness of modern medical knowledge in the elimination of tuberculosis.

QUESTIONS FOR CHAPTER 4

**1**   (*Objective 4.2*)

Reporting on the lecture given by Robert Koch on 24 March 1882, John Tyndall noted:

> Koch's last inquiry deals with a disease which, in point of mortality, stands at the head of them all. If, he says, the seriousness of a malady be measured by the number of its victims, then the most dreaded pests which have hitherto ravaged the world — plague and cholera included — must stand far behind the one now under consideration. Koch makes the startling statement that one-seventh of the deaths of the human race are due to tubercular disease, while fully one-third of those who die in active middle age are carried off by the same cause. (*The Times*, 22 April, 1882)

To what extent do statistics about deaths up to the end of the nineteenth century from TB and other causes support this judgement of the seriousness of tuberculosis?

**2**   (*Objective 4.3*)

Summarising major developments in tuberculosis pathology up to the 1960s, Esmond Long concluded:

> …the varying manifestations of this disease had been a stumbling block to physicians since the earliest times. Laënnec had finally reduced consumption to the rank of a single disease, and had gone on record against the prevalent view that it might be the sequel of a variety of inflammations. Virchow, the commanding figure of a later day, reversed this view, distinguishing two broad types of tuberculosis and tracing one of them to previous inflammation.

Another Frenchman, Jean-Antoine Villermin, however, soon brought forth the startling proof that tuberculosis could be transmitted from man to animals, and from animal to animal indefinitely, by simply injecting some of the material from the lesions into the normal animal. Koch completed the story by discovering the inciting micro-organisms, which had escaped his predecessors in the field, through a combination of patience and ingenious technique. (Long, 1965, pp. 148–9)

Why were both experiment and microscopy essential for confirmation of Laënnec's suggestion that tuberculosis was a unified disease?

3   (*Objective 4.4*)

In 1944 the head of the Emergency Public Health Laboratory Service maintained that

I should doubt whether BCG vaccination is likely to form a serious contribution to the control of human tuberculosis in this country. (Quoted in Bryder, 1988, p. 243)

Explain why British scientists were more reticent than their colleagues elsewhere to accept the importance of BCG vaccination.

4   (*Objective 4.5*)

Never in the long history of tuberculosis had there been any period to bear comparison with the [past]…30 years of high drama and revolutionary change that had seen the wonders of the past, artificial pneumothorax and [other techniques of gas injection] swept into oblivion together with the mutilating crudities of the surgery of pulmonary tuberculosis, so recently hailed as the ultimate in therapeutic endeavour. By the early 1970s intensive research work, backed in many instances by the financial resources of the major pharmaceutical firms, had produced such a sufficiency and variety of antibacterial agents that it had become possible to offer a guarantee of cure to any patient with tuberculosis — provided that the agents were correctly employed. (Keers, 1978, p. 243)

What has happened since 1978 to lead us to conclude that the author was heralding another false dawn?

# C H A P T E R 5

## Blood

### Study notes for OU students

This chapter builds on the discussion in Chapter 2 of holistic and reductionist approaches to understanding the structure and functioning of the human body. We do not assume any prior biological knowledge about blood, or about medical interventions involving blood (as in the case of transfusions and vaccination, which are mentioned in this chapter); a more detailed biological discussion can be found in *Human Biology and Health: an Evolutionary Approach* (Open University Press, second edition 1994; third edition 2001).

The historical development of views about blood — what it is, what powers and potentials it has, what it is made of, and how it functions in the life of animals and humans — will in this chapter be taken as an example of doubt and certainty in the context of changes over time in human thinking about nature. Blood is a particularly suitable instance to take, since while it has always been central to the Western medical tradition, it has also always been seen as a natural material full of special powers for affecting the world beyond the body itself. In this chapter certain critical moments have been selected in the transformation of blood from a 'spiritual' to a 'scientific' object, to indicate how successive new attitudes to blood have been the product of wider changes in attitude within society at certain times.

In particular, the case of blood will illustrate the change over time from a *holistic* to a *reductionist* attitude to understanding nature in general and the functioning of the human body in particular. In these respects, the story of blood illustrates the developments that permeated thinking about other medical matters.

## 5.1  The power of blood

'Blood is an entirely special juice' (*Blut ist ein ganz besonderer Saft*), as Mephistopheles says to Faust, insisting that they use blood to sign the contract over Faust's soul. Blood-contracts have greater force than any other kind, and the same extra force seems to be present across cultures wherever blood is invoked or ritually shed or used. For blood is widely, perhaps universally, thought to have special powers, both for good and evil, and these powers derive from the equation made between blood and life, between blood and the individual's being and identity, between blood and soul. The identity of a person and of a family is universally supposed to be passed on 'in the blood'. Blood has power because it is, or stands for, or embodies, the person and that person's powers. Loss of blood means loss of life, the life flows away as the blood flows away.

But, equally, shed blood still retains some of its powers, it is full of latent life and can influence persons or things in contact with it, and can be manipulated by others to enhance their own power. Thus the blood of a slain enemy, or of strong animals, can offer its strength to the fighter when smeared on his own body or drunk. 'Shed blood means mysterious soul-power let loose, for good or ill' (Wheeler Robinson, 1909, p. 715). Dangerous blood, or blood whose power one wishes to avoid, can have its power removed by shedding it in a sacred place, on some kind of altar. Sacrifice by shedding blood is the most powerful form of sacrifice to deities or spirits, and drinking the blood of the sacrifice can lead to possession and religious frenzy.

Women's blood is often regarded as most potent in defiling, and in many cultures there are taboos around women while menstruating and around menstrual blood itself.[1] Defilement supposedly also

*'Blood is an entirely special juice'. Here, in an engraving by Franz Stassen, Faust and Mephistopheles seal their contract in blood, giving it greater binding force. (Source: Mansell/Katz Pictures Ltd.)*

---

[1] There is a fuller discussion of menstrual taboos in Chapter 7 of this book.

*The shedding of blood in sacrifice has enormous power. In this twelfth-century picture, the sacrificial nature of Christ's death above is made explicit by the blood sacrifice of an animal below. (Source: The British Library)*

occurs to a woman from the blood shed in childbirth, such that she has to be ritually cleansed: a Christian ceremony of 'churching' women a month after childbirth in order to cleanse them so that they can re-enter society, was only transformed into a ceremony of thanksgiving in relatively recent times.

● Can you suggest any other examples of blood being used symbolically?

■ Blood is important in initiating and in bonding: in 'blooding' a child to initiate them into blood-sports; in bonds of 'blood brothership' where the self, in the blood, is mingled with the self of others in their blood in order to join them together in the strongest bond of loyalty and commitment, that of blood relationship.

As it is central to sacrifice to deities in many religions, so it is no surprise that blood played such a large role in the religious practices of the ancient Hebrews, as witnessed by the Old Testament, especially in the ritual sacrifice of animals. Many of these attitudes and practices were continued into Christianity, in which the concept of atonement through the shedding of blood is central. Christ, God-made-man, shed His blood in atonement for the sins of the world: He was a sacrificial lamb. Moreover the memory of Christ is invoked in the celebration of the most central Christian ritual, mass or communion, in which the blood of Christ is literally or symbolically drunk.

Thus blood not only has good and bad powers, but it can be used both to pollute and to purify, to sanctify and to desecrate. Such attitudes toward blood can be seen as a typical part of the world-view of traditional societies who believe the universe to be imbued with powers, both evident and hidden, which it is their role to co-opt for their own use and for the improved power of themselves as individuals. The aim is to get nature and the forces of nature onto one's own side, by making oneself go in nature's way. Somewhat different views of the nature and significance of blood are held by societies such as our own modern Western scientific society, where people see it as their role to turn nature to *their own* purposes, which are not necessarily those of nature. Yet modern scientific views of blood have much in common with these non-scientific views, though they are not directly derived from them. Some of the old views persist, not only in metaphor, beyond the advance of modern science.

● From your reading so far of this book, give some examples of the persistence of old views in present-day thinking about illness.

■ Humoral theory persists in lay explanations and remedies for colds and fevers; the Afro-Caribbean washout similarly reflects the persistence of old ideas, and the moral connotations of certain illnesses continue to be felt.

## 5.2   Blood and Western medicine, AD 200 to 1750

### 5.2.1  Galenic medicine

As you have seen in Chapters 2 and 4, in the early centuries of the Western tradition of 'bedside' medicine, blood was one of the four *humours*, together with black bile, yellow bile and phlegm. The balance of these humours supposedly produces health; their imbalance, where one or other is in excess or dominance, produces illness. Unlike modern medicine, this classical medical approach was a holistic one, taking into account the whole individual and the state of his or her whole body. Disease or illness was thought of as a particular imbalance in a particular person, and their personal state of health had to be understood in order to care for them medically. This model of health and disease derived from the Hippocratic writings, which date from the fifth century BC, and was developed in particular ways in a very large number of surviving books written by Galen of Pergamon, a prominent Greek physician active in Rome in the second century AD. As mentioned earlier, Galen's influence in medicine was to last into the eighteenth century, and certain features of his system of healing persisted in use even into the nineteenth century.

### 5.2.2  Pulse interpretation

In Galen's medical system blood plays a most important role. In the first place it was used as an indicator for the state of the whole body and of health. For, as you saw earlier, the blood was popularly thought to be or to contain the soul or vitality of the body. Galenic medicine[2] was adopted in the Christian society of Europe. It was certainly the case that, as the Bible taught, the soul was considered to be 'in the blood', following Deuteronomy 12.23, 'the blood is the life', and other Old Testament texts, though it was ambiguous whether the Christian immortal soul was localised in the body.

Working with the belief that there are two *independent* systems of blood vessels, the arteries and the veins, Galen thought that some almost immaterial vivifying substance (that is, a substance endowing life), *pneuma*, was brought in from the air when we breathe, taken to the lung and from there to the left chamber (ventricle) of the heart, where it was mixed with ordinary blood and was then drawn into the arteries. Its life-possessing and life-giving properties were evident to the senses when it was compared with the blood in the veins: arterial blood was bright, frothy, it spurted when the artery was cut, it needed the strong walls of the arteries to contain its natural tendency to expansion, and it had the pulse of life. Venous blood, by contrast, was dark and slow-moving, and the thinner walls of its vessels showed no pulse.

According to Galen, both kinds of blood were consumed in keeping the body alive: the venous blood was used up in keeping the body nourished, the arterial blood was used up in keeping it vivified. He believed that fresh supplies of nutritive blood were produced in the liver where the food was turned into venous blood. And in order to supply blood to the arterial system and keep it topped-up for its role of distributing vitality-giving *pneuma* to the body, there were, Galen believed, minute channels for small quantities of venous blood to pass through the central wall of the heart, from the right-hand chamber to the left.

[2] The terms 'Galenic medicine' and 'Galenists' were explained in Chapter 4 of this book.

In the Galenic practice of medicine the pulse of the blood in the arteries was regularly felt and assessed by the physician, since it was a reliable detector of the state of vitality of the patient. The state of the pulse, its relative hardness, rapidity, rhythm and motion revealed to the physician the current state of the patient and the direction in which his or her health was tending. The skilled Galenic physician learnt to distinguish dozens of different pulses, which indicated different states of health and illness and different trajectories of illness or recovery. He could recognise the pulse that leaps like a goat (*pulsus caprisans*), the pulse that moves slowly like a worm (*pulsus vermiculosus*) and the unequal pulse that crawls like an ant (*pulsus formicans*) and know what they meant about the state of the body and the course of the illness. The pulse indicated the state of the arterial blood, which was itself the indicator for the state of the body as a whole; thus the pulse indicated to the physician the state of vital strength. The pulse did not tell the Galenic physician anything in particular about the state of the heart.

Pulse interpretation became from Galen's time a whole area of practical medicine, and a skill proper to the physician, for feeling the pulse was one of the few ways in which the physician would touch the body of his patient, delicately holding the wrist with his fingers and thumb. For the reputation of the physician was built on the high-status *mental* skills of theoretical knowledge and not on the lower-status *manual* skills of practical knowledge.

**Figure 5.1**   *Diagram showing points for bleeding on the arm, from Berengario da Carpi's* Isagogae Breves, *published in Bologna in 1523. (Source: The British Library)*

### 5.2.3   Blood-letting

In the second place, blood was important for the Galenic physician because it was the humour most easy to regulate. From Galen's time, therefore, blood-letting (*phlebotomy*) was used as one of the main therapeutic procedures, and also in order to take precautions against the onset of disease (**prophylaxis**). A quantity of blood could be removed at certain stages of a disease in order to assist the course of nature in healing the patient.

In medieval and pre-industrial Europe (c. 1250–1750) the person on whose recommendation this would be done would usually be a physician, the person with access to theoretical knowledge; but as blood-letting was a manual procedure the person who usually performed it was a surgeon or surgeon-apothecary,[3] the person with the lower-status manual skills. Bleeding was usually performed from the forearm, from the basilic, cephalic or the communis vein (see Figure 5.1); the cephalic was thought to have particular sympathy with the head (*kephale*, in Greek); but at times it was performed from the legs or even from the head.

The first stage was to put a ligature on the limb, tying a bandage tightly around the arm or leg in order to make the veins near the surface of the skin swell up, and the selected vein was then incised with a lancet.

---

[3] Surgeon-apothecaries and other medical practitioners of this period are discussed in *Caring for Health: History and Diversity* (Open University Press, 2nd edn 1993; 3rd edn 2001), Chapter 2.

A predetermined quantity of blood (usually measured in ounces) was let into a bowl, and then the ligature was removed and the wound was bound up to staunch the flow. As the blood cooled in the bowl, the skilled physician could see it settle into layers with a skin or crust, the clotting blood separating from the clear liquid serum: he could often make inferences about the state of the blood in the body — and hence about the course of the disease — from inspection of the blood in the bowl.

An alternative procedure, to promote localised bleeding, was to apply a heated cupping-glass to the skin, thus raising an artificial blister as it cooled, which could be incised either with a lancet or, in later centuries, with the several little knives of a spring-loaded scarificator. Where only a small quantity of blood needed to be taken from a precise location, as when the physician wished to reduce certain kinds of swelling, leeches would sometimes be used.

In taking blood from the veins the physician was sometimes trying to reduce a perceived excess of venous blood itself, as in some fevers. More usually, however, he was removing blood in order to bring about some other change within the body or in a particular organ, such as the removal of some supposed obstruction, or compensating for suppressed menstrual periods in women in order to avoid dangerous complications that he believed would ensue.

Bleeding was performed prophylactically in the healthy patient (Figure 5.2) because in classical Galenic medical theory it was believed that the change from one season to another led to changes in the quantity and expansiveness of the humours of the body, especially the blood. Hence it was thought an especially wise precaution to have a certain amount of blood let from the arm at the arrival of spring in order to ward off the diseases, especially fevers, which were typical of spring and summer.

**Figure 5.2** *A woman is bled prophylactically c. 1635. Underneath the original etching is a poem: 'Courage, Sir, you have begun, and I'll be brave; tighten the bandage, puncture with confidence, make a good opening. Ah, the gush of blood surprises you! How phlebotomy purifes the spirits and cleanses the blood of great putrefaction!' (Source: Detail of picture of Bosse, Phlebotomy, from Ars Medica:* A Collection of Medical Prints Presented to the Philadelphia Museum of Art by the SmithKline Corporation; *reproduced by permission of the Philadelphia Museum of Art)*

As late as the 1760s the celebrated Italian pathologist Giovanni Battista Morgagni could give his considered opinion that an epidemic of apoplexy (what we would now call 'stroke') at Padua had been due to the fact that an unusually cold autumn, winter and spring were followed by sudden very hot weather, and hence the blood expanded more quickly than the blood vessels could: 'so that the blood, for this reason, expanding itself suddenly, the same thing happened as if the vessels were suddenly distended with a double quantity thereof' (Morgagni, 1761), and thus blood vessels in the brain burst and flooded the chambers (ventricles) there, producing an attack of apoplexy.

● How do the ideas of Galenic medicine, and the practice of bleeding, illustrate the features of the paradigm we have called *bedside* medicine, outlined in Chapter 3?

■ The use of Galen as a source illustrates the reliance on classical texts. The practice of prophylactic bleeding at certain seasons illustrates the idea that bodily states were intimately connected with the surrounding environment.

Bleeding, especially therapeutic bleeding, was central to the medical techniques that the ancient, medieval and pre-industrial physician had available, and it was very effective. For instance, a patient bled to *syncope* (fainting) on doctor's orders, in order to bring about some further change in the body, would not only faint but also feel much better afterwards, just as the doctor had foretold. Similarly in lesser bleedings, the patient would usually experience the relief that the doctor had anticipated. In such ways bleeding brought both immediate and indirect relief to symptoms, and also helped to cure diseases, both immediately and indirectly.

In other words, bleeding worked, according to all the important tests: patient and physician satisfaction, the removal or reduction of certain symptoms, and as a stage in the cure of diseases. It was not just a 'placebo', since its use really affected the state of the body and elicited important bodily responses, often of a dramatic kind. It was something that patients both expected and wanted to be performed on them, on the doctor's advice, when they were ill. Indeed, so important was bleeding in cure, and so sophisticated was the theory of blood-letting, that controversies over it often arose among medical men: controversies over whether or not blood should be let in a particular condition, over precisely how much blood should be let, from which particular vein, at which particular moments in the course of a particular disease in order to save a patient. Everyone recognised that a patient wrongly bled could die from the treatment, but they also all recognised that a patient could often only be saved or cured by being correctly bled. Pulse-feeling and blood-letting were integral parts of the coherent and rational Galenic approach to medicine.

Pulse-feeling gave the physician much important information, bleeding worked to the satisfaction of all concerned, and the role of all the blood and all the vessels was accounted for in the physiological and therapeutic theories of the Galenic physicians. No one therefore felt uneasy with this view of the flow, nature and function of blood, nor with the use of these diagnostic and therapeutic techniques. Although they argued about particular cases and points within this approach, there is no evidence of anyone within the Galenic tradition, over many centuries, questioning the importance and value of bleeding in general, or questioning the accounts of the motion and use of blood on which bleeding was built.

## 5.3  Blood in the seventeenth and eighteenth centuries

The discovery of the circulation of the blood was possibly the most important of all events in changing Western attitudes to the nature and functions of blood, and indeed to the understanding of the functioning of the human body. It was the English physician William Harvey (1578–1657) who discovered the circulation of the blood, publishing on it in Latin in 1628.

Harvey's work in this respect has been seen by historians as part of the **Scientific Revolution** of the seventeenth century, for historians have found in seventeenth-century Europe, especially in the north, a striking new enthusiasm and energy in investigating nature.

Although historians still argue about the precise origin and nature of this new intellectual movement, they are generally agreed that it was related to the great increase in the wealth of Europe at the time, and the expansion of trade. The intellectual innovations were first to be found in Italy, but in the course of the sixteenth and seventeenth centuries the focus of economic life moved to the north of Europe, and the focus of intellectual life, as one might expect, moved there also. Box 5.1 summarises its three interrelated characteristics.

> **Box 5.1   The nature of the 'Scientific Revolution' in Europe in the seventeenth century**
>
> 1   It involved a rejection of much of the book-learning of the previous few centuries, and a distinct preference for building one's opinions about nature on personal *experience* and on *experimentation*.
>
> 2   New kinds of *analysis* of nature, both practical and theoretical, were pursued, in which people sought to understand the behaviour and properties of natural objects through understanding the actions and characteristics of their component parts. For instance, at the practical level, *chemical* analysis was widely employed for the resolution of natural substances into their constituent parts. And, at the theoretical level, a great deal of energy was put into the mental analysis of nature into its supposed ultimate *physical* constituents, trying to work out the necessary nature and behaviour of the smallest particles of matter.
>
> 3   Underlying both the first two themes, there was a return to looking at the writings of ancient Greek philosophers who had investigated nature, in order to find *ancient models of research and explanation* which could be brought back into modern practice. The Greeks were thought to have developed their own views of nature on the basis of experience and experiment, rather than book-learning, and they had been the earliest to discuss the composition of natural objects in terms of their ultimate components.

As each ancient Greek philosopher of nature had often developed his own views in opposition to the views of some other Greek philosopher, it will be no surprise to find that some of the ancient research traditions revived in the seventeenth century were in crucial ways opposed to each other. You will find this to be the case with respect to blood. On the one hand, there was the revival of the research programme of Aristotle, one of the most important Greek philosophers, who was active in the fourth century BC. On the other hand, there was the revival of the explanatory model of the Greek *atomists*, who had tried to explain everything about the properties and behaviour of matter in terms of the properties of its supposed ultimate particles (atoms); it was partly in opposition to the atomists that Aristotle himself had developed his own views of nature.

But there was no contradiction in (a) rejecting 'Aristotelian*ism*', that is, the tradition amongst philosophers of the sixteenth and early seventeenth centuries of clinging to the truth of every *word* of the texts of Aristotle, while (b) at the same time modelling one's own new experimental research programme on the *research programme* of Aristotle himself, newly revived from antiquity. This in fact is precisely what William Harvey did with respect to the Aristotelian research programme into animals, and it is the primary reason why he discovered the circulation of the blood in living animals.

Thus the impetus to explore in a new way the motion of the heart and blood did not come from any desire on anyone's part to improve or replace the Galenic theory as such. For, although the Galenic medical system may appear erroneous to us now, it is important to remember that for its practitioners and the patients treated under it, this system was coherent and convincing and had no particular defects. Nor did it have any evident inconsistencies in it, nor was there a general sense that treatments (such as bleeding) based on Galenic understanding of the behaviour of blood in the body led to medical failure.

### 5.3.1 William Harvey and the circulation of the blood

The most important and radical elements of Harvey's discovery of the **circulation of the blood** in animals were the recognition of the following:

1   The blood vessels (the arteries and the veins) and the blood itself constitute a single system.

2   The blood circulates continuously (and rapidly) round the body, pushed out by the pumping action of the left chamber (ventricle) of the heart into the arteries, and returning to the right chamber of the heart via the veins, having been passed from the smallest arteries to the smallest veins through the tiny capillary veins which, Harvey reasoned, must exist throughout the flesh of the body (their existence was later confirmed by microscope study).

3   Part of the circuit in animals that possess lungs involves the passing of the blood through the lungs as well as through the heart; in the course of this passage the visible differences between arterial and venous blood are brought about — the slow dark red blood of the veins is turned into the lively bright red blood of the arteries.

●   In what important way does this description differ from Galen's?

■   Unlike Harvey, Galenists believed that the venous and arterial systems were separate.

*Harvey's work on the circulation of the blood was part of the wider intellectual 'Scientific Revolution' of the seventeenth century. In this artist's impression, Harvey demonstrates, on a dog, his discoveries on the circulation of the blood to his colleagues at the London College of Physicians. (Source: Mary Evans Picture Library)*

Harvey's own research projects on animals exactly followed those of Aristotle, both in topic and approach, with investigations of the generation of animals (the reproduction of their kind), the *respiration* (breathing) of animals, and the movement of the heart and blood vessels of animals among his main research fields, all of which had been areas of anatomical research conducted in antiquity by Aristotle himself. Harvey had learnt his approach in Italy (at the University of Padua) but practised it at his home in London, where he conducted private research in anatomy throughout his adult life.

In performing experimental research on the movement of the heart and blood vessels in animals, Harvey was undertaking a project which had not been pursued in precisely this way since Aristotle himself. The novelty of the project was that Harvey investigated the movement of the heart and blood vessels in *animals* — and that meant in *all* animals, not just in humans as the Galenist physicians and anatomists were accustomed to do. What, Harvey asked, were the roles and functions of the parts and movements of the heart and the blood vessels in all animals? What were they in those animals which (unlike humans) do not have a lung? What were they in animals that have a heart with only a single chamber, and what were they in animals that (like humans) have hearts with more than one chamber? (The human heart has two main chambers, or **ventricles**, and two lesser chambers, or **auricles**.) Were they the same in animals that are cold-blooded as in warm-blooded animals (like humans)?

As a consequence of such lines of investigation Harvey came to be especially concerned with two things: the sheer quantity of blood which must pass through the heart; and the presence in the veins, but not in the arteries, of small flaps. Eventually, and against his expectations, Harvey in 1628 came to ask himself whether the blood 'had a sort of motion as if in a circle, which afterwards I found to be true'. As a consequence of adopting this new view of the blood's motion, Harvey was able to see the 'flaps' in the veins as *valves* which stop the blood slipping backwards in the veins as it returns to the heart (Figure 5.3). Similarly he came to see the heart itself as acting like a *pump*.

**Figure 5.3** *Harvey's demonstration of the circulation of the blood, using the swollen blood vessels below a ligature tied round the arm. When blood is 'smoothed out' from a vein, the blood flow is revealed to be one-way, as valves stop blood slipping back towards the hand. From Harvey's* Exercitatio Anatomica de Motu Cordis et Sanguinis, *1628. (Source: The British Library)*

But Harvey's use of such mechanical metaphors as that of the heart as a pump and of the valves in the veins did not mean that he thought the whole system acted merely like a machine. Like a good follower of Aristotle, he still saw the blood as alive, and also as the *first principle* of life in the animal — the first material of the body to come into existence (he believed that the blood itself *constructs* the heart, and then the rest of the body). For Harvey the *soul was in the blood*. And one can almost feel his disappointment that he could not satisfactorily uncover the reason (the 'final cause' in Aristotelian terms) *why* the blood flowed in a *circle* — what was the *purpose* of the blood circulating? — having to settle for 'speculating' and 'likely reasons'.

## 5.3.2  Descartes' mechanistic account of blood

Harvey's view of the role and nature of blood was significantly different from that of Galen and seventeenth-century Galenists. For Harvey there was one blood system, not two; the blood was circulated constantly, rather than being consumed in nourishing and vivifying the body; and the blood could not be made from all the ingested food through some transformation in the liver. Given such novelties, it is therefore no surprise that the doctrine of the circulation of the blood received stiff opposition for a number of years, though by the time of Harvey's death in 1657 it had been accepted widely throughout society.

- What examples of opposition to new ideas did you read about in the chapter on TB, and what were the reasons for this?

- The BCG vaccine was subject to numerous obstacles in Britain, due to the existence of vested interests in other methods, and concerns about safety.

Some philosophers took up Harvey's scheme enthusiastically, since it could be used to extend their own novel programmes of investigation into nature. Chief amongst these was the French philosopher René Descartes (1596–1650), who rapidly adopted the theory but gave it a quite new reading, one with which Harvey could not agree at all.

Descartes' own preferred view of nature was, like that of Harvey, built on the resuscitation of an ancient Greek model. But in Descartes' case the ancient model was *atomism*, and the explanatory approach he created on this basis was a **mechanistic** one, known as the *mechanical philosophy*. Descartes' approach led him to seek to explain all physical events and change in the whole of nature in terms solely of *matter and motion*: limiting his explanatory terms to these two made Descartes' explanations both mechanistic and reductionist. It was to this theory that Descartes bent Harvey's discovery, and he made it the centre-piece of his account of the workings of the human body in his famous and very influential book, the *Discourse on Method* of 1637, and again in his *Treatise on Man* of 1651.

This way of explaining natural phenomena was taken up by many other researchers in later years. It is to Descartes (but not to Harvey) that the modern-day mechanistic understanding of the functioning of the body can be traced back, although Harvey had indeed used mechanical analogies.

- Which mechanical analogies did Harvey use?

- He saw the heart as a *pump* and the appearance of flaps in the veins as *valves.*

So Harvey's Aristotelian account of the motion of the blood was turned into a strictly mechanistic (and indeed atomistic) account by Descartes. Under Descartes' hand, the heart was turned into something like a heat engine and the blood was regarded as constituted by a host of tiny particles of different shapes, derived from the food eaten. The purpose of the circulation of the blood, for Descartes, was to distribute these tiny particles around the body, where they encountered different minute 'sieves' which passively strained off those particles that matched the shape of the holes in that particular sieve. In this way, Descartes thought, one could account for the way in which all the different fluids of the body were derived from the blood: they were strained off according to the shape of their constituent particles. Consequently, the perceptible qualities of the bodily fluids, such as the sharpness of tears, the yellowness of bile, and so on, were mere secondary characteristics, 'second qualities', incidental consequences resulting from their being composed of those particular minute particles in motion with respect to each other.

Descartes' aim in all this was to account for the characteristics of different matter, and the functioning of natural objects (including the human body) simply in terms of matter and motion, without having to use concepts such as 'faculties' (such as the blood-making faculty of the liver) or resort to talk of special active powers in each natural substance.

Over the next hundred years these two approaches, the *Harveian* and the *Cartesian* (named after Harvey and Descartes respectively), were further developed, sometimes in opposition to each other, sometimes as if they were complementary. Thus some people continued to see the body in **vitalist** terms, as Harvey did: as something whose essential vitality was beyond ultimate explanation, but where one could nevertheless study experimentally the way the vitality operated; for such people the blood was not only 'alive' but still the place where the soul was most active. Others went for an explanation that was both *mechanistic* and *reductionist*, following Descartes and others, using the assumption that all the operations of the live body can be reduced to (or be understood as simply being) the operations of lifeless matter in motion. The circulation of the blood was used by both camps for their physiological and medical explanations.

### 5.3.3  The first blood transfusion experiments

The discovery of Harvey and the theorising of Descartes and certain chemists on the constitution of the blood both played a role in a spectacular series of experiments conducted in the 1660s when the new Royal Society of London and that of France both attempted to transfuse the blood of one animal into another. Though when Harvey himself heard of the first plans to perform transfusions he thought the idea frivolous and the technique impossible.

It will be evident that what the experimenters hoped to achieve was the transmission of some *virtue* of one animal or person into another, so they were not seeing blood as some neutral substance, but one which still carried the characteristics of the person. The idea of attempting transfusion of blood between two animals arose from work by people in the circle of the physicist and chemist, the Honourable Robert Boyle, (1627–1691) on how poisons and medicines are absorbed into the blood and how they are spread by the circulation. Following Boyle himself, they were primarily concerned with applying the 'experimental philosophy' to the improvement of medicine, by exploring the causation of disease (especially poisons) and new means of cure (injected medicines and even foodstuffs). The architect, Christopher Wren (1632–1723) in his youth, injected a dog with 'wine and ale into the mass of blood by a vein, in good quantities, till I have made him extremely drunk, but soon after he pisseth it out' (Wren, 1750, p. 228).

*An idealised illustration of a transfusion from a lamb to a man from a German textbook published in 1705. (Source: The Wellcome Library, London)*

Richard Lower, an Oxford physician, wanted 'trials to be prosecuted to the utmost variety the subject will bear: as by exchanging the blood of old and young, sick and healthy, hot and cold, fierce and fearful, tame and wild animals' (Lower, 1666, p. 357). He hoped that medicine would profit from the experiments, since 'perhaps as much benefit is to be expected from the infusion of fresh blood as from the withdrawal of the old' in the traditional practice of prophylactic bleeding (Lower, 1669, p. 357). The two Royal Societies took this up and attempted experiments on humans, with the London Society in 1667 bleeding the blood of a docile animal, a sheep, into a 'cracked' Cambridge Bachelor of Divinity for two minutes; the man found he felt better (and presumably calmer) for the experiment. Such experiments were however soon discontinued because of a fatality and experimental difficulties.

### 5.3.4   Blood as a hydraulic fluid

In Descartes' scheme the blood, like all other fluids in the body, had been seen as a mass of small particles or corpuscles of different shapes, all in motion with respect to each other, and which together constituted a fluid. The analysis was 'mechanistic' but the blood was not considered in any significant way as acting *as a fluid* and having the characteristics of a fluid in motion, nor being under pressure, suffering resistance, and so on. But the blood did come to be considered in this way in the eighteenth century, particularly through the investigations of Stephen Hales (1677–1761), an English vicar and follower of Isaac Newton.

Hales investigated fluid pressure in dogs and horses, and extended his experiments to vegetables. These experiments were begun while Hales was a student at Cambridge, and then continued at his vicarage in Teddington, West of London. As a follower of Newton, the man who first recognised gravity to be a universally-acting force both on Earth and between the stars and planets, Hales was concerned with investigating the operation of *forces* in nature. Hales was building on some of the *hydrostatical* work of Newton and his immediate disciples. Hydrostatics studies the conditions under which fluids come to a state of *equilibrium*, that is, the conditions under which fluids which are moving as a result of some force come to a standstill because they are balanced against some other force, usually that of gravity.

Hales realised that one could assess the pressure of blood in the live animal by measuring the (average) height to which it rises against the force of gravity. His basic experiment was to tie down a dog or horse, and attach vertically to the crural artery (the large artery in the leg) a long, narrow, open glass tube. Blood rushed up the tube, and then came to an equilibrium at a certain height: this height was the point at which the force pushing the blood upwards was matched or balanced by the force of gravity pulling the blood downwards in the tube. This height could be used, Hales calculated, to give a reading of the force of the blood in the arteries, in other words, the contractive force of the heart. With a horse the blood rises to over eight feet in a narrow tube, so the size and scope of the experimental conditions can be imagined.

Hales also found ways of measuring the velocity of the blood leaving the heart, and the force within the heart itself. This new discipline of measuring the force of the blood Hales called 'Haemastaticks', and published a book under this title in 1733. While he drew from such experiments many deductions about the best procedure in bleeding humans therapeutically, this particular technique could not be applied to humans as the experimental animal always died in the course of the experiment. These experiments provided the first reliable quantitative information about the heart and blood pressure in the living animal.

Although as a result of the work and opinions of Harvey, Descartes, Lower, Hales and others, accepted medical knowledge of blood by about 1730 was considerably different from what it had been in 1600, there was no simple revolution in views about it.

●   What differences and similarities are there between the views of blood at these two dates?

■   By 1730, blood had come to be seen as something experimentally manipulable, it was under pressure, and made up of tiny particles together acting as a fluid. But it was also still believed by many to be alive in itself, and to have vital characteristics which, by their very nature, were not amenable to experimental enquiry, just as it had in 1600.

In eighteenth-century medicine, bleeding was still continued as a therapeutic practice: the fact that the blood was known to circulate, and that drawing off blood at one point was simply abstracting from a circulating mass of blood, seems to have had little if any effect on attitudes toward the importance of bleeding. For bleeding was known to work in practice. New, and usually mechanistic, theories were devised therefore to show, at the level of physiological theory, how and why bleeding led to the cure of the patient. This is a good example of how, at any given time, peoples' understanding of how the body works, and their views of good techniques of medical intervention vary. If people believe something works therapeutically, they will create a theory to match it; equally they will not easily abandon an established practice simply because it has no theoretical explanation or because its theoretical explanation is challenged or logically undermined.

## 5.4   Blood and clinical medicine

The next significant transformation in the way in which blood was considered, was part of the creation of *clinical medicine*, sometimes known as French *hospital medicine*. This kind of medicine was brought into existence in the throes of the French Revolution, which broke out in 1789. Indeed this new clinical medicine, as well as most other areas of intellectual enquiry, and the French Revolution itself, all had one of their origins in common in the speculations of the *philosophes*, French philosophers of the mid-eighteenth century, led in particular by the Abbé Condillac.

●   What were the main features of the paradigm we called *clinical medicine* in Chapter 3?

■   Clinical medicine was the culmination of a way of thinking that had been developing for some time, but important features included the relating of symptoms experienced while alive to pathological lesions identified at post-mortem, and the subsequent descriptions and classifications of diseases that developed from this technique.

### 5.4.1  Sensationalist thinking

Newton had stressed the need to build one's theories of the universe on observation of phenomena, and his friend the Oxford philosopher John Locke had argued at length in his *Essay Concerning Human Understanding* (1690) that we are not born with any knowledge, but all our knowledge is built up from sense-perception. The *philosophes* used these arguments from England, and claimed that the only trustworthy and reliable information accessible to humans had to be built on sense-perception: causes cannot be known, only phenomena. This **sensationalist** philosophy, as it was known, could be used politically to argue for the Rights of Man against monarchical government, or against the claims of the Catholic church. For, following sensationalist philosophy, one could say that such claims to authority were not built on any principles which had been or could be derived from sense-experience, but were mere claims and thus had no privileged status. But, as it was a general philosophical approach, sensationalism could equally be applied to medicine and other areas of human knowledge, especially as so many of Condillac's followers were medical men.

### 5.4.2  Clinical thinking

Its origin in sensationalist thinking accounts for the great stress on observation and the senses which was the leading characteristic of clinical medicine. Indeed, clinical medicine was 'sensationalist' philosophy applied to medicine. The development of a number of new techniques to *extend the senses* into the inside of the living body took place at the Paris hospitals under the leadership of *philosophe* physicians and surgeons, who had large numbers of poor patients in the hospitals on whom they could make their observations and, after the patients were dead, their dissections. For in this new approach medicine had to be learnt both in the clinic and in the post-mortem room (Box 5.2).

> **Box 5.2   Basic approaches of clinical medicine in the eighteenth century**
>
> 1   Systematic observation of the course of the disease in its 'natural' state (that is, without the doctor's intervention), with special emphasis on symptoms perceivable by the senses.
>
> 2   Dissection of the corpse after death (post-mortem) in order to correlate the symptoms that had been observed in life with the changes from the normal that were now visible in the organs inside the body. With sufficient correlations the physician could in time be in a position where, by simply inspecting the symptoms accessible to his senses, he could know what pathological lesions in the organs were occurring *inside* the body of the patient during life — for this constituted what was 'really' going on, in the view of the clinical physician.
>
> 3   And, in order to get sufficient correlations, another thing was desirable: the making of statistical assessments (*analyse numérique*).

By applying the three approaches of clinical medicine, one could discover the 'hidden causes' of disease, and of what pathological changes in the internal organs the disease symptoms were the visible effect.

●   Think back to Chapter 4. In what respect do later descriptions of TB reflect this way of seeing disease?

■ Observation of symptoms helped to distinguish different forms of TB (for example *scrofula* from *consumption*); descriptions of the development of tubercles in the lungs were based on post-mortem examination; Bayle in 1810 based his description of TB on 900 post-mortems.

Three kinds of physical examination were introduced that particularly helped the physician 'see' what was happening to the organs hidden inside his patient: **percussion** (tapping, especially the chest), **palpation** (feeling with the hands), and **auscultation** (listening, especially to the chest).

In all this radically new work, blood itself was not particularly an object of study: like anything else, only those of its properties which were directly accessible to the senses were of interest to good clinicians, and theorising about things beyond the evidence of the senses (such as the ultimate make-up of the blood) was anathema to them. But there were some significant developments in the concept of the blood — that is as a clinical entity — which were of great importance. Let us look briefly at three such developments, one in which it became possible to inspect the heart and respiratory organs during life, one in which the validity of blood-letting as a therapy came to be reassessed, and one in which the heat of the blood was turned into a fundamental clinical measurement.

### 5.4.3  Assessing the heart

Two leading French clinical physicians, Jean-Nicolas Corvisart in 1806 and then his pupil René-Théophile-Hyacinthe Laënnec in 1812, wrote books to expound the whole range of diseases of the chest, of the heart and of the great blood vessels, which they were able to distinguish or redefine using the new clinical methods. Laënnec was the inventor of the **stethoscope** or 'chest examiner', still today the emblem of the clinically-trained physician, which functioned to extend the senses in the clinical manner. Laënnec found that auscultation, placing his ear on the patient's chest, was not always convenient or polite. He rolled up some paper into a cylinder and thus invented the stethoscope, which made it possible to listen from a distance and, incidentally, amplified the sound. One effect of this clinical approach was that the pulse — long used to detect the relative vitality of a patient — now meant something different to the physician. From this time on the physician felt the pulse in order to learn something about the condition of the *heart*, not the state of the blood or the general vitality of the patient. One and the same act — feeling the pulse — had been transformed in its meaning.

### 5.4.4  Statistics and blood-letting

One use of statistical assessments by the Paris clinical physicians was concerned with trying to build disease **syndromes** — finding those constant and characteristic sets of symptoms, signs, and post-mortem findings that constitute particular diseases. Notable amongst such workers was Pierre-Charles-Alexandre Louis (1787–1872). But the statistical approach could also be applied to test the efficacy of customary treatments. And here Louis was also active, gathering and tabulating statistical evidence from the Paris hospitals to explore the efficacy of blood-letting in inflammations. The evidence led him to the unexpected conclusion that blood-letting, as currently practised, often had no effect, or a deleterious effect. His 1828 memoir on the subject did not lead to an immediate reduction in the practice, however, and disputes broke out among physicians over the issue, as in Edinburgh in the 1850s, with statistics being summoned on one side of the argument and the

*Blood-letting remains part of traditional medicine in some parts of the world. A traditional healer bleeds a patient from a blood vessel in the leg, Republic of Somaliland, 1998. (Photo: Hamish Wilson/Panos Pictures)*

personal experience of doctors' practice on the other. Physicians practising outside the orbit of Paris hospital medicine still found bleeding to be therapeutically effective and valuable. So, although blood-letting had now been shown, statistically, to be of no particular value, it did not fade out of use for this reason. In fact it seems to have largely declined in Europe in the second half of the century, for reasons not yet satisfactorily uncovered by historians, and then again revived in the period from 1875 to the 1920s, especially in Germany. However, it remains a part of traditional medical practice in some parts of the world today.

### 5.4.5  Measuring the heat of the blood

Finally we may glance at the introduction of the **thermometer** into regular medical practice as a diagnostic and predictive tool. What the thermometer measures in practice is the core body-heat — which is blood-heat. The thermometer was not a new instrument in the nineteenth century, having been first invented in the seventeenth century. But in the context of Paris-style clinical medicine, with its statistical analyses and its concern only with phenomena accessible to the senses, for the first time it made sense for anyone to try and assess the relationship to health and disease of this highly-measurable sensory phenomenon of the body. It was a Professor of Clinical Medicine, Karl Wunderlich at Leipzig, whose extensive statistical comparisons legitimated the use of the thermometer as a clinical instrument. He published on the subject in 1868, and his book was replete with graphs and charts.

Wunderlich found that the temperature of the body lies within a normal range in health; that it is constant in health, but varies in disease; and that it varies in regular ways in different diseases:

> …thermometry gives results which can be *measured*, signs that can be *expressed in numbers*, and offers materials for diagnosis which are incontestable and indubitable, which are independent of the opinion or the amount of practice or the sagacity of the observer — in one word, materials which are physically accurate. (Wunderlich, 1871, p. 48)

Thermometry was a technique which, in Wunderlich's words in 1868, 'gives us a peep, as it were, into a *scene of continual changes*', and thus excels all other physical methods of diagnosis. The 'vital heat' of the blood, which had been familiar for centuries, was thus turned into a numerical index of health and illness.

In the world of clinical medicine as originated in the Paris of the Revolution years, the blood came to be given new roles. The beat of the pulse had come to function as a sign of the state of the heart, thus making visible to the physician the heart hidden within the body; the heat of the blood was henceforth 'taken' by the thermometer and it signalled to the physician the state of health and the trajectory of diseases; and the traditional therapy of blood-letting had for the first time been questioned by the *analyse numérique*.

*Thermometers constructed by Santorio Santorio (1625). It was not until the nineteenth century that thermometers were introduced into regular medical practice. (Source: The British Library, London)*

## 5.5    Blood and laboratory medicine

Clinical, or hospital, medicine, as first developed in Paris in the years around 1800, is one of the two pillars of modern medical thinking and practice. The other pillar is *laboratory medicine*, which has had an even greater influence on the way we look at and understand the nature of blood today than the clinical method did.

The primary effect of blood being studied in the laboratory was that blood became *fragmented*, both conceptually and literally. Looking at it down their microscopes, laboratory researchers came to see blood as something made up of distinct *components*, and then particular *roles* in the economy of the body were given to each of the components. Thus, in the course of the nineteenth century, blood came to be seen as *consisting of* (rather than containing) cells of two main types (red and white), and minute 'platelets', all suspended in an almost colourless fluid, the plasma or serum, each of these components having *particular and distinguishable roles* in sustaining life and health. The red blood cells had been seen through (low-power) microscopes in the seventeenth century, and the white cells in the eighteenth century, and the serum had been familiar to physicians for centuries, as they saw it separate from the clotting blood in their bleeding bowls. But these distinct components of the blood had not hitherto been subject to the kind of concentrated study for which the laboratory was created.

Laboratory medicine is a creation of the mid-to-late nineteenth century and is established on and relies on a range of laboratories: for instance, *physiological* laboratories to pursue experimental work on animals to understand their functioning (and hence the functioning of the human), and *pharmaceutical* laboratories to develop and test new chemical drugs. With respect to the development of new ways of thinking about the blood, the most important initial kind of laboratory was the *bacteriological* (or microbiological) laboratory.

The microscope became the emblem of laboratory workers in bacteriology, as it was the instrument which allowed bacteriologists to inspect the growth and life cycles of micro-organisms cultivated in the laboratory **in vitro** (literally 'in glass', meaning in laboratory vessels). Blood particularly lends itself to microscope study, being convenient and easy to manipulate in the laboratory.

- How did the emergence of laboratory medicine (as described in Chapters 3 and 4) produce new knowledge of TB?

- Pasteur demonstrated the existence of bacteria that communicated disease, and Koch identified the causative agent of TB (later called *Mycobacterium tuberculosis*) by a process of inference from experiments and direct visual inspection through the microscope.

The rapid expansion of laboratory medicine was in part a result of the development of science as a state-supported profession and as a business and industry in mid-nineteenth century Europe and America. Both of these were consequences of the creation of capitalist, secular, centralised nation-states in the nineteenth century. The laboratory can be seen as a specialised factory for the production of scientific and medical knowledge for the direct or indirect benefit of modern industry and the modern state and its citizens. Its origin lies in the beginnings of large-scale industry in the nineteenth century.

France, the German states (before and after their unification in 1871), Britain, and the United States, were the places where laboratory medicine was developed, and the development occurred hand in hand with the creation of major chemical, brewing, textile and food production industries. The relationship was two-way. For instance, Louis Pasteur, one of the two individuals most directly responsible for the creation of bacteriological laboratories, worked to solve problems in the French brewing, silk-production and animal-rearing industries, in each of which he found micro-organisms to be agents impeding the flourishing of French industry. Techniques for cultivating and identifying **pathogenic** (disease-causing) **micro-organisms** (or **pathogens**) were developed by the other most important individual in the new science of bacteriology, Robert Koch. His work depended crucially on the development of synthetic dyes by the growing German chemical industry, especially methylene blue for staining micro-organisms so that they could be distinguished from each other.

### 5.5.1  The blood and tropical medicine

The development of bacteriology, more perhaps than that of any other science, was linked to the development of the tropical colonies which the Western capitalist powers were creating for themselves in the late nineteenth century. It was hoped and believed that bacteriology would provide the knowledge and techniques which would, in the language of the time, make the tropics 'safe for the white man' and his soldiers, animals and crops.[4] Most European colonising powers built schools of tropical medicine to train colonial doctors; some, such as France, developed bacteriological laboratories in their colonies. Moreover, bacteriologists went to the colonies to investigate: for instance, Koch went to Egypt and India to try to discover the causal agent of cholera in 1883–4, and to South Africa to try and discover a

---

[4] There is an extended discussion of the development of tropical medicine and the reciprocal influences on health and health care between Europe and its colonies in *Caring for Health: History and Diversity* (Open University Press, 2nd edn 1993; 3rd edn 2001).

microbial cause of rinderpest, a cattle disease, in 1896–8. (The photograph of Koch, which appears as Figure 4.4 earlier in this book, was taken in South Africa.) Pupils of both Pasteur and Koch went abroad to try and discover causal microbial agents for tropical and other diseases that threatened the safe colonisation of tropical climes, such as Alexandre Yersin (pupil of Pasteur) and Shibasaburo Kitasato (pupil of Koch), who in 1894 discovered the causal agent of plague in Hong Kong.

The blood was found to be a natural habitat of a number of disease-causing micro-organisms. Many pathogenic microscopic **parasites** (minute single-celled and multicellular animals, such as worms, as well as bacteria) were found to be moving around the body in the bloodstream, and/or to release **toxins** (poisons) into the bloodstream. Thus the blood came to be seen as the primary site and vehicle of infection in the human body. The central role of the blood in infection was highlighted within tropical medicine by the discovery of the role of blood-sucking insects as the vectors (carriers) of disease-causing micro-organisms. The work of Patrick Manson and Ronald Ross on malaria in the 1890s was particularly important in this respect, demonstrating dramatically to a fascinated public how the red blood cells of the human are used by the malaria parasites during part of their life cycle, and the stomach of the mosquito for the other part of the life cycle.[5] The investigative work of Ross was funded by the India Office because it was believed that the fight against malaria was so important for colonial policy. Ronald Ross received a Nobel Prize for his work on malaria, and both Manson and Ross were later knighted.

## 5.5.2  Immunity

As laboratory investigation into the cause and cure of infectious disease continued, it was found that blood was not only a major site of infection in the body, but also a major site of the phenomenon of **immunity** to infectious diseases.[6] It had long been known, especially in the case of smallpox, that anyone who survived an attack of the disease (for smallpox regularly killed, as well as disfigured), would not catch it again. They had acquired 'immunity'. Immunity could also be conferred *artificially*, by using **inoculation**. Smallpox inoculation had been widely practised in Europe from the beginning of the eighteenth century, when it had been introduced from folk medical practice in Turkey. Some matter from a pustule of someone with smallpox was introduced under the skin of a healthy person: the recipient received a slight case of smallpox, and then (usually) recovered. Then Edward Jenner from 1798 introduced a safer variation of this using cowpox material (hence called **vaccination**, after the Latin for cow, *vacca*). By undergoing a very slight, barely perceptible, episode of cowpox, a disease related to smallpox, a person would be far more resistant to attacks of smallpox itself.

Louis Pasteur spent much of his career developing vaccines to produce artificial immunity against infectious diseases. Pasteur's technique was to pass the causative micro-organism of a particular infectious disease successively through series of experimental animals until it had lost its ability to cause illness. It could then be injected into people and it gave them immunity from attack from the pathogen in its virulent state.

● How was this technique applied to TB?

[5] The life cycle of the malaria parasite is described (and illustrated) in *World Health and Disease* (Open University Press, 2nd edn 1993; 3rd edn 2001), Chapter 3.

[6] The immune system and the techniques of immunisation are discussed in *Human Biology and Health: an Evolutionary Approach* (Open University Press, 2nd edn 1994; 3rd edn 2001), Chapter 6.

An eighteenth-century caricature of Jenner vaccinating against smallpox. The caption reads 'The Cow-Pock — or — the Wonderful Effects of the New Inoculation!' (Source: Private Collection/ Bridgeman Art Library)

■ Calmette and Guérin commenced human trials with their BCG vaccine in 1921, having created a stable, non-virulent strain of the tubercle bacillus through its prolonged exposure to ox bile.

How did the understanding of what processes underlay 'immunity' occur? The history of the study of immunity is highly complex, so we shall limit ourselves to describing one moment in this history. In the 1880s and 1890s it was found that immunity was a phenomenon located in the blood itself (later research extended it to other sites). But there was dispute between researchers of the French and German microbiological schools over precisely what component of the blood was involved, and two rival theories were in existence for some three decades.

In 1883, the Russian zoologist Elie Metchnikoff, in connection with work originally on inflammation, saw with his microscope in the blood of a transparent water flea how white cells surrounded and then 'ate up' an invading yeast cell. He called these cells **phagocytes**, literally 'eating cells', and the phenomenon **phagocytosis**. He theorised that at all times the white cells are constantly patrolling in the bloodstream on the lookout for invading microbes, which they surround and absorb.

It followed that a person becomes subject to an infectious disease only when the phagocytes in his or her blood are overwhelmed in their attempt to absorb the invading pathogens. Thus the white cells in the blood had been given a very precise role, a *defensive* one, in keeping the whole body safe from harm from micro-organisms. Pasteur was sympathetic to this theory, and he invited Metchnikoff to the Pasteur Institute in Paris, where he spent the rest of his career.

The rival theory, which was originated less than a decade later, gave the central role in immunity not to the white cells, but to the **serum**, the almost colourless fluid in which the blood cells are suspended. It was in the rival great bacteriological laboratory, the one headed by Robert Koch in Berlin, that Emil von Behring and Shibasaburo Kitasato in 1890 discovered that the broth they used to cultivate tetanus and diphtheria pathogens in the laboratory itself became poisonous. Some poison, or toxin, was obviously being produced by the micro-organisms. After small doses of this toxin had been injected into healthy animals, they did not succumb to the disease when they were later injected with lethal doses of the virulent form of the toxin, but showed resistance to it; moreover, 'immune serum' taken from these animals induced increased immunity to the toxins when injected into healthy animals. Evidently, the capacity to produce immunity was in the serum, and the presence of the toxins in the blood somehow called specific resistant entities into being: these von Behring called 'antitoxins', and they were later called **antibodies** following the work of Paul Ehrlich. The joint paper by von Behring and Kitasato concludes with the quotation from Goethe at the beginning of this chapter: *Blut ist en ganz besonderer Saft*, 'blood is an entirely special juice' (von Behring and Kitasato, 1890, p. 1 114). Immunologists to this day refer to the protection conferred by molecules circulating in the blood and other body fluids as 'humoral immunity', an echo of Galenist thinking.

These two rival theories about the immunising agency in the blood (white cells or antibodies) were to a certain extent merged in the first decade of the twentieth century (although the importance of blood as *the* transporting fluid has declined), and today they are regarded as interacting processes, describing different ways in which different micro-organisms are disposed of. But at the time of their origination they were thought to be incompatible.

The teasing out of the multiple roles of the component parts of the blood continues today, and the physician owes to the laboratory medical scientist much new understanding of the nature, course and cure of diseases, from such work on the blood. The view is essentially of the blood fragmented, and is a typical instance of how the functioning of the body has come to be looked at in a reductionist way — in striking contrast to the holistic views of the Galenic medical tradition. And although the blood and its components are still seen to be alive, the soul is, for the laboratory medical scientist, no longer thought to be in the blood or relevant to laboratory thinking about blood or the body.

## 5.6  Transfusion of blood in the twentieth century

It was experimentally recognised at the end of the nineteenth century that there are a number of distinct 'types' of human blood, or **blood groups**, and that transfusions between people with *different* blood groups can, in some combinations, produce a fatal reaction. The different blood groups were distinguished through the work of Karl Landsteiner in the years around 1900. Together with the development of means of storing blood by adding citrate, this meant that blood transfusion now became a practical possibility. Five minutes was no longer the time within which the blood had to be transferred from donor to patient before it clotted: the blood could now be kept in a usable state for up to three days without refrigeration. But it seems to have needed the involvement of the State for blood transfusion to be put into practice on any significant scale. War provided the spur for the development of transfusion. It was first tried out in World War I by the allied forces in France, in cases of severe haemorrhage (blood loss) and shock.

Between the wars transfusion services were established, but only on a small scale. In England, a small-scale voluntary Blood Transfusion Service was set up in London in 1921, developed out of the Red Cross organisation, and built directly on war-time experience. A call was made for a panel of blood donors covering London, with details of their blood groups and addresses, who would make themselves available for immediate donation when called upon: in 1924, 26 of the donors were called upon, but within five years over 5 000 were being called upon each year. This non-governmental and relatively small-scale approach was adopted also in other British cities, such as Birmingham. But it was in the Spanish Civil War that the techniques of large-scale collection, storage and supply were developed, and in World War II full-scale transfusion services were established as part of the medical side of the war effort.

In the United Kingdom these services were regarded as a high priority because air raids were expected in the first months of war. It was relatively easy for the Emergency Transfusion Service, set up by the Ministry of Health and the Medical Research Council, to enrol a million donors, and to provide large supplies of blood and serum. With such resources available to it, and with medical scientists looking for new ways to use the blood, the availability of blood and blood products for therapy and research came to be taken for granted. Similarly, the *free* donation of blood for medicine and science came to be customary for the donors. Thereafter, war transfusion services could be adopted on a large scale into peace-time civilian health provision: in the United Kingdom the Emergency Transfusion Service was turned into part of the new National Health Service in 1948. Where, as in the United Kingdom, a socialised form of health service was created, the donors formed a voluntary system; in other countries the donors were paid for their services. Within such transfusion programmes, the tendency has been for the blood to be separated into its components for most effective use in a wide range of surgical operations, to which it is indispensable and which its free availability makes possible.

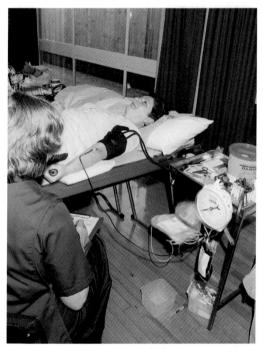

*Giving blood voluntarily and freely is symbolic of a social 'gift relationship' as well as providing a physical resource for medical care.*
*(Photo: Mike Levers)*

It might seem at first glance that the modern approach to blood has turned it completely into a 'scientific' object. But much of our traditional attitudes to it still persist, and not only in metaphor. Richard Titmuss, who was closely involved with the setting up of the National Health Service in the United Kingdom, published in 1970 a famous book on what he called 'the gift relationship', which is concerned with the nature of the act of donating blood for free. Here is this most precious and intimate part of ourselves, which is given freely in some societies, and sold as a commercial transaction in others. Such differences raise for Titmuss questions about the natures of these different modern societies, and of the attitude of their citizens to the society as a whole. The free donation of blood to strangers is in his view the most perfect example of altruism. But in order to be this, of course, blood needs to have very high personal and symbolic value in the eyes of the donor. As the publicity literature of the British blood transfusion service puts it: 'Give blood…the greatest gift of all', for to give blood is to give life — no matter how much it may be analysed into its component parts in the laboratory once it has been given.

It might also seem that the efficacy and desirability of blood transfusion is now self-evident from its results in the saving of life and the cure of disease. But transfusion brings its problems too. For instance a major threat to health occurred in the 1980s and 1990s when a rising number of people were infected with HIV as a result of contaminated transfusions and blood products to treat haemophilia: blood transfusion is the cause of such medical problems, not the cure. And although heat-treatment of blood in the developed world has made blood safe for future recipients, blood is increasingly infected in other parts of the world.

Moreover, one minority group in Western society has refused to accept a view of blood as a scientific object, and their insistence on seeing blood as sanctified continues to bring back to the surface questions about its identity and nature, as well as raising ethical questions. Jehovah's Witnesses' literal reading of the Bible leads them to insist that the Biblical prohibitions against eating blood mean that blood cannot be used for any secular purpose, and hence that blood transfusion is forbidden by God.

The law courts of Western countries are frequently called upon to decide whether Jehovah's Witnesses, their children and relatives, can be given blood transfusions against their will in order to fulfil physicians' views about necessary medical intervention. At one level, this is a dispute about the relationship of the moral and ethical codes of minorities to those of majorities in modern society. At another level, it is usually presented on the medical side as a dispute between enlightenment (scientific medicine) and primitive belief (Biblical literalism). But it is also of course a dispute over what kind of object the blood is: simply scientific or peculiarly sacred?

## OBJECTIVES FOR CHAPTER 5

When you have studied this chapter you should be able to:

**5.1** Define and use, or recognise definitions and applications of, each of the terms printed in **bold** in the text.

**5.2** Describe some of the ways in which blood has been and is interpreted as a religious and cultural symbol in different societies and historical periods, including our own.

**5.3** Describe how scientific ideas about blood have been determined by the paradigms of investigation current at particular points in history.

**5.4** Distinguish between the mechanistic and vitalist views of the body.

**5.5** Explain how laboratory medicine led to discoveries about the ways in which immunity is achieved.

## QUESTIONS FOR CHAPTER 5

**1** (*Objective 5.2*)

How are early vitalist beliefs about the sacred nature of blood maintained in modern times?

**2** (*Objective 5.3*)

Percussion, palpation and auscultation were all techniques of physical examination introduced in French hospital medicine in the late eighteenth and early nineteenth centuries. Why were they so important in the view of disease that was developing at that time?

**3** (*Objective 5.4*)

In what key respects did Descartes' view of the body differ from Harvey's?

**4** (*Objective 5.5*)

How did laboratory medicine contribute to an understanding of the working of vaccines?

# CHAPTER 6

## Hysteria

**Study notes for OU students**

During this chapter you will be asked to read an article specially written to accompany this chapter by Mary James, 'Hysteria and demonic possession'. This is contained in the *Health and Disease: A Reader* (Open University Press, second edition 1995; third edition 2001).

# 6.1   Introduction

The purpose of this case study is to show how medical categories may reflect broader cultural stereotypes. Thus medical knowledge may be *socially constructed* to suit purposes other than simply the objective advancement of scientific description. Taking **hysteria** as our example, we will consider how this 'disease', traditionally strongly associated with women and once explained in supernatural terms, later came to be understood scientifically and localised in the nervous system. The scientific approach was then revised so that now the diagnosis of hysteria, albeit rare, refers to a purely psychological condition with no identifiable physical correlates. An important aspect of this case study is to highlight the social and cultural features of hysteria. Not only are the manifestations of this disorder numerous, changeable and often dramatic, but in the great majority of cases they are associated with female behaviour. Yet no physical explanation can be found. For these reasons hysteria is well suited to reflect a range of non-scientific factors. It offers a potent insight into the *cultural relativism* of medical knowledge: descriptions vary significantly in different times and places, raising the question whether hysteria is, in any meaningful sense, a real disease entity.

Medical authors dating back to the seventeenth century have remarked upon the difficulty of defining hysteria. Indeed, except for a brief period in the late nineteenth century when the neurologist Jean-Martin Charcot (1825–93) imposed order on this concept by systematic observation and classification of the symptoms, doctors have always disagreed about the 'true' identity of this disease. Many doctors, through the generations, diagnosed as hysteria any 'nervous' malady, especially if associated with fits or convulsions or a feeling of strangulation. Other diagnostic criteria have been paralysis, anaesthesia (that is the loss of sensation on the surface of the body) and a whole variety of sensory disturbances. Hysteria, as we understand it today, is characterised by its ability to mimic the symptoms of a wide range of physical illnesses. Given the diversity of definitions in the past, it is likely that diseases now classified differently may once have been labelled as hysteria.

- In what way does the history of TB also illustrate the changing nature of systems for classifying diseases (Chapter 4)?

- What is now known as TB was once categorised under separate headings, such as scrofula or consumption. Bayle classified lung cancer as a form of TB.

In fact, whenever hysteria appears, broadly speaking, the form it takes reflects the attitudes and expectations prevalent in a cultural context in general, and of the medical profession in particular, concerning proper female conduct. Hysteria is inextricably bound up with the **gender roles** assigned to women.

In this chapter we will examine some of the many different strands of influence at play in the construction of hysteria as a diagnostic category by examining both lay and medical attitudes to women. Without assuming the existence of a single unchanging disease entity throughout thousands of years of medical history, hysteria may nonetheless illustrate general developments in the history of medical thought. It may also contribute to our understanding of the social construction of medical knowledge.

## 6.2   The quintessentially female malady

Hysteria, or at least what in more recent times has been interpreted as hysteria, has a very long history dating back to the medical papyri of ancient Egypt. A document known as the Kahun Papyrus, from around 1900 BC, described a series of morbid states, all attributed to displacement of the uterus or womb. The historian Ilza Veith has claimed that many of these are recognisable as hysterical disorders (Veith, 1965). Critics of this view, however, say that the conditions described in the papyri are often too vague to be recognisable, or else are indistinguishable from a range of gynaecological problems including premenstrual tension and puerperal fever (fever following childbirth caused by uterine infection) (Merskey and Potter, 1989).

Although we need to be cautious about assuming that the ancient Egyptians thought of 'hysteria' as a 'disease' in any meaningful sense, they nevertheless attributed certain capricious female behaviour to the upheavals and wanderings of the womb. This association was retained in the medical thought of ancient Greece and was given expression in the Hippocratic treatises of the fourth century BC. In these writings the exclusively *female* **aetiology** (assignment of a cause to a disease) was expressed by the term 'hysteria', deriving from the Greek word *hystera*, meaning womb.

The Hippocratic theory of the wandering uterus, causing mostly respiratory symptoms, was widely accepted in the ancient Mediterranean world. Aretaeus of Cappadocia, a Greek physician of the

*Women's behaviour has been subject to negative stereotyping of different kinds over the centuries. Witches flying on broomsticks from* Le Champion des Dames *by Martin le Franc, c. 1440 (Source: Bibliothèque Nationale, Paris)*

*'Extase', a photograph by P. Regnard from the* Iconographie Photographique de la Salpêtrière, *1878, of Augustine, one of Jean-Martin Charcot's 'hysterical' patients in the hospital of Salpêtrière (Source: The British Library)*

second century AD, incorporated the thought of Hippocrates into his writings and described the movements of the uterus as follows:

> In the middle of the flanks of women lies the womb, a female viscus, closely resembling an animal, for it is moved of itself, hither and thither, also upwards in a direct line to below the cartilage of the thorax, and also obliquely to the right or to the left, either to the liver or spleen; and it likewise is subject to prolapse downwards, and, in a word, it is altogether erratic…and, on the whole, the womb is like an animal within an animal. (Quoted in Palis, Rossopoulos and Triarhou, 1985, p. 226)

The womb's propensity for movement was apparent to doctors from uterine *prolapses*, when the muscles that hold the womb in place become slack, causing it to bulge into and even out of the vagina.

In Hippocratic texts it was noted that hysterical women tended most often to be single or widowed, deprived of sexual relations. Feelings of strangulation before the onset of a seizure were explained as the rising of the womb to the throat. The prescription for this condition was marriage, if possible, otherwise the womb had to be lured back to its rightful place by fumigation. Unpleasant odours inhaled by mouth could, it was thought, repel the womb downward, whereas sweet-smelling odours applied through the vagina might entice the womb back to its correct position.

## 6.2.1  Hysteria and sexual abstinence

However, the theory of uterine movement described above was not held by all doctors. Soranus of Ephesus and Galen of Pergamon, writing in the second century AD, related hysteria to the womb, but emphasised a strong sexual cause. Thus Soranus recommended a regime consisting of such erotic remedies as gentle massage and olive oil applied to the genitals. Galen put forward a theory that women produced a secretion similar to semen which, if not released, could produce hysterical complaints. Galen also believed that this could lead to analogous disorders in men. However, although Galen's teaching on hysteria was subsequently influential, this aspect of it was largely ignored by his contemporaries, for whom the relationship with the womb, and therefore with women, was implicit in the term hysteria itself.

## 6.2.2  Women as mutilated men

Galen's belief that women produced a secretion analogous to semen implied that women played an active role in reproduction, with both men and women contributing. In this respect he was more egalitarian than Aristotle who taught that women played only a passive role in the begetting of children, namely as the receptacle for male sperm, from which alone children were thought to be formed. He believed that women were defective versions of the male prototype and described them as 'mutilated males'. They were not just *biologically* inferior, they were, accordingly, *morally* weaker too.

If Galen was influential, so was Aristotle, his views on women being cited for generations afterwards. In the Middle Ages, Aristotle's ideas became the foundation of Islamic philosophy, and were also incorporated into Christian theology in the synthesis carried out by Saint Thomas Aquinas (*c.* 1226–74) who, following Aristotle, referred to women as 'misbegotten men'.

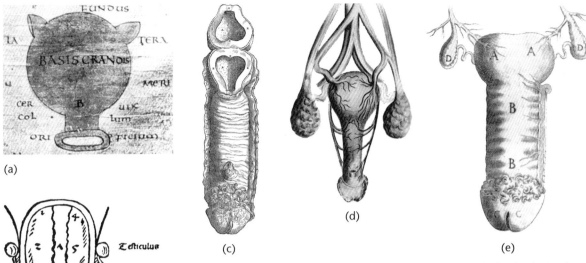

(a)

(b)

(c)

(d)

(e)

**Figure 6.1** *(a) The uterus in a ninth-century manuscript, with the 'fundus' or base, the cervix, the neck or vagina (collam) and the vaginal mouth (orificium), all roughly labelled. (Source: The Royal Society of Medicine) (b) A sixteenth-century illustration of the uterus copied from the* Anathomia *(1316) of Mondino dei Luzzi. (Source: The Wellcome Library, London) (c) The uterus, vagina and external genitalia, from Andreas Vesalius, 1543. (Source: The Wellcome Library, London) The female reproductive organs according to (d) Georg Bartisch, 1575, (Source: The Wellcome Library, London) and (e) Scipione Mercurio, 1595. (Source: The Wellcome Library, London)*

● Consider the anatomical illustrations in Figure 6.1. These appeared originally in documents written by male physicians between the ninth and the sixteenth centuries. Compare them with the modern illustration in Figure 6.2. What differences can you spot between the old and the new versions? What might have been the model for the traditional anatomy?

■ Several errors are detectable in the earlier illustrations: for example, the womb appears to *include* the cervix and vagina (Figure 6.1a and b). The ovaries are labelled 'testiculus' (Figure 6.1b) after the male sexual glands, and there can be no mistaking the masculine appearance given to the female reproductive organs in Figure 6.1c, d and e. This would suggest that male physicians believed women to be formed on the pattern of men's anatomy, either because of male prejudice, or because, in the absence of detailed anatomical investigation, the only *visible* model was that of the male reproductive organs.

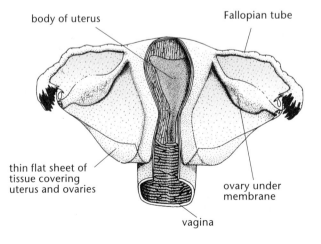

body of uterus

Fallopian tube

thin flat sheet of tissue covering uterus and ovaries

ovary under membrane

vagina

**Figure 6.2** *A modern anatomical drawing of the female reproductive organs.*

### 6.2.3  Medieval attitudes to women and sexuality

Many male writers in the medieval period took a particularly anti-female or *misogynistic* stand. One commonly cited work is the anonymous fourteenth-century compendium *De Secretis Mulierum* ('On the Secrets of Women'). This was allegedly written at the request of a priest who sought guidance in assigning appropriate penances to women for their sins given that they were 'extremely venemous [*sic*] during their menstrual periods'. The text warned, for example, that the retention of menstrual fluid in old women could produce dreadful results. A malevolent glance from such a woman might, apparently, kill a young child. It drew widely on the European folk tradition as well as on more academic sources and was incorporated into a work known for centuries as *Aristotle's Masterpiece* (though it had little to do with Aristotle). This went through hundreds of editions in English between 1684 and 1930, and was a most important source of popular information about sexual matters and childbirth.

Besides academic and folklore traditions, a third important source of theory about the character of men and women was that of religion. Christianity became the official religion of the Roman Empire under Constantine in the early part of the fourth century AD. In the Old Testament, in particular, women are inferior to men. In the Book of Genesis, for instance, it was Eve who persuaded Adam to eat the apple from the Tree of Knowledge, which God had expressly forbidden. As punishment God expelled them from the Garden of Eden and condemned them to lives of sorrow and hardship. On the basis of this account it was possible for those who wished to do so to ascribe the more painful features of human existence to the failings of a woman.

Furthermore, elements of the Christian tradition gave credence to *supernatural* theories of disease, which were a standard part of European folklore, and this too was sometimes used against women. Hysterics frequently fell into extravagant paroxysms with bursts of terrifying frenzy and rage, lending credence to the notion of demonic involvement. They were regarded as sinful creatures who either had wilfully allowed themselves to be possessed or, through carnal lust, had entered into league with the Devil. Women, as 'the weaker vessel' (I Peter, 3.7) were considered to be so much more prone to possession by evil powers that they were designated the 'gateway of the Devil' by Tertullian, one of the Church Fathers.

According to Saint Augustine (AD 354–430), sexual lust was the source of original sin in Adam and Eve. Sexuality was fraught with evil and hysteria was the product of demonically inspired lust. Whereas Galen and others had seen sexual *fulfilment* as the cure for hysteria, some of those in a more Christian tradition recommended sexual *abstinence*. Both these traditions continued to have a powerful influence throughout the Middle Ages (a period roughly from the latter part of the fifth century AD to the middle of the fifteenth century).

## 6.3  Women and witchcraft

The stereotype of the demonic witch was the product of the end of the Middle Ages. It involved the idea of a detestable and threatening creature who flew by night to meet others of her kind at great assemblies presided over by the Devil (see Figure 6.3). Only when such a stereotype was in being did it make sense to worry about **witchcraft** as an alternative,

**Figure 6.3**  *Witches and spirits flying to sabbath on a pitchfork, from Ulrich Molitor,* De Laniis et Phitonicis Mulieribus *(1489). (Source: The British Library)*

**Figure 6.4** *The burning of Anne Hedriks for witchcraft at Amsterdam in 1571. During the pre-industrial period of European history (c. 1450 to 1750, generally referred to by historians as the 'early modern' period), over 100 000 people, mostly women, were prosecuted by secular and ecclesiastical courts for allegedly practising harmful magic and worshipping the Devil. About half were executed, usually by burning. (Source: Rijksmuseum-Stichting, Amsterdam)*

anti-Christian religion. Although, throughout the history of Christianity, magic had been viewed as the work of the Devil and a form of heresy, by the late fifteenth century the heresy of the witch was seen as much more organised and dangerous. The emergence of the belief that witches were not merely magicians but Devil-worshippers changed the nature of the crime, making it a much more serious offence (see Figure 6.4).

Intellectual support for the persecution of witches was heavily influenced by some of the Church's teaching. In 1484 Pope Innocent VIII issued a Papal Bull denouncing the treacheries of witchcraft and this gave *carte blanche* to the Inquisition. Among those appointed to stamp out witchcraft were two Dominican monks, Heinrich Kramer and James Sprenger, authors of a treatise entitled *Malleus Maleficarum* (*The Hammer of the Witches*). This treatise, first published in 1486, was reprinted 14 times before 1520, and assumed a major role in disseminating the new ideas about witchcraft, such as could not have occurred before the invention of printing in the mid-fifteenth century. For more than two hundred years it served judges and magistrates in Europe as an 'encyclopaedia' of witchcraft, making them more conscious of the crime and probably more credulous of its reality. Kramer and Sprenger believed with Saint Augustine that since the 'first corruption of sin…came to us through the act of generation,…greater power is allowed by God to the Devil in this act than in all others', and concluded:

> All witchcraft comes from carnal lust, which is in women insatiable. … There are three things that are never satisfied, yea, a fourth thing which says not, It is enough; that is, the mouth of the womb. Wherefore for the sake of fulfilling their lusts they consort even with devils…. It is no matter for wonder that there are more women than men found infected with the heresy of witchcraft. And in consequence of this, it is better called the heresy of witches than of wizards, since the name is taken from the more powerful party. (Quoted in Summers, 1971, pp. 47–8)

● Why were women more likely than men to be prosecuted for witchcraft?

■ Women were believed to be morally weaker than men, a point of view backed up by biblical references, so they were considered more easily persuaded into witchcraft by the Devil. Furthermore the sexual appetite of women was believed to be insatiable, inclining them to copulate with Satan.

Hysteria overlaps with the phenomenon of witchcraft in highly complex and controversial ways. Church doctrines about the evils of sexuality, particularly female sexuality, are one obvious example. It might also be that some of the women tried as witches were themselves hysterical. Descriptions of some of the characteristic signs of witches, as well as the afflictions of their alleged victims, parallel some later descriptions of the symptoms of hysteria, such as local immunities to pain, mutism, blindness, convulsions and false pregnancies. Women were twenty times more likely than men to be accused of witchcraft (Figure 6.5). In the nineteenth century this same ratio was applied to the diagnosis of hysteria. Although witches tended typically to be women over 50, rather older than the commonest age for hysteria, they were most often widows and spinsters, the same category of women whom classical writers had stressed were most prone to hysteria. Finally it could be argued that those who perpetrated the witch-hunts themselves furnish a tragic example of hysteria in its *collective* form, known today as **mass hysteria**.

### 6.3.1 The challenge to witchcraft beliefs

Despite the fact that Kramer and Sprenger boldly claimed that those who denied the reality of witchcraft were themselves heretics, witchcraft beliefs did not pass unchallenged. One of those who questioned the doctrines of the *Malleus Maleficarum* was the Dutch physician Johann Weyer (1515–88) who, though he believed in the Devil and magic, took a tolerant attitude towards those accused of witchcraft. He argued that the ignorant and lonely women who confessed to this crime were suffering from delusions and in fact had a disease of the uterus. He also gave natural medical causes for the symptoms of those who claimed to be the victims of witches' spells.

Figure 6.5 *Matthew Hopkins, the English witchfinder of Manningtree, Essex, who was active in 1645, with one of the women he accused and her supposed 'imps'. Women were twenty times more likely than men to be accused of witchcraft. From Matthew Hopkins,* The Discovery of Witches, *1647, London. (Source: The British Library)*

An explicit distinction between hysteria and possession by evil spirits was made by the English physician, Edward Jorden (1569–1632) in his book entitled *Briefe Discourse of a Disease Called the Suffocation of the Mother* (1603). Jorden, who was one of the first physicians to write about hysteria in English, produced this work in the wake of the case of a fourteen-year-old girl, Mary Glover, who claimed she had been bewitched. Glover fell ill after a dispute with an old woman, Elizabeth Jackson, in 1602. Her spectacular fits and accusations of witchcraft against the old woman resulted in a dramatic trial that aroused considerable popular interest. Jorden and another physician who were called upon to defend Jackson, claimed that Glover was the victim of a natural disease. They were, however, unable to make a convincing case and Jackson was found guilty. Jorden's *Briefe Discourse* was written in response to the humiliating repudiation of his testimony in court and aimed to restore his credibility by documenting the scientific reasoning behind his argument. In this treatise he steadfastly maintained that hysteria was the cause of Glover's symptoms. Since Mary Glover had not yet reached puberty, Jorden could not apply the ancient model of hysteria as a disease of the uterus caused by the deprivation of sexual relations. Although he agreed that menstrual problems and sexual abstinence were causes of hysteria, he argued that the brain, too, played a part in producing hysterical symptoms and that these might be purely the result of psychological stresses.

## 6.4 The search for natural causes

### 6.4.1 The Renaissance

The historical period in which the *Malleus Maleficarum* was published and witch mania reached its peak is known as the *Renaissance*. Paradoxically, this intellectual movement, which spanned the period from the fourteenth to the sixteenth century, is usually associated with the revival of Greek and Latin classical culture in Europe.

Among the outstanding characteristics of the Renaissance was the growth of *scepticism* and free thought, and the work of men such as Weyer and Jorden was influenced by this context. This intellectual climate led to questioning of the ultimate authority of the Church.

● Think back to Chapter 5. How does William Harvey's work on blood and its later interpretation by Descartes reflect the growth of scepticism about the classical view of nature and the decline in religious authority?

■ Although he lived after the period of the Renaissance, Harvey's discovery of the movement of the blood involved the revival of Aristotelian methods of experimental enquiry into nature. Although Harvey held a *vitalist* view of the blood as containing the soul, his description of circulation was used by later thinkers (for example, Descartes) as part of a more secular understanding of the body as a mechanism.

The fact that belief in witches should have reached proportions of such magnitude at the very time when natural science began to flourish as never before shows that the designation of historical periods inevitably involves considerable oversimplification. It also reminds us that what we may now see as 'progress' is rarely a straightforward matter.

● How does the history of the treatment of TB also illustrate this last point?

■ The enthusiasm for surgical treatments for TB between the two world wars is now regarded as being based on inadequate evidence of effectiveness. The earlier emphasis on the curative powers of physical labour is another example.

During the Renaissance the classical emphasis on rational explanation and the search for *natural* causes began to regain ground over *supernatural* accounts of phenomena. Naturalist theories influenced medical thinking in several areas and promoted the systematic exploration of the human body. This new approach was to have profound consequences for theories of hysteria.

● How did anatomical investigation contribute to a new conception of disease?

■ Through locating the pathological lesions associated with symptoms, thus supporting the notion of *localised pathology* underlying disease.

Renaissance scientists explored the womb and some startling discoveries were made. For instance, until 1315–16 when Mondino dei Luzzi (c. 1275–1326) dissected two female corpses, anatomists were largely ignorant of the structure of the female reproductive organs (look back at Figure 6.1). In the fifteenth century the *hymen* was described for the first time, then in the sixteenth century it was discovered that the womb is divided into two parts, the upper part consisting of a single cavity. During the sixteenth century descriptions of the *mons veneris* and the *clitoris* were produced and the first encyclopaedia, or 'system', of gynaecology was published. In the seventeenth century the 'female testicles' came to be known instead as the *ovaries* and the traditional method of describing the female genitalia from the inside out, beginning with the womb, was reversed. Anatomical writers now began with the external genitalia and worked from the outside in. The modern linguist Ian Maclean, commenting on these new developments, has noted that

> By 1600, in nearly all medical circles…one sex is no longer thought
> to be an imperfect and incomplete version of the other. Indeed,
> far from being described as an inferior organ, the uterus now
> evokes admiration and eulogy for its remarkable role in procreation.
> (Maclean, 1980, p. 33)

However, the new knowledge was not accepted uniformly and many of the old
anatomical beliefs still lingered on. For instance, in 1636 John Sadler, a 'doctor in
physicke' at Norwich, published a gynaecological handbook for women entitled
*The Sicke Woman's Private Looking Glass*. Referring to the womb, he noted that:
'the form or figure of it is like a virall [virile] member, onley this excepted, the
manhood is outward, and the womanhood within' (Sadler, 1636, p. 5). Moreover,
like the vast majority of seventeenth-century physicians, Sadler believed that the
condition of the womb determined a woman's physical and emotional well-being.
The influence of the womb on the general health of women was stated by Sadler
as follows:

> For through the evill quality thereof, the heart, the liver, and the
> braine are affected; from whence the actions vitall, natural, &
> animal are hurt; and the virtues concoctive, sanguifficative,
> distributive, attractive, expulsive, retentive, with all the rest are all
> weakened. So that from the womb comes convulsions, epilepsies,
> apoplexies, palseyes, hecticke fevers, dropsies, malignant ulcers,
> and to bee short, there is no disease so ill but may procede from
> the evill quality of it. (Sadler, 1636, preface)

## 6.4.2 Cerebral influences emerge in the seventeeth century

Despite the fact that many seventeenth-century physicians stuck to the uterine
theory of hysteria, some still maintaining that the womb could move about the
body, in the context of the new understanding of anatomy ideas began to change.
Post-mortems had revealed precisely how the womb was held in place and, when
carried out on patients who had suffered from hysteria, but died of other causes,
indicated that the uterus was untouched by any disease. It became more difficult
to claim that it wandered at will.

Thomas Willis (1622–75) is usually credited with the first major critique of uterine
theories. As Professor of Natural Philosophy at Oxford, Willis carried out some
important studies on the anatomy of the brain and central nervous system by post-
mortem investigations. In 1666 he moved to London where he established a
successful and fashionable medical practice, whilst continuing to pursue his studies.
Among his clientele were many patients with hysterical complaints and his expertise
in neuroanatomy was brought to bear upon them. This resulted in the formulation
of a new theory of the *cerebral* origin and seat of hysteria.

Willis proposed that 'the Distemper named from the Womb is chiefly and primarily
Convulsive, and chiefly depends on the Brain and nervous stock [system] being
affected' (quoted in Veith, 1965, p. 132). According to Willis, hysterical fits were
the result of 'Spirits inhabiting the Brain, being now prepared for Explosions' (Veith,
1965, p. 132). Although he said the point of departure was usually in the head, he
still saw the uterus as occasionally playing a role in the production of hysteria, but
no more so than any other organ of the body. Willis's clinical practice furnished
him with the evidence he needed to disprove the link between hysteria and the
womb. Not only did Willis find hysteria in women of every age and condition,

including young girls and old women, but also sometimes in men. If hysteria was not limited to the female sex, it could not truly arise in the womb. Nevertheless, he was aware that women were far more likely to be hysterical than men and this he explained as the result of their weaker physical constitution. He wrote, 'Women, from any sudden terror and great sadness, fall into mighty disorder of spirits, where men from the same occasion are scarcely disturbed at all' (Veith, 1965, p. 133).

Willis's contemporary Thomas Sydenham (1624–89) also developed new insights. Among the causes of hysteria he noted 'over-ordinate actions of the body; and still oftener over-ordinate commotions of the mind, arising from sudden bursts of anger, pain, fear and other similar emotions' (quoted by Veith, 1965, p. 143). Because Sydenham emphasised disturbances of the emotions as a significant cause he recognised, as Willis had, that men too could be afflicted with this disease. To avoid implicit reference to the uterus he called male hysteria 'hypochondriasis'.

Willis and Sydenham's ideas were not widely accepted. Hippocratic and Galenic conceptualisations of the disorder proved to be remarkably durable and ancient genital theories continued to be maintained by all but a small minority of more 'progressive' medical men at the end of the seventeenth century. In the eighteenth and nineteenth centuries, the separation of hysteria from the uterus and the recognition of its symptoms in men persisted alongside the uterine theory. Furthermore, this latter view led, in the nineteenth century, to numerous operations removing the uterus, fallopian tubes and ovaries of perfectly healthy women. Common to these different theories, however, was the idea of a relation between hysteria and female sexuality. Even when hysteria was admitted in men, it was understood as, nevertheless, an affliction to which women were especially prone. A generalised association of hysteria with female behaviour, constitution, temperament and so on, was the single unifying theme of the various medical conceptualisations.

## 6.5    A disease of female delicacy

For those medical men who accepted that hysteria was located in the brain and nervous system, the susceptibility of women to become hysterical had to be explained along the lines that Willis and Sydenham had taken, namely in terms of the greater delicacy of female physiology. The association of nervous disorders with delicacy and a soft existence was by no means new in the 1680s when Sydenham advanced his theory of hysteria. Indeed, as the medical historian Mark Micale has shown, in much of the literature dating from a century and a half before Sydenham's observations, manual labour was specifically recommended to counteract nervous complaints (Micale, 1990). In the eighteenth century, the tendency of hysteria to afflict celibate well-born women was frequently documented in the medical literature. In *A Treatise on Female Disease* (1717), Henry Manning wrote of the 'hysteric passion' among London high society. He observed that:

> This disease chiefly seizes women who are delicate and endowed with great sensibility. The unmarried and widows are more subject to it than those who have husbands, in so much that many have been relieved from it by entering into conjugal life. (Quoted in Shorter, 1992, p. 101)

●    Which other disease has been associated with refined sensibility in the past?

■ TB acquired this reputation, particularly in literary circles of the eighteenth and early nineteenth centuries.

However, Mark Micale (1990) has argued that this picture of hysteria as a disease of refinement in the eighteenth century may be a misleading one since during this period the wealthier strata of society were far more likely to seek medical advice from expensive specialists, and it was these prominent physicians who tended to publish medical texts. In fact other sources suggest that in the late eighteenth century hysterical convulsions were experienced in all social classes. This suggests that the medical theories that were expressed in books were not always in line with medical practice.

### 6.5.1 Hysteria and culture in the eighteenth and nineteenth centuries

Nevertheless, the medical stereotype of women as inherently frail and emotional creatures whose wellbeing depended upon marriage and raising children, resonated profoundly with ideas about female gender roles permeating the broader European culture of the eighteenth and nineteenth centuries. It has been suggested that representations of women in the literature of this period both derived from and contributed to, medical expectations, and may have influenced the way in which hysteria, itself, was manifested. 'One had the hysteria one was expected to have' (Heath, 1982, p. 32).

The work of the French writer and philosopher, Jean-Jacques Rousseau (1712–78), for instance, captures the climate of eighteenth-century thought. In *Emile* (1762), his widely disseminated treatise on education, Rousseau characterised the sexes as follows:

> In the union of the sexes each alike contributes to the common end, but in different ways. From this diversity springs the first difference which may be observed between man and woman in their moral relations. The man should be strong and active; the woman should be weak and passive; the one must have both the power and the will; it is enough that the other should offer little resistance.

> When this principle is admitted, it follows that woman is specially made for man's delight. If man in his turn ought to be pleasing in her eyes, the necessity is less urgent, his virtue is in his strength, he pleases because he is strong. I grant you this is not the law of love, but it is the law of nature, which is older than love itself. (Rousseau, 1933 edn, p. 322)

For Rousseau this was both natural and a moral imperative, concurring with the eighteenth-century medical view of women's delicate nervous system. However, his views did not go unchallenged. Mary Wollstonecraft (1759–97) the feminist writer and educationalist, was determined to cast doubt on the idea that the frailty of middle-class women was natural. Her main contention in her treatise *Vindication of the Rights of Woman* (1792) was that social environment, not nature, was responsible for the differences in the characters of men and women. Upper- and middle-class women were, she claimed, socialised from birth into an artificially constructed 'femininity' that made them submissive, overly-emotional and irrational.

With marriage virtually the only means for a woman to gain respectability and to survive economically, these women were

> Confined, then, in cages like the feathered race, they have nothing to do but to plume themselves, and stalk with mock majesty from perch to perch. It is true they are provided with food and raiment, for which they neither toil nor spin; but health, liberty and virtue are given in exchange. (Wollstonecraft, 1986 edn, p. 146)

Excelling in femininity, as social pressure required, inevitably meant, to some degree, cultivating frailty. Furthermore hysteria was linked to the *essence* of cultural definitions of femininity through its vast and variable range of emotional and physical symptoms. Fits, fainting, laughing, sobbing, paralysis and general malaise were just part of its repertoire — and the swift transition from one symptom to another seemed to reinforce the instability and capriciousness traditionally associated with feminine nature. By the end of the nineteenth century the term 'hysterical' was almost synonymous with 'feminine' in literature, where it indicated any expression of excessive emotion.

In the eighteenth and nineteenth centuries there was in practice little scope for rebellion against this role, largely due to the social and economic dependency of women on men. Rebellion, if it took the form of unconventional or aggressive behaviour, or rejection of the norms of marriage and motherhood, was liable to be interpreted as pathological, i.e. as a sign of hysteria. Passive rebellion was more common, namely a refusal to perform daily 'duties', but this only served to reinforce the stereotype of female frailty. Some feminist historians (for example, Carroll Smith-Rosenberg, 1972) have suggested that hysteria was a powerful mode of protest for women deprived of other social or intellectual outlets or opportunities for self-expression. The hysterical woman is seen as being engaged in a power struggle with a male-dominated social order in an attempt to redefine her social role.

However, others argue that hysterical behaviour was tolerated precisely because it posed *no* threat to the prevailing patriarchal order. Thus Elaine Showalter, in *The Female Malady,* comments:

> It is difficult to escape this sobering view. In its historical contexts in the late nineteenth century, hysteria was at best a private, ineffectual response to the frustrations of women's lives. (Showalter, 1985, 1991 edn, p. 161)

Showalter points out, moreover, that women who campaigned for access to the universities, professions and the vote in the early days of the women's movement were liable to be labelled hysterics on account of their rebellious behaviour (Figure 6.6). By defining their behaviour as *pathological*, the hysteria diagnosis served as a means of social control to keep women in their 'rightful' place.

**Figure 6.6**    *Suffragettes force-fed in prison, 1909. (Source: By Achille Beltrane, Mary Evans Picture Library)*

## 6.6  Nineteenth-century science

### 6.6.1  The search for universal laws

During the eighteenth century, *observation* and *experiment* became the driving forces of contemporary advances in the physical and natural sciences, building on the earlier Renaissance emphasis on the power of reason and natural (rather than supernatural) explanations for phenomena. This led to an expansion of what became known as **scientific methods** of investigation, which aimed to discover genuine and practically useful knowledge, drawn from observation and stated in terms of universal laws.[1]

The application of this approach to medicine resulted, during the nineteenth century, in the rapid development of medical science. Increasingly emphasis was placed upon discovering universal laws governing the causes of disease by correlating clinical observations of symptoms with detection of pathological lesions discovered either at post-mortem or in the living body of the patient. Thus, during the nineteenth century, the shift begun in the Renaissance in the medical notion of disease was complete: medical ideas had moved entirely away from seeing disease as an affliction of the whole body, to seeing diseases as highly *localised* disturbances of anatomical structure. (You have already traced this development in the case study of TB in Chapter 4.)

●    What methods were developed to allow doctors to search for and locate lesions within the patient's *living* body (as described in earlier chapters)?

■    *Percussion* (tapping especially on the chest); *palpation* (feeling with the hands), and *auscultation* (listening, especially to the chest).

By observation of the facts of numerous particular instances, recurrent patterns of symptoms and pathological lesions could be identified. This revealed the 'regularity of nature' in the development of specific diseases such as TB. The corollary of this was that doctors gained the power to *predict* future outcomes when similar facts were presented. Thus *universal laws* apparently governing the development of pathological phenomena could be identified. In this new climate, professionally trained doctors were anxious to ensure that their practice was securely founded on a scientific basis. This meant a recognition of the *organic seat* of the complaint, that is to say its *biological* basis, as well as the laws of its development.

### 6.6.2  Hysteria and scientific methods

Hysteria was widely regarded by nineteenth-century doctors to be unsatisfactorily defined. To gain the status of an objectively real disease-category, the physical cause and its law-governed nature had to be revealed by observation and experiment. Thus hysteria had to have distinguishing features that followed a particular *course* of development.

Pierre Briquet (1796–1881) was the first to identify a law-governed regularity in hysteria. Between 1849 to 1859 he made detailed clinical investigations of around 450 patients at the Hôpital de la Charité in Paris. Roughly two-thirds of these patients

---

[1] Scientific methods are discussed in detail in *Studying Health and Disease* (Open University Press, 2nd edn 1994; colour-enhanced 2nd edn 2001), Chapter 2.

suffered from fits of *gradual* onset. Briquet described four successive phases and named this type of hysteria *hystero-epilepsy* on account of its resemblance to the classical epileptic fit. Briquet, whose observations were published in his *Treatise on Hysteria* (1859), understood hysteria as an invisible but real organic disease of the nervous system, and was the first to establish definitively that it afflicted both sexes, albeit twenty times more likely in women. This propensity was explained with reference to the more delicate nervous system of women which caused them to *feel* rather than to *think*. Briquet said that to feel was almost to *be* hysterical and thought that this tendency had been bestowed upon women by providence in order to furnish them for their social role.

For hysteria to be studied scientifically a population of working-class hysterics was required. These could be used rather like guinea-pigs, being experimented upon and demonstrated for teaching purposes, in a way that was not possible with genteel, fee-paying 'ladies'. In the latter part of the nineteenth century, it was to the lower classes that the diagnosis of hysteria was most frequently attached. This shift in class emphasis occurred in the context of the theory known as **hereditary degeneration**, which, during this period, gained widespread acceptance. According to this theory, crime, madness and all forms of socially aberrant behaviour could be explained as being passed from parents to offspring. The lower classes were said to be degenerate on account of their frequent ill-health and dissolute habits; hysteria (at least in part) was attributed to hereditary factors. Thus, from the mid-nineteenth century, far from being a sign of 'good' breeding, hysteria was now claimed to be more commonly a disease of the poor. Nevertheless, the association with refinement persisted in popular culture.

● How did the theory of degeneration affect medical attitudes towards TB towards the end of the nineteenth and early twentieth century?

■ Because of the association of TB with poverty there was little sympathy for those afflicted. They were regarded as the victims of their own idleness and moral decay.

## 6.7   Jean-Martin Charcot and the Salpêtrière

In 1862 Jean-Martin Charcot (1825–1893) was appointed chief physician of one of the largest sections of the Salpêtrière hospital in Paris. This vast and ancient hospital housed at that time some 5 000 female patients suffering from a great variety of largely unclassified, chronic illnesses, particularly diseases of the nervous system. Charcot recognised the enormous potential the Salpêtrière held for medical research and aimed, by the clinico–pathological method, to identify each ailment as a specific clinical entity. Until Charcot, this method had been little employed in neurology (the study of the nervous system). By the late 1860s Charcot had identified several major diseases, hitherto undifferentiated, for example constructing the clinical and pathological picture of multiple sclerosis. In 1882, in recognition of his achievements, a Chair in Diseases of the Nervous System was created for Charcot by the French government. It was the first of its kind in the world. As a result Charcot became one of the great public figures of his time and was in a pre-eminent position to mould medical opinion.

*Jean-Martin Charcot examining a brain, from a sketch made by Brissaud in 1875.*
(*Source:* Nouvelle Iconographie de la Salpêtrière, *Vol. II, 1898, Masson, Paris*)

## 6.7.1 Functional lesions

In 1872 Charcot took charge of the section for Epileptics and Hysterics at the Salpêtrière. Until that time these patients were housed together on account of the observed similarity between these two convulsive conditions. His work addressed head-on the problem that hysteria posed for medical authority at that time. For hysteria to be a matter of scientific concern it had to be shown to be well differentiated as a clinical entity and for this the identification of a physical cause was important.

Charcot classified hysteria as an inherited **neurosis** (*névrose*), using this term in its strictly neurological, late nineteenth-century sense to mean an *organic* disorder of the nervous system, that is one with an anatomical and physiological basis. In neuroses, lesions were *assumed* to be present even though they might not be studied directly at post-mortem. However, since there was no direct evidence of lesions in any *specific* location, the lesions associated with a neurosis were assumed to be widely *diffused* or scattered defects in the nervous system. They were termed **functional lesions**, since their existence was demonstrated solely by disturbances in the patient's ability to function. Charcot was convinced that, in time, the functional lesion in hysteria would be confirmed by advances in microscopic and chemical examination. Present-day medical science, however, has not fulfilled his expectation and the term *functional* is now reserved for conditions where no lesion of *any* kind can be found.

## 6.7.2 Regular patterns and pure types

For Charcot, Pierre Briquet's study of hysteria as a law-governed neurological disease was particularly influential and was often referred to in his lectures. During the 1870s, extending Briquet's work, Charcot described regular patterns of symptoms characteristic of what he called **la grande hystérie**, comprising four distinct stages. Pure types of *la grande hystérie* were very rare. Indeed, in ten years only *twelve* cases were found. The majority of patients who came for consultation were diagnosed as suffering from variations of this disease. In such cases stages might be missed out, or appear with varying degrees of intensity. Charcot asserted that it would nevertheless be easy for those who possessed the basic formula to recognise an intelligible order to the symptoms. (Open University students should now read 'Hysteria and demonic possession' by Mary James in *Health and Disease: A Reader*[2] and answer the following question.)

● Describe a frequently occurring variation of the four-stage *grande attaque hystérique* and say what was most significant about this diagnostic label.

■ The *attaque démoniaque* as described by Charcot was a common variation of the classical attack. It consisted in the predominance of the second stage known as *grands mouvements* (great movements, Figure 6.7) and was characterised by enormously increased muscular strength, agility and suppleness. This diagnostic label was important because it allowed Charcot to draw a comparison with the signs that had historically been interpreted as indications of demonic possession, showing these to have a scientific explanation.

**Figure 6.7** Three *sketches of aspects of the grande attaque* hystérique, *from Charcot, J.-M. and Richer, P.,* Les Démoniaques dans l'Art, *1887, Paris. (Source: The British Library)*

[2] *Health and Disease: A Reader* (Open University Press, 2nd edn 1995; 3rd edn 2001).

He also distinguished between *grande* and *petite hystérie*, the latter the non-convulsive variety of hysteria, which, as Briquet had said, constituted about a third of all cases. Diagnosis depended upon the identification of certain signs known as *permanent stigmata* including phenomena such as ovarian pain, hemianaesthesia (the loss of sensation in one half of the body), and disturbances of sight, smell, hearing and taste. Hysterics, whether *petite* or *grande*, could also be recognised by their propensity to *paralyses* and *contracture*, often brought on by a trivial injury. Contractures were the result of violent muscle spasms in which the affected part became rigid for prolonged periods.

### 6.7.3 Clinical experimentation

Charcot devoted much of his attention to distinguishing genuine from deceitfully-simulated hysterical symptoms.

● Suggest why this was important to him.

■ Requirements made of medical scientists at the time emphasised the discovery of biological causes and the universal laws governing diseases. Without such proof, hysteria could not be clearly differentiated from wilful malingering.

**Figure 6.8** *Experiment intended to verify the reality of the contracture of the hand, from Charcot, J.-M.,* Lectures on Diseases of the Nervous System, *translated by Sigerson, G., New Sydenham Society, 2nd series 1877–81. (Source: The British Library)*

An example of one of Charcot's experiments to distinguish 'real' symptoms from malingering is shown in Figure 6.8. Here, patients were strapped to various purpose-built apparatus and weights were attached to contractured parts. Breathing and heartbeat were recorded on a graph, which was compared with graphs produced for healthy subjects simulating hysterical symptoms, whose fatigue in feigning a contracture under such conditions generated a different pattern (Figure 6.9).

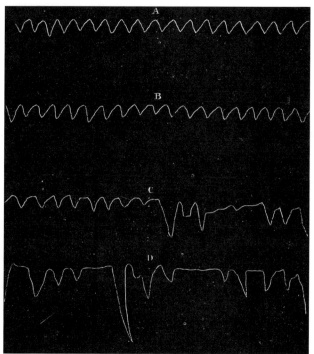

**Figure 6.9** *Graph showing breathing and heartbeat. The lines A and B represent the respiratory movements of the patient; the lines C and D those of a simulator. From Charcot, J.-M.,* Lectures on Diseases of the Nervous System, *translated by Sigerson, G., New Sydenham Society, 2nd series 1877–81. (Source: The British Library)*

### 6.7.4  Male and female stereotypes

For Charcot, as for Pierre Briquet, an important feature of the study of hysteria was the application of this diagnosis to the male.

● Why should this have been important to him?

■ Because he conceptualised hysteria as a disorder of the *nervous* system, which is common to both sexes.

Nevertheless, it was young women who provided the vast majority of his cases. Again following Briquet, Charcot explained this in terms of the more sensitive nervous system of the female. Women, he said, like the symptoms of hysteria from which they so often suffered, tended to be unstable, changeable and capricious (Charcot, 1878). By comparison Charcot was at pains to depict his *male* hysterics as virile, robust and hard-working whose hysteria was provoked by *physical* rather than emotional trauma. Male hysterics were at first seen at the hospital only as out-patients, mainly because Salpêtrière was a women's hospital but also because, Charcot said, their symptoms, like their characters, tended to be more stable. Thus the prevailing gender stereotypes of masculinity and femininity were represented as biologically based and were given scientific credibility by being related to the physiology of the nervous system. Though presented as objective, Charcot's scientific study of hysteria was in fact riven with cultural stereotypes.

### 6.7.5  Theatrical appeal and the doctor–patient relationship

Once admitted to Charcot's ward, those patients who best exemplified his description of *la grande hystérie* in its 'pure' four-stage form were most likely to be selected for demonstration at his lectures. These patients were mostly young, working-class women with grievously disturbed backgrounds. If Charcot took a special interest in their case, they could achieve a kind of celebrity. Indeed they often vied with one another to appear 'on stage' with him. This effect of patient celebrity became particularly pronounced when in 1878 Charcot began to use *hypnotism* to investigate the psychic mechanism underlying hysterical symptoms. Demonstrations of hypnosis were incorporated into his bi-weekly lectures, imbuing them with such a broad theatrical appeal that they became a fashionable event (Figure 6.10). The lecture theatre was always packed, not just with doctors and medical students, but with the leading lights of Parisian society. Actors, artists, authors and journalists were reputed to attend. Charcot's demonstrations also received considerable coverage in lay as well as medical journals, bringing his *grandes hystériques* strikingly before the public eye.

**Figure 6.10**    *'Un Leçon Clinique à la Salpêtrière' ('A clinical lesson at Salpêtrière') by André Brouillet, 1887. (Source: Mary Evans Picture Library)*

Although Charcot provided his 'best' patients with their moment of stardom, this is not to suggest that they consciously simulated their crises in order to please him. It is likely, however, that in the psychologically charged environment of the hospital, where Charcot's word was law, both doctors and patients were anxious to receive his approbation. The pattern of hysteria, once set, recurred as a result of their collective expectations. In addition, Charcot recommended that the patient should be removed from the environment in which the hysteria arose and he prohibited all visits from family and friends. To inhibit the propensity of hysterics to imitate one another (itself understood as a sign of their extreme impressionability) efforts were also made to isolate patients from each other, although in practice this was difficult to achieve because of lack of space. Isolation was favoured by Charcot for its enhancement of the doctor's power of persuasion over the patient, which was at times so strong that a seemingly intractable hysterical paralysis could be suddenly removed by an authoritative command, especially when using hypnosis.

The system of rewards and punishments that operated in the clinic may also have helped to shape the pattern of 'acceptable' hysterical behaviour. For the patient who behaved well, the reward sometimes took the form of promotion to nursing assistant, with the financial and status increment that this entailed. On the other hand violent outbursts were controlled by the threat of removal to the section for the insane.

### 6.7.6  Outside the hospital

The example of Charcot demonstrates the capacity of doctors to shape the symptoms of their patients in certain conditions. However, we need also to look outside the hospital walls to the socio-cultural climate of the day. During the 1870s and 1880s, Charcot's example converted many other physicians to his view of hysteria as an inherited neurological disease. Although most visible at the Salpêtrière, *la grande hystérie* was found wherever there were physicians well versed in his doctrines, or where there were patients who had read colourful accounts in the press. Thus the number of recorded cases of hysteria dramatically increased, not only in France, but all through Europe.

France, at this time, was engaged in a struggle for scientific and cultural supremacy. Having lost political and military prestige after its humiliating defeat by the Prussians in 1871, the emphasis was placed instead on glorifying the State through intellectual and cultural achievement. The result was that during the last decades of the nineteenth century there was an unprecedented upsurge of artistic, literary and scientific talent centred on Paris (as you have already seen in Chapter 4).

It was also a time of modishness and exhibitionism. Fashionable life revolved around the café and the theatre, and Charcot's fame rivalled that of any actor. Theatricality was the order of the day, and among society women it was *à la mode* to behave like his hysterics, who themselves were often recognisable by their theatrical appearance, 'their flippant air and taste for finery' (Charcot, 1889, p. 39). The nearest, however, that a working-class woman was likely to get to playing a leading role at a fashionable event was to be selected as one of Charcot's *grandes hystériques*. Hysteria, in fact, became known as 'the sickness of the century' by writers who, at the time, recognised the influence of culture on medical thinking. One author, Jules Clarétie, in his 1882 portrayal of Parisian life, described it as the need to make an appearance, to stand out, to be seen and to create an uproar. This, he said, was inflaming the brains of his contemporaries. This description tacitly reveals the double-bind in which women were caught. Exhibitionist behaviour by males was never questioned. But expressed by a woman it was evidence that hysteria was not confined to the hospitals. Hysteria was the culturally unacceptable expression of feelings and frustrations, defined as a medical condition. During this period almost any female behaviour, conventional or otherwise, was likely to be interpreted in this way.

- ● From your reading of the article 'Hysteria and demonic possession', say what socio-cultural influences might have had a bearing on the form taken by Geneviève's attacks.

- ■ Geneviève was born and raised in Loudun and spent much of her childhood and adolescence at the Ursuline convent there. This was the scene of a demonic possession in the seventeenth century and the stories were well known. Her contact with the nuns and the religious emphasis of her education may have shaped the manifestations of her hysteria.

## 6.8   Freud's theory of the unconscious

With the passing of Charcot in 1893, the hysterical behaviour he had described ceased to be fashionable and within a generation *la grande hystérie* had ceased to exist at all. This illustrates the extent to which hysterical symptoms had been shaped by Charcot's medicine. Hysteria as a disorder did not disappear, but its form of expression changed.

The prime mover in developing a new approach to hysteria was Sigmund Freud (1856–1939). His importance in establishing current concepts of mental function and its disturbances has been immense and has indeed influenced Western thought as a whole. However it is not within the scope of this chapter to take more than a cursory glance at his theory of hysteria, let alone to do justice to the revolution created by him in psychiatry.

In 1885 the young Freud was awarded a travelling bursary that enabled him to spend some time studying at the Salpêtrière under Charcot. Here, he extended his interests to hysteria and hypnosis. On his return to Vienna he became more and more engaged in the treatment of the neuroses. It was this work which brought him into contact with Josef Breuer, a distinguished Viennese doctor, whose flourishing practice included patients suffering from hysteria. In collaboration with Breuer, Freud began to formulate a new therapeutic method based on the assumption that hysterical symptoms were the product of early psychical trauma. The hypnotised patient was induced to recall the trauma and express the concomitant emotions. In 1895 Freud and Breuer published jointly a work entitled *Studies on Hysteria*, containing case histories and a description by Freud of his technique. Before very long, however, Freud began making changes to both the method and the underlying theory. This led to a breach with Breuer and ultimately to the development by Freud of the system known as **psychoanalysis**.

What was most significant about Freud's psychoanalytic approach was that it shifted the emphasis away from clinical *observation* as the means of understanding the symptom, to *listening* to what the patient had to say. Central to this method was Freud's concept of the *unconscious*, mental processes of which the person is unaware. Freud postulated that some unconscious processes could easily become conscious, whilst others, such as fantasies, wishes and painful memories, because they are unacceptable, were subject to the defence mechanism of *repression*. These, nevertheless still remain active, indirectly influencing experience and behaviour, and producing neurotic symptoms. Freud regarded the symptom as a *symbol*, a kind of bodily metaphor for the expression of acute psychological distress. By 'reading' the symptom in this way, Freud was able to conceptualise neuroses such as hysteria, not as diseases of the nervous system, but as disorders of the *personality*. Psychoanalysis, by encouraging the patient consciously to confront repressed impulses, memories and emotions, helps to resolve them and thence to remove the symptom.

● What significant departure from Charcot's theory of hysteria was developed by Freud?

■ He offered an explanation of hysterical manifestations in purely psychological terms, giving meaning to symptoms and dispensing with the need to identify physical pathology.

## 6.9 The twentieth century

Changes in hysterical manifestations cannot be explained exclusively in terms of changing medical attitudes towards the conceptualisation of this condition. They need also to be understood in the context of major changes in the role of women in society, particularly in developed countries.

### 6.9.1 Changing social attitudes to women

During the twentieth century the rights of women in developed countries were enhanced. Both politically and economically women ceased to be invisible and to some extent their role was extended from the purely domestic sphere. During the First and Second World Wars female labour became a necessary commodity and women were able to show that they were capable of performing tasks usually reserved for men. During subsequent periods of economic prosperity women were again needed in the job market. Currently it is accepted as legitimate for women to be economically active.

The development of improved methods of contraception, concurrent with changing economic circumstances, has made greater choice possible for women with respect to child-bearing, allowing them to compete with men in the public sphere in a way that would have been unthinkable in the nineteenth century. Better contraception also brought with it a shift in attitudes towards sexuality. A greater freedom of sexual expression is now sanctioned for women, who no longer have to fear countless pregnancies and the dangers of childbirth. The role of vulnerable invalid is no longer as appropriate as it may have been for earlier generations.

### 6.9.2 Modern parallels with hysteria

Throughout the twentieth century there was considerable controversy over the diagnosis of hysteria. Some doctors argued that it is no longer a valid disease category and it has been dropped from some medical encyclopaedias. It may be that patients who at one time would have been labelled hysterics, may now be diagnosed as suffering from one of a range of mental disorders such as schizophrenia, multiple personality syndrome or personality disturbances — diagnoses that were not available in the days when hysteria was said to be rife.

Certain disorders of modern times resonate profoundly with the hysterical complaint. One such relatively common phenomenon is **anorexia nervosa**. This eating disorder, which is characterised by self-starvation, was in fact understood in the nineteenth century as a variant non-convulsive form of hysteria. Significantly its incidence among girls is currently about twenty times higher than among boys, the same ratio as was said to be the case for hysteria generally in the nineteenth century. Anorexia nervosa now, and hysteria as described by Charcot and Briquet, are found to occur most frequently in adolescence. It has been interpreted as a crisis reaction to sexual and emotional changes. Severe anorexia requires expert medical attention, usually in hospital, where it is treated as a psychiatric disturbance.

Another contemporary echo of the construction and reconstruction of hysteria is the condition which in recent times has come to be known as **chronic fatigue syndrome (CFS)**. Also known as 'postviral fatigue syndrome' and *myalgic encephalomyelitis* or ME, it is characterised by extremely low energy levels that are so debilitating that a normal pattern of life becomes impossible. Again there is no consensus of medical opinion. Chronic fatigue syndrome, which affects rather more women and girls than boys and men, is dismissed by some doctors as malingering and as a result, like hysteria, it has tended to carry pejorative connotations. Unlike anorexia, which is medically understood as a psychiatric condition, there is a dispute about whether CFS is a physical rather than a mental disorder. People with CFS and an increasing number of doctors believe that it is a consequence of an earlier infection by a virus. However, scientific evidence of disturbances to cell function which might explain the chronic fatigue remains controversial. Thus there is medical uncertainty as to the true nature of the complaint. The debate surrounding CFS demonstrates that it is still the case that the surest route to medical 'respectability' for a new disease category is to identify an underlying physical cause. In spite of the contributions of Freud and others, purely psychological diseases are of doubtful status.

## 6.10   Conclusion

Hysteria has always been the cause of considerable dispute. It is the classic 'fashionable disease' that has fluctuated and varied throughout the ages, making the question as to whether it constitutes a 'real' disease both complex and controversial. Descriptions of hysteria have changed enormously over time and a wide variety of criteria have been used historically for its diagnosis. Some instances of hysteria recorded in the past were almost certainly cases of diseases now found to have organic causes. It has been dismissed by some doctors as the wilful malingering of attention-seeking women, an example of the feminine penchant for deceit.

There is now no general agreement among doctors as to whether hysteria should be considered as a disease entity. Contemporary psychiatric criteria of hysteria, no less than those of former times, are shifting and controversial. Nevertheless the many and various theories of hysteria share one thing in common. They reflect professional and popular views of women and consequently reveal the importance of the prevailing socio-cultural context in the construction of this disease concept.

In the twentieth century, analyses of the significance of gender roles in the production of hysteria gained ascendence. Before this time medical inquiry was still focused primarily on the body, although as you have seen, the site of its investigation underwent major changes. Although the rise of the methods of natural observation and experiment were problematic, they led, most importantly, to the decline of religious and supernatural interpretations of the condition. By the nineteenth century, hysteria was localised in the brain and nervous system. This view ended for good the claims of gynaecologists and obstetricians to authority over the subject. However, the neurological view of functional lesions of the nervous system as the seat of hysterical symptoms, was not substantiated and was motivated by the desire to legitimate disease categories by finding a physical correlate.

Charcot's work in particular illustrates the attempt to make mental phenomena conform to the disease model developed for physical diseases. Although Charcot's theory amply satisfied the prevailing view of science, his approach, as you have seen, shaped and moulded the hysterical phenomena that he studied. Not until Freud developed his theory of the unconscious would hysteria be understood in purely psychological terms. Although such non-physical theories of disease are now much more widely accepted than in Charcot's time, the case of CFS shows continuing scepticism by some doctors about diseases for which they have been unable to find a convincing physical cause.

Comparison with TB highlights major differences in the manner in which different diseases may be shaped by biological as opposed to social factors. In the case of hysteria the social factors are paramount, and it is this non-medical feature of the disorder that makes it so intractable to medical certainty. The cultural relativism and flexibility of the concept 'hysteria' emphasises most starkly that medical knowledge and practice cannot be dissociated from the socio-cultural context in which they occur. As you have seen, the 'meaning' of hysteria is altogether different in the ancient Egyptian world, the world of demonology in the Middle Ages, in nineteenth-century neuroscience and in late twentieth-century psychiatry. By the start of the new millennium, 'hysteria' had become an everyday shorthand for mass excitement at rock concerts and sporting events. We cannot foresee how it might evolve in the future.

## OBJECTIVES FOR CHAPTER 6

When you have studied this chapter, you should be able to:

**6.1** Define and use, or recognise definitions and applications of, each of the terms printed in **bold** in the text.

**6.2** Demonstrate how medical science has been influenced by cultural stereotypes of women, using examples from the history of hysteria.

**6.3** Using examples from the history of hysteria, illustrate the decline of religious interpretations and the rise of naturalistic and secular views.

**6.4** Illustrate how the experimental and therapeutic approach to the investigation and treatment of hysteria could influence the form it took.

**6.5** Discuss the extent to which the modern conception of disease has been formed by the requirement to find physical correlates of clusters of symptoms.

**6.6** Outline the possible reasons why the hysteria diagnosis has declined during the twentieth century.

## QUESTIONS FOR CHAPTER 6

**1**  (*Objective 6.2*)

How did hysteria become associated with a stereotype of female refinement in the seventeenth and eighteenth centuries?

**2**  (*Objective 6.3*)

What form did early challenges to religious interpretations of hysteria take and how were these consistent with Renaissance thought?

**3**  (*Objective 6.4*)

How did the climate Charcot established at the Salpêtrière influence the production of *la grande hystérie*?

**4**  (*Objective 6.5*)

To what extent were Willis, Charcot and Freud intent on discovering or rejecting physical causes for hysteria?

**5**  (*Objective 6.6*)

Suggest why hysteria is rarely used as a diagnostic category nowadays.

# CHAPTER 7

## Medical knowledge and medical practice

**Study notes for OU students**

This chapter includes an analysis of the representation of the female reproductive system in medical textbooks. No prior knowledge of biological terms is assumed here; a more detailed account of biological and sociological processes in human reproduction is given in another book in this series, *Birth to Old Age: Health in Transition* (Open University Press, second edition 1995; colour-enhanced second edition 2001). During Section 7.4.1 of this chapter you will be asked to read an extract from an article by Sarah Nettleton entitled 'Protecting the vulnerable margin: towards an analysis of how the mouth came to be separated from the body', which can be found in *Health and Disease: A Reader* (Open University Press, second edition 1995; third edition 2001).

# 7.1 Cultural stereotypes in modern medicine

The rise and fall of the diagnosis of hysteria is an example of how medical science has been influenced by cultural stereotypes about women. You should understand by now that the scientific ideals of objectivity and rationality have developed gradually, over time; they are not fixed. In modern times, an appeal to scientific ideals is often made in boundary maintenance disputes (as discussed in Chapter 2), involving the claim that medicine is 'free from overriding social values and political bias' (BMA, 1986). The purpose of this chapter is to assess this claim.

First, we will continue from the last chapter's focus on the medical view of women by examining the extent to which *modern* medical accounts reflect cultural stereotypes about women, particularly in textbook descriptions of the female reproductive system. The discussion will then broaden out to consider the extent to which irrational elements enter clinical practice as well as medical knowledge. The clinical interview, a method of examining patients which all modern doctors are trained to use, will then be described. You will be invited to consider views that challenge the idea that this method is an objective means of scientific enquiry, free from the influence of cultural factors. We will touch on the problems as well as the insights given by these challenging views. The chapter ends with a discussion of the place of ritual in modern medical practice.

# 7.2 Menstruation

## 7.2.1 Medical metaphors

We will start with a feminist account of modern medical descriptions of the female reproductive system. As you read this, try to decide whether modern medicine has shaken off the negative images of women contained in the earlier medical accounts of hysteria described in the previous chapter. Here are two extracts from a modern American medical textbook on human reproduction describing, in turn, menstruation and spermatogenesis (the development of sperm cells).

> **Extract 1**
>
> The fall in blood progesterone and estrogen, which results from *regression* of the corpus luteum, *deprives* the highly developed endometrial lining of its hormonal support; the immediate result is *profound constriction* of the uterine blood vessels due to production of vasoconstrictor prostaglandins, which leads to *diminished* supply of oxygen and nutrients. *Disintegration* starts, and the entire lining (except for a thin, deep layer which will regenerate the endometrium in the next cycle) begins to slough.... The endometrial arteries dilate, resulting in *hemorrhage* through the weakened capillary walls; the menstrual flow consists of this blood mixed with endometrial *debris*....
>
> The menstrual flow ceases as the endometrium *repairs* itself and then grows under the influence of rising blood estrogen concentration. (Vander *et al.*, 1985, p. 577, quoted in Martin, 1989, p. 49, emphasis added by Martin)

**Extract 2**

The mechanisms which guide the *remarkable* cellular transformation from spermatid to mature sperm remain uncertain. Perhaps the most *amazing* characteristic of spermatogenesis is its *sheer magnitude*: the normal human male may manufacture several hundred million sperm per day. (Vander *et al.*, 1980, p. 483–4, quoted in Martin, 1989, p. 48, emphasis added by Martin)

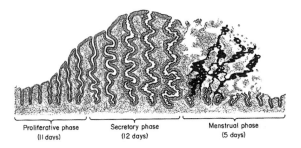

Proliferative phase          Secretory phase          Menstrual phase
   (11 days)                     (12 days)                (5 days)

**Figure 7.1**  *Changes in the endometrium during the monthly cycle. (Source: Guyton, A. C., 1981, Textbook of Medical Physiology, 6th edn, W. B. Saunders, Philadelphia, Figure 81–6, p. 81)*

● In what way might these descriptions, and the picture given in Figure 7.1, be seen as value-laden?

■ The words emphasised in italics suggest that menstruation is viewed as the *failure* of a process whose purpose is reproduction. The picture captures the imagery of disintegration. Spermatogenesis, on the other hand, is described in terms of awesome triumph.

Emily Martin, a social scientist from whose book (*The Woman in the Body: A Cultural Analysis of Reproduction*) these examples are taken, argues that modern medical texts are laden with *metaphors* about the body. Thus in the case of female reproduction a dominant metaphor is that of a signalling system in which parts of the body are seen as transmitting messages to each other, stimulating processes to occur. The imagery used to describe cells is often that of a factory producing substances. The image of the body as a machine is also a popular **medical metaphor**.[1] Menstruation is particularly subject to *evaluative* (or value-laden) metaphors in medical thought. Words that Martin found in other descriptions of menstruation were 'degenerate,' 'decline,' 'withdrawn,' 'lack,' 'weakened,' 'leak,' 'deteriorate,' 'discharge,' 'ceasing,' 'dying,' 'losing,' 'denuding' and 'expelling'.

● What objection might there be to seeing these extracts as value-laden?

■ Many people might feel that menstruation just *is* in some objective sense a process of breakdown and deterioration. The words fit the reality. The comparison of spermatogenesis with menstruation is unfair: the logical equivalent to spermatogenesis in men is the production of ova (egg cells) in women.

In fact, Martin *does* analyse descriptions of the production of ova. Ovarian *follicles*, which contain all the cells from which ova will develop after puberty, are already present at birth. They do not elicit the same enthusiasm as does spermatogenesis for medical writers. There is no stress on the vast excess of follicles produced in a female fetus compared to the number needed, rather an image of eggs that 'merely sit on the shelf, as it were, slowly degenerating and aging like overstocked inventory' (Martin, 1989, p. 74).

Martin also points out that the regular shedding of the stomach lining to protect the stomach from self-digestion is a bodily process analogous to menstruation, yet medical textbooks describe this as a positive event of renewal and replenishment, without the negative connotations of deterioration that are applied to menstruation. Nor is the fact of shed cellular material being a constituent of *seminal fluid* (semen) mentioned in the medical texts that Martin analysed.

[1] As you saw in Chapter 5, Descartes, in the seventeenth century, originally used mechanical metaphors to describe the human body.

The strength of Martin's work is that it sensitises us to the subtle messages that lie behind apparently objective scientific explanations. When we examine the thought of people in past times, or in other cultures, it is often very easy to 'see' apparently irrational elements, because the contrast with our own common sense is obvious. This is normally more difficult when looking at knowledge produced in our own culture because of our attachment to 'our' way of thinking.

● What is the process of standing back and analysing our own cultural beliefs called? (Think back to Chapter 2.)

■ Making things anthropologically strange.

## 7.2.2  Menstrual taboos

Anthropological studies of menstrual symbolism in a variety of cultures have often uncovered **menstrual taboos**. Some of these were described in Chapter 5. The word 'taboo' is derived from the Polynesian *ta*, which means 'to mark,' and *pu*, which means 'thoroughly'. Menstrual taboos are practices that set menstruating women apart from normal social life involving, for example, restrictions on the preparation of food, or sexual relations. They are associated with views of menstruation as dirty or shameful, a process to be hidden. The function of these taboos may be to guard against *symbolic pollution*, and many anthropologists argue that they are promoted by men to assert dominance over women. Martin's work draws attention to the parallels between such practices and modern medical knowledge which, she argues, maintains its historical allegiance to male interests.

However, recent anthropological work has been critical of the view that menstrual taboos are always associated with women's subordination. Sometimes, indeed, they are associated with the opposite. Until recently, among the Yurok Indians of California, a menstruating woman was segregated to a special shelter where food was prepared and eaten separately from the rest of the family. Yurok women perceived this as an opportunity for the renewal of energy and the concentration of power. Similarly, there are a variety of taboos amongst the Beng of the Ivory Coast. Far from being oppressive, these practices are an assertion of the special relationship that Beng women are felt to have with the fertility of the earth. A Beng man said about this:

> Menstrual blood is special because it carries in it a living being. It works like a tree. Before bearing fruit, a tree must first bear flowers. Menstrual blood is like the flower: it must emerge before the fruit — the baby — can be born. Childbirth is like a tree finally bearing its fruit, which the woman then gathers. (Buckley and Gottlieb, 1988, p. 58)

This metaphor of a tree contrasts with the medical metaphor of menstruation being a failure in a factory-like production process, identified by Martin. Martin presents her own alternative description of menstruation to show how the process might be presented in a more positive light in modern medical textbooks.

> A drop in the formerly high levels of progesterone and estrogen creates the appropriate environment for reducing the excess layers of endometrial tissue. Constriction of capillary blood vessels causes a lower level of oxygen and nutrients and paves the way for a vigorous production of menstrual fluids. As a part of the renewal

of the remaining endometrium, the capillaries begin to re-open, contributing some blood and serous fluid to the volume of endometrial material already beginning to flow. (Martin, 1989, p. 52)

By proposing a metaphor of renewal and replenishment to replace the metaphor of disintegration, Martin hopes to encourage a more positive view of menstruation in both doctors and women.

## 7.3   Variations in medical practice

If medical knowledge is influenced by cultural beliefs, as Emily Martin argues, this undermines the modern view of science as an objective, value-free way of thinking. The medical practitioner's task is often seen as the rational application of medical knowledge; problems arise when that knowledge is influenced by non-rational factors, or when doubt replaces certainty, giving an insufficient basis for consistent practice.

### 7.3.1   Surgical rates

In the early 1980s there was a growing awareness among doctors that there were variations in medical practice across countries that were difficult to explain. Table 7.1 compares rates of use of some common surgical procedures in New England (USA), Southern Norway and a British health authority in the 1970s.

**Table 7.1**   Surgical rates per 100 000 population in three New England States, Southern Norway, and the West Midlands Regional Health Authority (RHA) between 1974 and 1978.[1]

| Surgical procedure | New England | Norway | West Midlands RHA |
|---|---|---|---|
| hernia repair | 276 | 186 | 137 |
| appendectomy | 128 | 150 | 177 |
| cholecystectomy (removal of gall bladder) | 238 | 86 | 89 |
| prostatectomy (removal of prostate) | 264 | 236 | 132 |
| hysterectomy | 540 | 118 | 220 |
| hemorrhoidectomy (removal of rectal piles) | 76 | 45 | 28 |
| tonsillectomy | 289 | 64 | 172 |

[1] The rates are adjusted to allow for differences in the age and gender profiles of the populations. (Source: McPherson *et al.*, 1982, p. 1 311, Table 1)

● In which country was a person most likely to undergo surgery?

■ The New England rates were the highest for all the operations except appendectomy (known as appendicectomy in the United Kingdom).

● What might explain the variation?

■ Two explanations are possible: first, there may have been variation in clinical need (e.g. more people had appendicitis in the West Midlands than in New England); second, there may have been variation in the clinical judgements of doctors (perhaps influenced by patients who preferred surgical solutions).

In fact, the second explanation is generally accepted to be the one that best explains variations such as these, because the health profiles of these nations are fairly similar. Variation in clinical judgement occurs because of the lack of agreement between doctors on appropriate indicators for intervention. This allows fashion and cultural preference to influence decisions about treatment.

Various attempts have been made to explain why there is such a high volume of surgery in the USA. One possible explanation relates to the way in which medical services are paid for. In the USA doctors are paid for what they do (known as **fee-for-service medicine**), so there is an incentive to over-treat people, the majority of whom pass the costs on to third-party insurance companies. In the United Kingdom, the NHS doctor is paid the same amount however much he or she does, so there is an incentive to under-treat.

Rosemary Stevens, a historian of medicine, explains the difference as arising from the different organisation of American and British medicine during the nineteenth and twentieth centuries.[2] In the USA, an oversupply of doctors and an absence of regulatory bodies ensured intense competition between doctors for patients. A system of referral from GP to specialist became institutionalised in British medicine in the early part of the twentieth century, but this could not occur in the USA as referral of a patient to another doctor meant a loss of income. The American doctor was therefore under pressure to cover all aspects of patients' care, so participation in surgery was desired by most doctors and became a part of medical culture. In the United Kingdom, surgery remained the preserve of the few.

Others prefer explanations that draw upon notions of national character. Lynn Payer, a journalist, describes the American view of medicine as part of a national 'can-do' attitude.

> This medical aggressiveness reflects an aggressiveness of the American character that has often been attributed to the effect the vast frontier had on the people (mostly Europeans) who came to settle it…. Disease…could be conquered, but only by aggressively ferreting it out diagnostically and just as aggressively treating it, preferably by taking something out. (Payer, 1990, p. 127)

The aggressive treatment approach of American surgeons, compared to other doctors, is summarised in the comment of a leading American surgeon:

> A surgeon knows nothing, but does everything. An internist[3] knows everything but does nothing. A psychiatrist knows nothing and does nothing. A pathologist knows everything, and does everything, one day too late. (A. Schwartzbart, quoted in Katz, 1985, p. 155)

---

[2] See Rosemary Stevens, 'The evolution of health-care systems in the United States and the United Kingdom: similarities and differences' in *Health and Disease: A Reader* (Open University Press, 2nd edn 1995; 3rd edn 2001). This article is set as essential reading in connection with *Caring for Health: History and Diversity* (Open University Press, 2nd edn 1993; 3rd edn 2001), Chapter 4. This book also reviews contemporary methods of financing health care around the world (see Chapter 9).

[3] Internist is an American term for a specialist in internal medicine.

Decisions on how to treat illness are normally based upon what doctors have been trained to do, or upon what, during their clinical careers, they have come to believe to be effective. David Eddy, an American cardiothoracic surgeon and professor of health policy, has estimated that only about 15 per cent of medical interventions are supported by solid scientific evidence (Smith, 1991). Early in his medical career Eddy became concerned about the evidence to support what he and other doctors were doing. He began his investigation of this by selecting the treatments for glaucoma[4] that were commonly advocated in medical texts and found that there had been no trial of the effectiveness of the standard treatment for this condition. Treatment practices had simply been handed down from one generation of doctors to another. He did the same analysis for a number of other standard treatments, and his figure of 15 per cent was the eventual product of this research.

Eddy became a speaker much in demand at international **consensus conferences**, which are meetings of doctors and other interested parties trying to establish agreement on the best method of treating particular diseases. Such conferences usually start by summarising the available scientific literature concerning the effectiveness of treatments, with leading experts in the field contributing. Treatment protocols are produced, which represent the most up to date view on the best way of treating particular diseases. Consensus conferences are part of a wider strategy (termed **evidence-based medicine** in the 1990s) which encouraged doctors to adopt scientifically tested treatment protocols, thus increasing effectiveness and eliminating the grosser variations in clinical practice.[5]

● Why should doctors be concerned about variations in clinical practice?

■ It is a waste of resources to treat people when it is not necessary, and wrong to treat with therapies that are less effective than alternatives. Evidence of clinical variation is also embarrassing to a profession concerned to promote an image of scientific rationality.

## 7.3.2 Medical fashions

If some medical activity is based on tradition and belief rather than on proven effectiveness, the door is open for **medical fashions** to influence practice. You saw in the example of hysteria (Chapter 6) that certain disease categories may come and go and equally ephemeral treatments whose rationale depends on the category currently in vogue are constructed. Some of the treatments advocated for TB (Chapter 4) also demonstrate irrational attachment to particular methods (for example, surgical treatments). The history of medicine is littered with rejected disease categories. The advocates of particular diagnoses compete for inclusion, sometimes supported by vocal groups of sufferers anxious to gain the medical legitimacy of a disease label and the comfort of associated treatments. In recent years diseases such as hyperactivity, chronic fatigue syndrome, and post-traumatic stress disorder have achieved partial medical recognition.

[4] In glaucoma, the pressure within the eye rises and destroys the visual nerve fibres, causing blindness if untreated.

[5] Evidence-based medicine and other initiatives by practitioners to set agreed standards of health care are discussed in several chapters of *Dilemmas in UK Health Care* (Open University Press, 2nd edn 1993; 3rd edn 2001).

There is also some international variation in modern medical disease categories. Until the mid-1970s, *crise de foie* (liver problems) was commonly invoked by French doctors to explain a variety of conditions, ranging from migraine headache to tonsillitis. Drug prescribing practices reflected the targeting of the liver as the site of disease. The decline of the French medical interest in the liver resulted from a growing awareness of its culture-bound nature among liver specialists exposed to foreign influence. By contrast, German doctors exhibit a unique concern with low blood pressure, which they identify as a cause for feelings of tiredness and fainting and treat in a variety of ways. The British diagnosis of chilblains has no clear equivalent in other countries.

Medical fashions in treatment have also been revealed in studies of medical education. Training to be a doctor inevitably involves discussion between teachers and students of reasons for doing things. Here are some extracts from the field notes of Paul Atkinson, a sociologist observing clinical teaching in an Edinburgh medical school in the late 1970s.

> They discussed the problems of high blood pressure and reducing it. Dr Cowan told us that on admission, the patient had a palpable fourth heart sound, and they had been afraid he'd go into failure. 'The question is,' he said, 'What drug do you use to reduce blood pressure?' The students suggested a number of possible treatments, and Dr Cowan commented, 'You get used to one drug. Propalanol is used a lot in Edinburgh.'...
>
> ...The surgeon had explained to the [students] the difference between 'simple' and 'radical' mastectomies. Returning to the patient who had provided the starting point for the more general discussion, the surgeon told us, 'In this city, she'd have a simple mastectomy; in Edinburgh it's accepted that most units do a simple mastectomy...' (Atkinson, 1981, p. 111)

● What do these extracts reveal about medical fashions in treatment?

■ They may have a local character, based on the traditions that have built up within particular medical schools.

*Medical schools can pass on local fashions in treatment to students and so can individual consultants. (Photo: Mike Levers)*

## 7.4 The clinical method

Being a doctor involves an overriding orientation towards action. Students must learn how to interview patients, how to take blood samples, and how in general to achieve a medical appearance. Superficially, this may be gained by wearing certain items, such as a white coat and a stethoscope, and the significance of such objects will be discussed later in this chapter in a section on ritual. However, actual experience in dealing with patients is sought after hungrily by medical students, because such clinical experience is thought of as a stock of personal legitimacy, rivalling the book-learning that is supposed to underlie medical practice. At the core of medical practice is the **clinical method**, that is the method used by practitioners to arrive at judgements about the patient.

One of the first things that medical students have to learn is the way in which doctors discover what is wrong with their patients. The basis of this is in the process known as **diagnosis**. This is the art of distinguishing one disease from another, and finally naming the disease presented. In diagnosis a high degree of skill is required, and a number of techniques are involved.

As the first step in making a diagnosis, the young prospective doctor is taught to **take a history**. This involves the patient describing their experience in their own words, from which the doctor is expected to select only those elements that are of medical significance (i.e. those that indicate the presence of a disease). These significant items of information include the **symptoms** of which the patient complains. The taking of a history should include an account of the patient's past medical career, and in some cases may also include his or her history family and social background. In addition, a **physical examination** may be performed using a variety of tools for listening and looking within the body.

● What were the techniques of physical examination discussed in Chapter 5?

■ Pulse-feeling, percussion, palpation and auscultation (for which the stethoscope was developed), the measurement of blood heat (for which the thermometer is used).

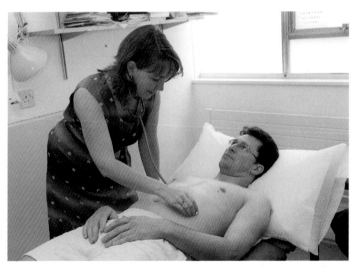

*Physical examination forms an important part of the clinical method.*
*(Photo: Mike Levers)*

**Diagnostic tests** requiring special support, such as laboratory analysis, may also be called upon. Examination and testing may reveal clinical **signs**, which are abnormalities of the body (for example, high blood pressure) which the patient is not aware of (at least initially) and so cannot report, but which may nevertheless be indicative of a disease. The process of assembling this information is increasingly informed by *provisional* diagnoses, which are like the *hypotheses* in a scientific experiment. They are the doctor's best guesses about what might be wrong with the patient, to be accepted or rejected on the basis of further investigation until, ideally, a single diagnosis is logically isolated. Diagnosis is to be distinguished from **prognosis**, which is a forecast of the probable course and result of an illness, particularly with regard to the prospect of recovery. Once a diagnosis is formulated, treatment may then proceed.

Underlying a diagnosis is an implicit statement about a *pathological lesion*, which is some disturbance in the normal structure or function of the body. As you saw in Chapter 2, the requirement that *disease labels* be related to pathologies is crucial in maintaining the modern scientific medical view of disease. Old age, chill, abdominal pain and headache are frowned upon as diagnoses because they do not relate to a precisely identified underlying pathology, and therefore cannot be taken as identifying diseases.

● What are the components of the modern medical definition of a disease? (Recall Chapter 2.)

■ A disease should have a physical cause, involving a disturbance to a part or parts of the body's structure, and follow a recognisable course with characteristic symptoms.

● How did Charcot seek to define hysteria in these terms (see Chapter 6)?

■ He was unable to locate a specific pathological lesion, and suggested that the lesion was *functional*, or diffused through the nervous system in a way that could not be directly detected. He claimed that hysteria typically passed through four distinct stages, although not all cases exhibited all four (indeed, he only observed twelve that did).

## 7.4.1  Discovering or constructing disease?

The clinical interview is characteristically thought of as a process of *discovery* in which the identity of the disease is *revealed* through the process of taking a history and identifying symptoms and signs. There is, however, another view that regards the doctor, in applying the clinical method, as *constructing* the disease. The origins of this view, sometimes called the **social constructionist** approach to medicine, lie in a particular reading of history, which is summarised by David Armstrong, a doctor and sociologist.

> I doubt if it ever occurred to me or my fellow medical students that the human body which we dissected and examined was other than a stable experience. It was therefore with considerable surprise that years later I learned that it was only since the end of the eighteenth century that disease had been localised to specific organs and tissues, and that bodies had been subjected to the rigours of clinical examination.

At first it seemed strange to me how the apparent obviousness of disease and its manifestations inside the body had eluded scientific discovery for so long. How had pre-Enlightenment generations failed to see the clearly differentiated organs and tissues of the body? Or failed to link patients' symptoms with the existence of localised pathological processes? Or failed to apply the most rudimentary diagnostic techniques of physical examination? My disbelief grew until it occurred to me that perhaps I was asking the wrong questions: the problem was not how something so obvious today had remained hidden for so long, but how the body had become so evident in the first place. In dissecting and examining bodies I had come to take for granted that what I saw was obvious. I had thought that medical knowledge simply described the body. I argue…that the relationship is more complex, that medical knowledge both describes and constructs the body as an invariate biological reality. (Armstrong, 1983, p. xi)

Figure 7.2 and its caption illustrate Armstrong's point that modern medical teaching *constructs* the way doctors see the body.

In the historical chapters of this book you saw that the modern medical view of how the body works, and indeed the modern conception of disease, emerged in *opposition* to previous ways of seeing the body. The distinction between signs and symptoms was not always made in the past, since this required the development of the idea of localised pathology underlying disease. Wherever 'bedside medicine' has been the dominant medical paradigm (see Chapter 3), physical examination for signs was restricted to the most detailed observation of the patients' external appearance and behaviour, and the patients' reports of symptoms were heavily relied upon. The search for underlying physical pathology was of marginal concern to a physician whose theories about the causes of disease were based primarily on readings of classical Greek writers, rather than on anatomical dissection. The whole

**Figure 7.2** *'The anatomical atlas stands between ignorance and medical knowledge. The atlas enables the anatomy student to see certain things and ignore others. In effect, what the student sees is not the atlas as a representation of the body but the body as a representation of the atlas.' (Armstrong, 1983, pp. 1–2) (Source: Warwick, R. and Williams, P. L., 1973, Gray's Anatomy, 35th edn, Churchill Livingstone, p. 624)*

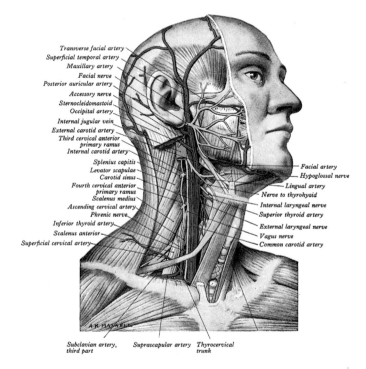

patient and their physical, emotional and spiritual world was seen as an *expression* of the disease, not as *distinct from* the disease. The concept of disease having characteristics independent of the unique character of the patient is a construction associated with the later paradigm of clinical or hospital medicine.

Armstrong sees no reason to give privileged status to the modern medical view of disease as located in physical pathology. In this respect, he shares the view of the British Holistic Medical Association reported in Chapter 2, to the effect that 'Science is not an objective reality, it is constructed as a social entity by persons' (BHMA, 1986, p. 69). This is the position of *cultural relativism,* and you should by now be familiar with some of the moral and conceptual problems that this philosophical stance raises. The social constructionist view, in essence, denies the idea that movement from one paradigm to another represents progress in the development of accurate accounts of the body. Disease categories are not neutral discoveries of facts, but are symbols of successful 'lobbying' by their advocates to get the categories accepted and used by doctors. Notions of medical progress are illusory and all that observers should try to do is to explain how it is that some systems of knowledge dominate in particular places or at particular periods in history.

● When it is said by sociologists that doctors *construct* disease, does this mean that their activities make patients ill?

■ No. For the social constructionist the issue is not whether patients are or are not 'really' ill. What is of interest is the way in which illnesses are described and categorised at a particular point in history.

In a sense, social constructionism is the ultimate end-point of making our own culture appear anthropologically strange. You may be feeling by now that the denial of medical progress by social constructionists is absurd. What point could there be in adopting such an extreme position; what sort of insights could it possibly give? The work of Sarah Nettleton, a social constructionist writer on the history of dentistry, shows the value of this approach. An extract from her article, 'Protecting the vulnerable margin: towards an analysis of how the mouth came to be separated from the body', is reprinted in the Reader.[6] (Open University students should read it now.)

● How does Nettleton describe the official medical view of the development of dentistry?

■ The official view is that increases in dental disease were caused by increased sugar consumption during the nineteenth century. This led to a greater need for more effective intervention, and dental knowledge duly developed.

● How is her view at variance with this?

■ Rather than dentistry being a response to conditions in mouths, she regards dentistry as having constructed a particular view of the mouth, based on thinking of it as the point of entry for contagion. The disciplines of oral hygiene, such as toothbrush drill, were ritualised ways of keeping out germs, an extension of the Victorian interest in public health and hygiene. This, and the regular dental check-up, were also ways of promoting discipline in the population — particularly in children — and encouraging a sense of what was 'normal'.

[6] *Health and Disease: A Reader* (Open University Press, 2nd edn 1995; 3rd edn 2001).

Writers within the social constructionist tradition usefully alert us to the influence of cultural factors in medicine. However, many accuse them of exaggerating the degree to which these, rather than the reality of the natural world, determine the shape of medical knowledge. Social constructionists are able to argue their case because their position involves a (usually implicit) denial of the possibility of knowing about the world independently of the language used to describe it. Whether we agree with this or not, the usefulness of adopting this position is the subsequent ease with which a sense of anthropological strangeness is achieved, and the insights that then flow from this.

## 7.5    Ritual

Less extreme than the social constructionist position is the view that distinguishes elements of medical practice that serve a **ritual** function from those that serve a *technical* function. Rituals perform symbolic acts of transformation, often being concerned with a passage from one status in life to another, such as the well-known ritual of male circumcision. This may on the one hand be regarded as ritual that transforms boys into men, or affirms a cultural identity (e.g. Jewishness). On the other hand it has sometimes been explained as a technical act (it keeps the penis free from infection) and is thus freed from ritual connotations. The distinction between ritual and technical realms implies a degree of acceptance that medical knowledge can describe reality in an objective and value-free manner. Cecil Helman uses this distinction in defining ritual:

> …for those that take part in it, ritual has important social, psychological and symbolic dimensions. A key characteristic of any rituals is that they are a form of repetitive behaviour that does not have a direct overt technical effect. For example, brushing one's teeth at the same time each night is a repetitive form of behaviour, but not a ritual. It is designed to have a specific physical effect: the removal of food and bacteria from the teeth. (Helman, 1990, p. 192)

● If brushing teeth is not a ritual for Helman, why is it one for Nettleton?

■ Helman may not be aware of the early history of dentistry, where other, less rational, purposes were given for the brushing of teeth; but even if he did, he believes it is possible to describe and act upon an external reality in a rational manner. Nettleton would not recognise the distinction between actions done for technical reasons and those done for symbolic reasons, and would argue that 'external reality' is in fact socially constructed.

An important function of ritual is to mark in a symbolic way what is considered dirty, polluting or bad. You saw earlier that this was often a function of menstrual taboo. (Remember, literally, taboo means 'to mark thoroughly'.) Ritual also marks out individuals who are designated with powers to control pollution. Modern medical theories depend heavily on the idea of contagion, and medical practice may depend on its control.

The sociologist Julius Roth, writing in 1957, observed the wearing of protective clothing by medical and other staff in a hospital treating people with tuberculosis. Masks, gowns and hair coverings were supposed to be worn whenever staff came into contact with patients. However, Roth observed that these items were not always worn. He recorded compliance with the regulations according to the grade of staff, and according to the purpose of the contact (whether socialising or work).

*Ritual clothing and symbols of authority mark out individuals who are designated with powers to control pollution and heal the sick: a witchdoctor from the Aymara people in Bolivia and an anaesthetist in an English hospital. (Sources: (left) David Mercado/Reuters/Popperfoto; (right) photo: Mike Levers)*

● The results are presented in Tables 7.2 and 7.3. What do the two tables show?

**Table 7.2**  Wearing of protective clothing by doctors and nursing personnel in hospital.

| Staff grade | Times entered room | Percentages wearing: | | |
|---|---|---|---|---|
| | | Cap | Gown | Mask |
| doctors | 47 | 5 | 0 | 5 |
| professional nurses | 100 | 24 | 18 | 14 |
| practical nurses[1] | 121 | 86 | 45 | 46 |
| aides | 142 | 94 | 80 | 72 |
| students | 97 | 100 | 100 | 100 |

[1] Practical nurses were of a lower grade than professional nurses. (Source: Roth, 1957, p. 312, Table 2)

**Table 7.3**  Wearing of protective clothing by practical nurses when carrying out duties and when 'socialising' with patients.

| Purpose of contact | Times entered room | Percentages wearing: | | |
|---|---|---|---|---|
| | | Cap | Gown | Mask |
| carry out duties | 39 | 97 | 75 | 80 |
| socialising | 23 | 91 | 17 | 9 |

(Source: Roth, 1957, p. 314, Table 4)

■ The wearing of protective clothing is more common in lower staff grades, with doctors rarely and students always wearing the clothes. Practical nurses are less likely to wear the items when socialising, more likely when carrying out duties. The cap is the item least likely to be discarded.

Roth says that higher grade staff broke the clothing rule more often because they were more likely to know that there was little scientific evidence to justify the wearing of the clothes. Higher grades were also less likely to be chastised for failure to obey the rules. Of the results in Table 7.3 he remarks wryly: '[This] suggests that the tubercle bacillus works only during business hours' (Roth, 1957, p. 314).

Later authors have made similar observations about the wearing of protective clothing in operating theatres, particularly the wearing of masks. Nicholas Fox, a sociologist observing surgery in a British hospital in the 1980s, noticed (as did Roth) that many wearers of masks drew them down below the nose for comfort. This was done particularly by anaesthetists, and also by many surgeons, but rarely by nurses. He asked a theatre sister about the scientific justification for wearing masks.

> *Theatre sister:* These things work for two minutes, and then have no effect. At the Children's Hospital they've stopped wearing them. There's no evidence that they work.
>
> *Fox:* So it's traditional and symbolic?
>
> *Theatre sister:* Yes. You do what the boss says, so here we do some things which are not done elsewhere. (Fox, 1992, p. 27)

If the technical function of surgical masks is so openly acknowledged to be doubtful, there must be some other purpose. There are in fact two ritual functions to the wearing of specialised clothing.

● Can you suggest what they are?

■ First, the wearing of ritual clothing serves to mark out status distinctions, in particular the right of particular individuals to assess the implications of medical knowledge for themselves (and, in this case, display their status by pulling down the mask). Second, the wearing of ritual clothing is a sign that the wearer may engage in a special type of activity, that would otherwise be prohibited.

Surgery is an assault on the body, which if it occurred in any other social setting would be regarded with horror. Hence consultant surgeons often wear expensive suits on ward rounds, the absence of a white coat perhaps indicating that they are

*Surgery is an assault on the body which would be regarded with horror if it occurred in any other social setting. (Photo: Deep Light Productions/Science Photo Library)*

not just 'butchers'. This second function of operating room ritual was described by the anthropologist Pearl Katz. She notes the profound effects that rituals concerning antisepsis have on the participants. She observed the doctors whom she had seen operating watching a film about different techniques for draining and lancing pus-filled abscesses.

> The boundaries which separate the operating room from the outside contribute to a particular mental set for the participants, which enable them to participate in a dispassionate manner in activities they would ordinarily view with strong emotion. For example, in the operating room, they look dispassionately upon, and touch internal organs and their secretions, blood, pus and feces. Outside of the operating room context, these same objects provoke emotions of embarrassment, fear, fascination and disgust in the same persons…. The reactions observed for the surgeons watching this movie were unlike any reactions observed for the same surgeons while they drained abscesses in the operating room. They uttered comments and noises indicating their disgust. They looked away from the screen…. Outside of the operating room there are no rituals to diffuse their concentration. The operating room, with its focus on precise rituals, permits diffusion of emotions and encourages discontinuity from everyday life. (Katz, 1981, p. 345)

Medical students learn that a variety of ritual objects, such as the wearing of a white coat and stethoscope, can help them to achieve the social transition from student to doctor. Achieving this transition is not just a matter of how doctors appear to others, but also how they feel about themselves. In this sense, people act as their own audience.

Identifying the ritual aspects of medical practice exposes some of the mystery that surrounds this powerful group of practitioners. This may be profoundly unsettling for people who like to rely on certainty and believe in the objective nature of science. For others it may be used to legitimate a destructive attitude towards medical power that fails to recognise the benefits that medicine has brought. The social science of medicine treads uneasily along this path.

## OBJECTIVES FOR CHAPTER 7

When you have studied this chapter, you should be able to:

**7.1** Define and use, or recognise definitions and applications of, each of the terms printed in **bold** in the text.

**7.2** Identify cultural influences on modern medical knowledge.

**7.3** Define the terms used to describe the modern clinical method, including history taking, symptoms, signs, diagnostic tests, disease labels, diagnosis, treatment and prognosis.

**7.4** Distinguish between accounts of the clinical method as a social construction, or as a process of discovery of external reality.

**7.5** Distinguish ritual from technical aspects of medical practice, and comment on their symbolic meaning.

## QUESTIONS FOR CHAPTER 7

**1** (*Objective 7.2*)

Figure 7.3 is an attempt by a *Time* magazine artist to show how the human immunodeficiency virus (HIV, then known as HTLV, Human T-cell Leukaemia Virus), which causes AIDS, reproduces. What metaphors are being used, and what type of medical practice might be associated with such metaphors?

**Figure 7.3**  *A contemporary image of cells as factories. (Source:* Time *magazine, 30 April 1984, Vol. 67, Figure 6, p. 38; reprinted by permission from* Time*)*

**2** (*Objective 7.3*)

Identify the taking of a history, signs, symptoms, physical examination and diagnosis in the following account.

> [The doctor] asked him what had made him come into the hospital. He replied...that he had pain, indicating his abdomen. [The doctor] asked if he had had any trouble with his stomach previously; he said that he had had 'a lot of gas' over the previous year and had hiccoughed a lot. The surgeon asked him if he had been taking any pills or powders for his stomach. The patient said he hadn't. [The doctor] asked him if he was in pain now, and the patient told us that he was.... [The doctor] then palpated the abdomen.... [The doctor] then turned to the [X-ray] films and asked the students what they could see.... Somebody volunteered, 'a burst duodenal ulcer', while [another student] muttered 'ruptured viscus.'... [Another student] suggested that it might be the bladder.... [The doctor] pointed out that the bladder is outside the peritoneum and doesn't contain air anyway...[he] said he would put his money on this patient having a ruptured diverticulum. (Atkinson, 1981, p. 92)

**3** (*Objective 7.4*)

Are the students in the extract above constructing the patient's disease, or discovering it?

**4** (*Objective 7.5*)

To what extent is the brushing of teeth a ritual activity?

# CHAPTER 8

## Medicalisation and surveillance

**Study notes for OU students**

During this chapter you will be asked to read two articles from *Health and Disease: A Reader* (Open University Press, second edition 1995; third edition 2001). In Section 8.3.2 you should read 'Malingering' by Richard Asher, and in Section 8.4.1, 'The epidemics of modern medicine' by Ivan Illich. A third article, 'The mode of state intervention in the health sector', by Vicente Navarro, is optional reading for Section 8.4.2 of this chapter.

*Uniformed warders at Horton Asylum, 1907. Medicine and therapeutic institutions can have a significant part in controlling the 'sick'. (Source: Hulton Getty Picture Collection)*

## 8.1   Introduction

By now, you should be familiar with the idea that medical knowledge and practice are thoroughly bound up with other forms of knowledge and practice in society. That is, you should by now appreciate the mutual influence between medicine and its *social context*. This chapter will take you further along this road. First, you will be invited to consider the view that the modern medical profession — as well as alleviating and preventing illness — performs a specific social function in maintaining social order, by regulating the conduct of the sick. Medical knowledge is ever-expanding, and this chapter will describe the fears of some that this expansion into ever more areas of social life — a process known as **medicalisation** — may have harmful consequences. The counter-argument, that medicalisation represents progress, will also be considered. Finally, an account of medicine as a system of *surveillance* of the population will be given.

Initially, however, we shall consider the origins of the medical specialist in less developed societies than the United Kingdom. Through this, we can approach some of the fundamental issues involved in interpreting the role of modern doctors.

## 8.2   The origins of medical specialism

When people live together in groups a division of labour emerges. Individuals become specialists at the various tasks that face the group and expertise develops as a result. Specialists may then be regarded as having knowledge and powers that can be passed from one person to another, perhaps by technical training, perhaps by magical ceremony. The idea that harm can be done by those possessing special powers lies very deep in the roots of our social consciousness.

Horacio Fabrega, to whose work you were introduced in Chapter 2, has described the emergence of specialist healers in societies with elementary systems of medicine. In some of the groups he studied, there were no such healers. However, in groups where medical systems of thought were more complex, there was a need for specialists, or *shamans*, who had the knowledge or experience deemed necessary to influence illness. In particular, shamans increasingly came to direct healing rituals, which themselves involved fewer people — typically members of the immediate family and an apprentice to the healer. Shamans were often seen as having the power to communicate with the spirit world from which illness was believed to originate.

Fabrega found that accusations of sorcery as a cause of illness were only found in groups where shamans had developed as specialist healers. This was because the power to heal was perceived as the personal possession of the shaman, rather than as generally diffused through the group. The shaman's capacity to communicate with the spirit world could then be used to harm as well as to heal (Fabrega, 1979).

## 8.3  Doctors, social order and the sick role

Accounts of sorcery and witchcraft are familiar to us in children's stories, but we rarely consider our own society to possess shamans, except in the lurid accounts of bizarre magical practices that appear in many tabloid newspapers. However, we do live in a society where there is a complex division of labour, and where an enormous variety of specialist healing roles are recognised. We attribute to our modern healers a great deal of power, and trust that they will use it for our benefit rather than to harm us. Professional codes of ethics are basically promises that doctors will use their knowledge to benefit patients. There is a generally recognised contract between doctors and the people they serve, that consists of rights, obligations and privileges for both doctors and patients. The sociologist Talcott Parsons, writing in 1951, described what he considered to be the key points of this contract; these are summarised in Box 8.1. These rights, obligations and privileges are standards of behaviour, which Parsons felt people in American society believed desirable in the 1940s. The sociological term for such a standard of behaviour is a **norm**.

---

**Box 8.1  Parsons' analysis of the roles of patients and doctors**

*Patient: sick role*

*Obligations and privileges*

- Must want to get well as quickly as possible
- Should seek professional medical advice and cooperate with the doctor
- Allowed (and may be expected) to shed some normal activities and responsibilities (e.g. employment and household tasks)
- Regarded as being in need of care and unable to get better by his or her own decisions and will

*Doctor: professional role*

*Obligated to*

- Apply a high degree of skill and knowledge to the problems of illness
- Act for welfare of patient and community rather than for own self-interest, desire for money, advancement, etc.
- Be objective and emotionally detached (i.e. should not judge patients' behaviour in terms of personal value system or become emotionally involved with them)
- Be guided by rules of professional practice

*Rights*

- To examine patients physically and to enquire into intimate areas of physical and personal life
- Considerable autonomy in professional practice
- Position of authority in relation to the patient

*(Source: adapted from Scambler, G. (ed.), 1991, Sociology as Applied to Medicine, Baillière-Tindall, London, p. 50, Table 1)*

Sociologists distinguish between the physical and emotional manifestations of being 'sick' and the norms of behaviour considered proper for a sick person to adopt — the so-called **sick role**. To gain the right to be in a role such as the sick role, a person must conform to the norms attached to that role, otherwise other people will regard the claim (in this case, to be 'sick') as illegitimate. A person who does not abide by the norms of seeking medical advice, or wanting to get better, may be regarded as not 'really' sick, or at least as breaking the rules, and will not be accorded the privileges of the sick role. Entry to the sick role, then, is like entering into a bargain or negotiated contract.

### 8.3.1  Critics of Parsons

Later writers have been critical of Parsons. They argue that the obligations and privileges outlined for patients do not fit people's experience of illness. For example, the chronic, degenerative diseases associated with old age, which are incurable by medical science, are more common now than they were a hundred years ago.

● How well does Parsons' ideal fit the situation of a person disabled by chronic disease?

■ Not very well. A chronic disease, by definition, is one where the patient cannot expect to get better. Medical science may only be able to alleviate symptoms rather than cure the disease. The obligation to want to get well as quickly as possible would be unrealistic, and medical advice would be of limited use. The disabled person may have a better knowledge of his or her illness than the doctor and therefore be justified in deviating from some medical advice.

Parsons' model also seems to overlook the fact that there is a great deal of tension between doctors and patients over consultation for 'trivial' illnesses. General practitioners sometimes complain that they see too many of these; conversely, patients often hesitate to consult for fear of bothering the doctor unnecessarily. Thus patients in Parsons' ideal model are to some extent in a 'double bind' situation; they are expected to have sufficient medical knowledge to know whether something is trivial or not, but are also expected to relinquish claims to medical knowledge once they enter the surgery. Many people, these days, like to think of themselves as more able to take responsibility for their own health than the rather passive 'model patient' that Parsons describes.

Another criticism is that Parsons' ideal covers up the conflicts of interest that can exist between doctors and patients.

● Can you think of any such conflicts?

■ You may have thought of a number of these, but here are three:

1   It may be in a patient's interest to conceal a sexually transmitted disease, but the doctor may feel a responsibility to disclose it for the benefit of others.

2   It may be in a patient's interest to receive some very expensive treatment, but the doctor may feel responsible for rationing scarce resources, giving priority to others.

3  Medical students and junior doctors must learn their trade by gaining clinical experience, but the patients on whom they practise may get better treatment from doctors with more experience. (In fact, one enquiry into deaths associated with surgery has shown that these were more common where surgeons were of a more junior grade.)

However, although these criticisms can be made of Parsons, his view that the medical profession plays a key role in maintaining *social order* is an important one. There is a sense in which doctors act as moral guardians or gatekeepers, deciding who may enter the sick role and benefit from its privileges.

● From your reading of Chapter 2, who else might be involved in deciding that people are sick?

■ Most health care occurs in the *lay* sector. For example, parents may act as gatekeepers to the sick role for their children.

### 8.3.2  Doctors as moral guardians

The labelling of people as 'sick' establishes a blameless category, distinct from a general class of behaviour that would otherwise been seen as deviant or morally reprehensible. Failure to perform normal duties threatens the smooth working of social institutions, such as the work place. This is particularly evident in the issuing of sick notes by doctors, and the passionate debates that sometimes occur over whether a person is faking illness in order to avoid work responsibilities. A classic contribution to this theme can be found in the Reader article, 'Malingering' by Richard Asher, a doctor.[1] (Open University students should read it now.)

● How does Asher distinguish between malingering, hypochondria and hysteria?

■ It is difficult to distinguish clearly between these conditions, although he considers clear malingering to be rare. Whereas the malingerer deliberately imitates illness, merely pretending to be ill, hypochondriacs worry obsessively that they really are ill; so much so, in fact, that they would seemingly almost prefer to be ill. Hysteria is different again. The hysteric actually experiences the major physical symptoms described in Chapter 6, all without any observably faulty biology. To the sufferer, however, the illness is no less real than if the symptoms were produced by a 'real' biological malfunction.

## 8.4  Medicalisation and social control

The issuing of sick notes is something about which many doctors have mixed feelings. While they are concerned to do the best they can for their patients, this practice suggests a rather overt role in maintaining social order. This is an example of medical *practice* serving a function of **social control**, whereby people are ordered in a manner that allows a social system to function. However, medical *knowledge* also has a role in social control, and the **medicalisation thesis**, which is the subject of this section of the chapter, emphasises this.

---

[1] *Health and Disease: A Reader* (Open University Press, 2nd edn 1995; 3rd edn 2001).

### 8.4.1  The medicalisation thesis

The idea that society was becoming excessively medicalised gained currency in the 1970s when considerable scepticism was growing about the benefits of modern medicine. One of the leading proponents of this view was the philosopher and theologian Ivan Illich. An extract from Illich's article, 'The epidemics of modern medicine' appears in the Reader.[2] (Open University students should read it now.)

● What part has medicine played in improving health during the twentieth century, according to Illich?

■ In some areas it has been crucial, for example in pernicious anaemia and polio, but its overall effect has been far less important than the changes in the wider environment, such as better housing and working conditions, and in nutrition.

● What part does he claim medicine has played in creating new types of disease?

■ A major one. He lists as harmful the side-effects of many new drugs and the consequences of unnecessary surgery. For Illich, surgery and chemotherapy (drug treatment) are new forms of epidemic. Together, he calls these harmful effects of medical practice **iatrogenesis** (*iatros* is a Greek word for physician, thus iatrogenesis means 'generated by physicians').

● What other harmful effects does he feel the rise of scientific medicine has had?

■ It has made all of us patients. We are now subordinate to medicine instead of medicine being our servant. Our capacity to deal with health problems ourselves has been undermined. This he calls **social and cultural iatrogenesis**.

*The medicalisation of childbirth is seen by some as turning a natural event into an illness. This baby, however, has been born by Caesarean section, which may have been life-saving, and modern anaesthetics enable the mother to remain conscious. (Source: Science Photo Library Ltd.)*

There is a parallel to be drawn between Illich's view of modern doctors and the fear of healers' special powers in the traditional societies that Fabrega describes. Unlike the social constructionists, whose ideas were explained in the last chapter, Illich does not hesitate in ascribing external reality to the natural world, and medicine's capacity to influence it. Illich is claiming that medical powers frequently damage patients, both directly, by affecting their bodily health, and indirectly, by weakening their tolerance to suffering, and creating over-dependence on technical 'fixes'. This contrasts with Parsons' ideal model of smoothly-functioning reciprocity between doctors and patients.

[2] *Health and Disease: A Reader* (Open University Press, 2nd edn 1995; 3rd edn 2001).

As well as the notion that medicine is more likely to be harmful than not, the medicalisation thesis includes the idea that more and more areas of life are being subjected to medical jurisdiction. Problems are defined in medical terms and medical treatments are put forward as solutions. Alcoholism, for example, used to be thought of as caused by sin but is now seen as an illness. Childbirth, in particular, is seen as having become excessively medicalised; here the highly technical and impersonal hospital environment has been criticised as turning what should be a natural and healthy event into an illness. Feminist writers have argued that the diagnosis of premenstrual syndrome is an aspect of medicalisation that is detrimental to women. Symptoms of this 'condition' include irritability and hostility, which Emily Martin (1989) for example, whose analysis of medical textbook accounts of menstruation you met earlier, sees as often being a natural response to the specific stresses of women's roles.

'The pledge', 1890. Alcoholism, once thought of as primarily caused by sin, is now considered an illness. (Source: Courtesy of the Institute of Alcohol Studies, London)

Supporters of the medicalisation thesis say that the penetration of everyday life by medical knowledge is analogous to, and in some cases directly replaces, the power of the Church and religious knowledge in previous times. Doctors are the new priesthood, from whom guidance is sought for an ever-increasing number of moral questions. Their judgements are influenced by their orientation towards supporting the social order. To illustrate this, consider the following description, taken from a report in the *Lancet,* assessing the influence of diet in causing a disease in children known as *hyperkinetic syndrome.*

> The children had a more than one-year history of short attention span, distractibility, impulsivity, and poorly organised overactivity. In addition, children had to have a score of more than 15 on [a scale which consisted of] ten items of behaviour: restless or overactive; excitable, impulsive; disturbs other children; fails to complete tasks, short attention span; constantly fidgeting;

inattentive, easily distracted; demands must be met immediately, easily frustrated; cries often and easily; mood changes quickly and strikingly; temper outbursts, explosive and unpredictable behaviour. Each is rated on a four-point scale: 0, not present; 1, mild; 2, moderate; 3, severe... (Egger *et al.*, 1992, p. 1 150)

● The researchers suggest that certain foods provoke this disorder. What alternative explanations might there be?

■ The children may simply be 'naughty'; they may have suffered some earlier psychological trauma; they may be reacting to oppressive treatment at home or at school.

The drug Ritalin is increasingly used to control such children's behaviour, particularly in the USA, but also in the UK in recent years. One psychiatrist who studied this phenomenon found an eight-year-old boy who referred to his drug as his 'magic pills which make me a good boy and make everyone like me' (Wender, 1971). Supporters of the medicalisation thesis would suggest that by providing a *medical* interpretation of the children's behaviour, doctors collude with parents and teachers who wish to resist more challenging interpretations.

## 8.4.2 Doctors and the state

The medicalisation thesis is allied to more overtly political ways of assessing the role of medicine. This can be seen in critical assessments of the **medical model** of disease. For example, some people claim that the way in which most doctors are trained to see disease blames individuals unfairly for becoming ill. This is because there is an excessive emphasis in medical thinking on the internal workings of the body, or of organisms that enter the body and interfere with its functions. Doctors tend to focus on how *individuals* can behave to preserve their health, promoting the idea that, for example, personal decisions about diet and exercise are the key to avoiding illness. This, it is argued, underemphasises factors such as poverty, pollution and occupational health hazards as explanations of the cause of disease.[3] If doctors would only admit these as being of overriding importance, it would be but a short step towards recognising that the interests of capitalists, big business, the drug companies and so on, are served by this individualising of health problems. This view has been most forcefully put by the Marxist writer and doctor, Vicente Navarro. In 1976 he argued that the medical profession was the agent of the modern state, and of the ruling class that controlled the state. (An extract entitled 'The mode of state intervention in the health sector' appears in the Reader; Open University students can usefully read it if you have time.)

● How might an individualised explanation of smoking-related disease differ from Navarro's perspective?

■ An individualised explanation would regard smoking as a dangerous habit indulged in out of personal weakness.

---

[3] These arguments are central to *World Health and Disease* (Open University Press, 2nd edn 1993; 3rd edn 2001) and are also discussed in *Caring for Health: History and Diversity* (Open University Press, 2nd edn 1993; 3rd edn 2001), and *Dilemmas in UK Health Care* (Open University Press, 2nd edn 1993; 3rd edn 2001), Chapter 9.

*(Source: Kevin Kallaugher)*

The counter-argument to this would point to the reluctance of governments to curb cigarette advertising for fear of losing revenue and harming the profits of cigarette companies. It might also suggest that poor people smoke more because it is one of the few 'luxuries' that they can afford. These arguments are not just put forward by people who call themselves Marxists, but have influenced the thinking of many people who reject other aspects of Marxism.

The view that the medical profession acts simply in the interests of the state has itself been criticised as being a rather crude representation of affairs. A more sophisticated view is one that recognises the relative *autonomy* of the medical profession from the state. Although the long-term interests of doctors and government often coincide, in that both benefit from social control, in the short term doctors are often in conflict with the state. The relationship of the British Medical Association (BMA) with various governments is a case in point. The BMA hierarchy initially opposed the setting up of the National Health Service (NHS) in 1948, and mounted a vigorous advertising campaign against government plans to create an 'internal market' in the NHS in 1991.[4] This was because they perceived both reforms as threatening professional interests.

● In what way is Navarro's view different from that of Ivan Illich?

■ Illich's criticisms make no reference to institutional interests that lie beyond the medical profession. For him, it is enough to denigrate the 'expert', opposing this with an implied utopia of natural health. For Navarro, doctors are minor players in a larger drama, involving wider social interests, such as government and business.

It could also be claimed that Illich is wrong not to recognise the technical usefulness of medicine in curing disease. Navarro, for example, feels that the very effectiveness of medicine is what makes it such a powerful tool in keeping the otherwise oppressed masses satisfied. The state, however parsimoniously it may provide for health services, has been forced by pressure from the working classes to make public provision of doctors' services. Navarro is ambivalent in his attitude towards such provision. On the one hand, he is critical of the medical model that is thus promoted; on the other hand he regards the establishment of institutions such as the NHS as a significant victory, worth defending against attempts to cut provision.

[4] The opposition of the BMA to government plans for the NHS is discussed in *Caring for Health: History and Diversity* (Open University Press, 2nd edn 1993; 3rd edn 2001), Chapter 5.

Some of the most glaring examples of doctors acting in the interests of an authoritarian state come from the former Soviet Union. When Stalin led a drive to industrialise the USSR faster than any other country had previously managed, doctors were not allowed to give sickness certificates to more than a limited number of factory workers.

● What effect did this have on the construction of the sick role?

■ The doctors' obligation to their partients as gatekeepers sanctioning entry to the sick role was subject to explicit state control, which made it harder for sick people to gain entry; the sick role became much more narrowly defined.

Soviet psychiatry was also used to control political dissidence in the 1970s. Individual protestors, often members of the intelligentsia, were harassed, brought in for psychiatric investigation, diagnosed as being mentally disturbed (typically, schizophrenic) and then incarcerated in mental hospitals. What to Western eyes appeared to be a political protest was thus turned into a non-political question about illness. It may be, however, that the sense of scandal that Western observers experience when hearing about such stories is misplaced. You have learned in the course of this book that it is much easier to see the irrationality in other cultures, or in our own culture in past times.[5]

## 8.5   Problems with the medicalisation thesis

### 8.5.1   The benefits of medicalisation

The medicalisation thesis involves the idea that medicine is expanding its scope to include aspects of life previously deemed outside medical knowledge. Although writers like Illich usually regard this as a bad thing, it is debatable that this is so. Take, for example, the psychiatric view of *battle fatigue.* In World War I, soldiers who ran away from the battle, or refused to go 'over the top', were shot as cowards. Observation of soldiers in Britain who had returned from the front, however, led people to understand the effects of combat as *shell shock.* Psychiatrists became interested, taking the view that what was previously seen as cowardice was a natural response to the stress of battle, a mental illness rather than a moral failing. The symptoms of men with shell shock in many respects paralleled those of female hysterics. Elaine Showalter (1987) has suggested that the appalling conditions of the front challenged men's ability to conform to popular stereotypes of masculinity. However, to call such men hysterical would have too openly suggested that men possessed feminine qualities, so the more 'manly' disease label of shell shock was developed.

During World War II and in subsequent conflicts, American and British army psychiatrists evolved treatment programmes for soldiers thus affected. Recently, there have been calls to engrave the names of soldiers shot for cowardice on World War I memorial stones. Thus public perceptions have changed, in part because of the medicalisation of the problem, which has turned 'cowardice' into a medical condition.

---

[5] Arguments that question the role of psychiatry in the United Kingdom in controlling deviance are discussed in another book in this series, *Experiencing and Explaining Disease* (Open University Press, 2nd edn 1996; 3rd edn 2001).

● What other example was mentioned earlier where, what was previously regarded as a personal weakness or sin, is now seen as a medical problem?

■ Alcoholism and other drug addictions are now treated by psychiatrists.

Similarly, the categorisation of chronic fatigue syndrome as a medical condition 'protected' sufferers from accusations of malingering, as Chapter 6 pointed out. Medicalisation, then, may be experienced by individuals as a welcome relief from personal blame. You may feel that it is right not to shoot deserters any more. The right of drug addicts to be absolved from personal responsibility for their condition is less easily won: medical staff themselves are often rather ambivalent when dealing with addiction. However, these examples serve to illustrate the point that medicalisation can benefit some people, as well as harm others.

## 8.5.2 The limits of medicalisation

The power of medical thinking to penetrate lay thought can be overestimated. This is demonstrated in the work of Emily Martin, to which you were introduced in Chapter 7.

● How did Martin characterise medical thinking about menstruation?

■ As potentially oppressive, in that menstruation was viewed as failed production.

Martin found that the middle-class American women she interviewed about menstruation all gave accounts of internal organs, their structures and functions, accepting the view that the purpose of the process was to conceive, and seeing menstruation as a failure to conceive. By contrast, almost all the working-class women described menstruation in terms of their own bodily experience, or as a part of a life change. Thus she gives examples of two working-class women who said, in response to a question asking them to say how they would explain menstruation to a daughter:

> I don't know, it's part of mother nature I guess. I guess I would explain it the same way my mother explained it to me…. It's just part of life, your body's changing and you're becoming a woman. (Martin, 1989, p. 109)

> With it comes displeasure because one, your period makes me sick because the blood, it ain't got the best odor in the world and I would tell her to check with the pharmacist for the best thing to use…. And you feel it close to you and it is an icky feeling. Just like having sex and not going to wash up. (Martin, 1989, p. 108–9)

American working-class women also engaged in extensive discussion of menstruation with female family members:

> Mothers, grandmothers, sisters, and friends give these women the detailed information and practical knowledge they need: 'My mother just told me how to use everything and that was it'…. 'My mother talked for hours the whole day about it'… (Martin, 1989, p. 110)

Martin concludes that the middle-class women had taken on the medical model to a greater extent than the working-class women, who had retained a view that left them with a greater sense of control over the process. Thus she claims that working-class women are more effective in resisting medicalisation than middle-class women — at least in the USA. (This judgement is rather different from what appears to be the case in the television programme and audiotape for Open University students associated with Chapter 2 of this book, 'Why me? Why now?', in which researcher Jocelyn Cornwell finds little evidence of discussion of menstruation among female family members in her study in London's Bethnal Green.)

### 8.5.3  De-medicalisation

Writers like Ivan Illich tend to overlook the fact that **de-medicalisation** has also occurred in certain areas of life. There is a great deal of popular resistance to medicalisation, and this has sometimes born fruit. For example, many people have been critical of the medical management of childbirth for a number of years. Hospital birth has been seen as impersonal and highly technical, treating women as if they were ill, rather than experiencing a natural event. Women's freedom to decide how to manage their experience, ranging from birthing position to pain control, was felt to have been taken away by medical technique. Partly as a result of this sustained and sometimes bitter dispute, the medical management of childbirth

*A low-technology home birth — in some parts of Britain medical management of childbirth relaxed in the 1990s. (Source: Science Photo Library Ltd.)*

has become considerably more relaxed in recent years, paying greater attention to women's views. Supervision of childbirth has increasingly passed to midwives — an (almost) all-female profession (there were 12 male midwives in England in 1999–2000, among 1720 females).

There are other examples of de-medicalisation. The community care of people who would formerly have been treated as hospital psychiatric patients has been actively promoted in government policies in a number of countries, supported by medical opinion, as a reaction to the negative consequences of long-term institutional care. Critics of mental hospitals had argued that institutions actually made patients more dependent on medical care, because they were no longer under any constraint to adapt to life in the community. The policy of closing mental hospitals has been pursued vigorously in a number of European countries as well as the USA, to be replaced by various forms of community provision.[6] However, inadequacies in the support for people with mental disorders in the community in the 1990s led to campaigns for greater medical supervision and restraint for certain categories of patients.

## 8.6  Surveillance

There are those who argue that the development of apparently more humane and progressive methods of treatment can be deceptive, as new arrangements for **surveillance** of the population may serve to control behaviour in a more subtle

---

[6] Community care policies are discussed in *Caring for Health: History and Diversity* (Open University Press, 2nd edn 1993; 3rd edn 2001), Chapter 7, and *Dilemmas in UK Health Care* (Open University Press, 2nd edn 1993; 3rd edn 2001), Chapter 4.

manner. Proponents of this view are associated with social constructionism, which you met in the previous chapter. Their inspiration is the work of a French social philosopher, Michel Foucault. In the 1960s, Foucault wrote extensively on an earlier shift in the treatment of people regarded as mad in the eighteenth century, focusing particularly on the liberalisation of asylum regimes that occurred in the late part of the century. Previous to this change, people thought to be mad had not been separated from other types of deviant:

*William Norris, a lunatic, in his chains in Bethlem, 1814, from an etching by G. Arnauld. (Source: The Wellcome Library, London)*

> In 1690 a survey of 3 000 internees at *Salpêtrière*...revealed that the majority of them were paupers, vagabonds and beggars, while the rest were, in the terminology of the survey, 'ordinary folk', 'prisoners of *lettres de cachet*', 'decrepit women', 'infirm and dotty old women', 'epileptics', 'innocent dwarfs and deformed', 'feeble minded', 'violent mad', and 'incorrigible girls'. Almost a century later, in 1781...in a Berlin workhouse 'idlers', 'rogues and libertines', 'infirm and criminals', and 'destitute old women and children' all mixed together. (Foucault, quoted in Cousins and Hussain, 1984, p. 110)

Although there was some medical involvement with these people, the religious authorities played a large part in determining their treatment, which involved making little distinction between sin, disease and violation of social norms. The distinction between mental and physical illness at this time was hardly established. Inmates were often treated punitively, houses of internment being closer in character to prisons than hospitals. If it was distinguished from other disorders, madness was seen as an ethical choice made in favour of Unreason in preference to Reason. This justified the incarceration and punishment of the mad.

Foucault points to a period in history when a new conception of the mad replaced these views, associated with new regimes of treatment. These new regimes were not solely promoted by medical practitioners. One of the reformers of this period was William Tuke, a Quaker who in 1796 set up a house for the insane in York, known as the Retreat. Here the Quaker virtues were practised; a system of rewards and punishments controlled behaviour, rather than the chains and whips of the old madhouse, and cure was based on an appeal to the small core of Reason that was held to persist even at the heart of madness. Thus Foucault describes the arrival at the Retreat of a maniac:

> ...young and prodigiously strong...loaded with chains; he wore handcuffs; his clothes were attached by ropes. He had no sooner arrived than all his shackles were removed, and he was permitted to dine with the keepers; his agitation immediately ceased...the keeper explained that the entire house was organised in terms of the greatest liberty and the greatest comfort for all, and that he would not be subject to any constraint as long as he did nothing against the rules of the house or the general principles of human morality.... At the end of four months, he left the Retreat, entirely cured. (Foucault, 1967, reprinted in Rabinow, 1984, pp. 144–5)

Similar developments were taking place in France under medical guidance, and a famous picture of Dr Philippe Pinel releasing the chains of the mad in order to begin a moral regime similar to Tuke's is reproduced in Figure 8.1. However, far from regarding this as a liberation, Foucault observes that:

> …liberation of the insane, abolition of constraint, constitution of a human milieu — these are only justifications. The real operations were different. In fact Tuke created an asylum where he substituted for the free terror of madness the stifling anguish of responsibility; fear no longer reigned on the other side of the prison gates, it now raged under the seals of conscience.

> …The asylum, which it is Pinel's glory to have founded, is not a free realm of observation, diagnosis, and therapeutics; it is a juridical space where one is accused, judged and condemned, and from which one is never released except…by remorse. (Foucault, 1967, reprinted in Rabinow, 1984, pp. 145, 158)

**Figure 8.1** *Pinel freeing the insane from the hospital of Salpêtrière, from a painting by Tony Robert-Flemming (1837–1912). (Source: Roger-Viollet, Paris)*

In a sense, the mad people under the new regime were being encouraged to become their own jailers, monitoring their behaviour according to moral judgements that they had taken upon themselves. The paradox that Foucault points out in his phrase 'the free terror of madness' is that under the old regime the mad in their chains were subject to physical rather than moral constraint. The new form of surveillance — which was promoted by both medical and non-medical interests — was much more pervasive and detailed in its effects.

### 8.6.1 Panopticism and normality

In subsequent work, Foucault relates this change in disciplinary technique to developments in wider society. Increasingly the various institutions of society — schools, prisons, hospitals — adopted a form of surveillance over their charges which has been described as **panopticism** ('all-seeing'). This term is derived from the word that the English philosopher and social reformer, Jeremy Bentham (1748–1832) used to describe his plan for a model prison, the Panopticon, shown in Figure 8.2. The design of this prison is such that the guard in the central tower could observe the inmates' actions, without being seen by the prisoners themselves. Each cell has two windows: one to allow the guard to see in, another to allow light in from the other side. For Foucault, this picture symbolises a form of disciplinary power based on surveillance.

The idea of medicine and allied professions such as dentistry as a part of a broader apparatus of surveillance is expressed by later writers who draw on Foucault's ideas. Sarah Nettleton, whose article on the history of dentistry you read with Chapter 7, expresses this theme.

● What techniques of surveillance does Nettleton identify?

■ The mouth is 'policed' and 'normalised' through a training in toothbrush drill and regular dental checkups. This creates a view of the normal mouth, which individuals carry with them as a way of assessing how closely they conform to this concept of normality (Figure 8.3).

In fact, the concept of **normality** is central to medical surveillance.

● What instances have you experienced so far in your life of being assessed for evidence of normal health?

**Figure 8.2** *Jeremy Bentham's plan of the Panopticon (Source: University College, London)*

■ When you, or any children you may have had, were born you would have been checked carefully against a rating scale that assesses whether vital functions (such as breathing and heart rate) were normal. At school you were probably measured and weighed at regular health checks and had your eyesight and hearing tested and your teeth inspected, to assess whether your growth and development were normal for your age. Pregnant women are also monitored closely, for example, by routine sampling of their blood and urine. You may have undergone a medical check-up for insurance purposes or before starting a new job.

**Figure 8.3** *Is this an extension of medicalisation and surveillance? A routine dental check in a British school is combined with an inspection of how effectively children are brushing their teeth. (Photo: Mike Levers)*

This view of medicine as an apparatus of surveillance and discipline can be applied to almost any reform or new development. From this perspective, the closure of mental hospitals could be interpreted as the demise of a particular form of disciplinary power. Whatever arrangements or exhortations are applied to the discharged patients might be analysed as a new form of surveillance. Care in the community, in the form of hostels for the mentally ill or handicapped, or even return to families, might be regarded as a further intricacy in the development of what Foucault has called the *medical gaze* ('*le regard*'), penetrating still further into everyday life.

Indeed, as a final elaboration of the story, David Armstrong, who has written extensively on modern medicine as a form of surveillance, proposes that some of the academic disciplines allied to medicine, including sociology, are a part of the surveillance industry. This is particularly shown by the use of social surveys, in which sociologists enquire into the lives of the population.

> Sociology made its principal contribution in the post-war world when its mastery of survey techniques made it of value to a medical gaze intent on exploring the surveillance possibilities of this new technology. Sociologists, in close alliance with medicine, opened up areas of the health experiences of 'ordinary' people through survey of health attitudes, of illness behaviour, of drug taking and of symptom prevalence. More recently, as the medical gaze has focused on individual idiosyncrasies, personal meanings and subjectivity, sociology too has turned its attention to fresh possibilities. (Armstrong, 1983, p. 114)

● If a social constructionist says that some programme, such as community care of the mentally ill, involves a form of surveillance, does this mean that it is a bad thing?

■ Social constructionism is based on *cultural relativism* (see Chapter 2). This allows for no firm basis for moral or evaluative judgements. Something is right or wrong only from a particular perspective, which itself may be judged right or wrong from some other perspective. For many people, this is the fundamental problem of the social constructionist position.

Furthermore, the medical gaze, in Foucault's sense, is not simply an instrument of repression and control. It also *constructs* our view of the objects it surveys (such as 'the mouth' or 'the body'), and these objects may themselves be the site of competing sets of ideas (as, for example, in rival theories of mental illness).

## 8.7  Postscript

We began this chapter with the finding of Horacio Fabrega that accusations of sorcery arise only in societies where healers are perceived to have gained special powers. We live in a world of extreme medical specialisation where there are constant reminders of the power of medical technology. This chapter has focused almost exclusively on what might be thought of as modern equivalents to the accusation of sorcery: the medicalisation thesis, the view of medicine as social control, and of disciplinary power exercised through surveillance. Part of your task as you learn more about modern medicine will be to assess the extent to which you accept these as criticisms of medical power.

## OBJECTIVES FOR CHAPTER 8

When you have studied this chapter, you should be able to:

**8.1** Define and use, or recognise definitions and applications of, each of the terms printed in **bold** in the text.

**8.2** Describe Parsons' theory of the roles of doctors and patients, and some of its limitations.

**8.3** Give examples of ways in which the interests of the medical profession are in conflict with those of patients.

**8.4** Assess the argument that society has become excessively medicalised, giving examples that either support or undermine the medicalisation thesis.

**8.5** Describe how medical knowledge and practice can be viewed as an apparatus of surveillance.

## QUESTIONS FOR CHAPTER 8

**1**   (*Objective 8.2*)

In the context of a discussion of Parsons' sick role, Eliot Freidson has described 'voodoo death' and the abandonment of the sick in some traditional groups:

> In extreme cases — as in the 'magical fright', where a person who believes that powerful black magic has been invoked against him obliges the magician by dying, and in the…response to an individual's inability to eat by assuming he is a hopeless case and abandoning him on the trail to starve and be eaten — 'exemption' from ordinary obligations is so thoroughgoing that death is the consequence. (Freidson, 1970, p. 229)

In what ways do these examples reveal a limitation of Parsons' theory of the sick role?

**2**   (*Objective 8.3*)

Look at Figure 8.4, which shows data collected at the time of the Vietnam War. Describe these patterns of conscription and suggest three possible explanations for them. Does this study show the mainly white medical profession acting against the interests of patients? What does it tell us about medical surveillance and the sick role?

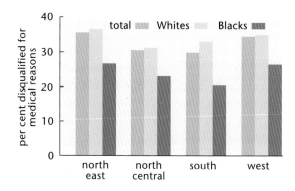

**Figure 8.4**  *Variations in the proportion of conscripts from white- or black-skinned ethnic groups who were disqualified from service in the American army for medical reasons in different geographic areas of the USA in 1968. (Source: Waitzkin, H., 1971, Latent functions of the sick role in various institutional settings,* Social Science and Medicine, *5(67), Pergamon Press, Figure 8.3)*

**Questions 3 and 4**

First read the following extract from the French essayist Montaigne (1533–92) and answer the questions below.

> At the foot of our mountains called Lahontan the inhabitants lived a peculiar sort of life, their fashions, clothes and manners distinct from other people, ruled and governed by certain particular laws and usages, received from father to son, to which they submitted, without other constraint than the reverence to custom. The little state had continued from all antiquity in so happy a condition, that no neighbouring judge was ever put to the trouble of inquiring into their doings…nor was ever any of them seen to go a-begging. They avoided all alliances and traffic with the outer world, that they might not corrupt the purity of their own government…

> [But then a physician comes amongst them]

> …This man first of all began to teach them the names of fevers, colds, and imposthumes; the seat of the heart, liver, and intestines, a science till then utterly unknown to them; and instead of garlic, with which they were wont to cure allmanner of diseases, how painful or extreme soever, he taught them, though it were but for a cough, or any little cold to take strange mixtures, and began to make a trade not only of their health but of their lives. They swear till then they never perceived the evening air to be offensive to the head; that to drink, when they were hot, was hurtful, and that the winds of autumn were more unwholesome than those of spring; that since this use of physic, they find themselves oppressed with a legion of unaccustomed diseases and that they perceive a general decay in their ancient vigour, and their lives are cut shorter in half. (Montaigne, 1952 trans., p. 375)

**3**    (*Objective 8.4*)

What similarities are there between Montaigne's story and the medicalisation thesis expressed by Illich and others?

**4**    (*Objective 8.5*)

Identify elements of surveillance in the above account of Lahontan, and draw parallels with the social constructionist analysis of shifts in the nature of medical surveillance in the past.

# CHAPTER 9

## Doctor–patient interaction

**Study notes for OU students**

In Section 9.2.1 of this chapter you will be asked to read an article in *Health and Disease: A Reader* (Open University Press, second edition 1995; third edition 2001), entitled 'Truth, trust and paternalism' by Thurstan Brewin. A television programme on doctor–patient interaction, 'Brief encounters', and an audiotape, 'The consultation' are also associated with this chapter. You will be asked to listen to the audiotape in Section 9.2 of this Chapter; you can watch the TV programme at any convenient time during this study week. They both look critically at the way in which doctors and patients relate to each other in medical consultations, which is the focus for study here. Full details of these programmes can be found in the *Audiovisual Media Guide*.

## 9.1  Introduction

> ...dilemmas become particularly acute, or are experienced with special force, during the fateful moments of an individual's life...the individual feels at a crossroads.... Fateful moments are phases when people might choose to seek refuge in pre-established beliefs and in familiar modes of activity [but they] also often mark periods of reskilling and empowerment...at fateful moments individuals are today likely to encounter expert systems. (Giddens, 1991, pp. 142–3)

You have by now been exposed to a range of views about medical knowledge. The material in previous chapters has had the underlying theme of showing some of the difficulties that are involved in maintaining certainty in the face of alternative views. The history of medical knowledge demonstrates that people have often been certain about diseases and their treatments in the past, only to have their certainties overthrown by subsequent knowledge. Regarding present-day society as anthropologically strange involves the suspension of certainty, and a readiness to live with doubt.

With such a mental attitude, however, it may be difficult to know who to trust when seeking help. Anthony Giddens, the sociologist who wrote the words quoted above, says elsewhere in his book, *Modernity and Self-Identity,* that people's use of abstract systems, such as medicine, 'depend on trust, yet they provide none of the moral rewards which...were often available in traditional settings' (Giddens, 1991, p. 136). The modern individual tends to gather as much information as possible about the risks and rewards of certain actions (such as following a doctor's advice) in an attempt to eliminate reliance on trust. Yet a degree of trust at 'fateful moments', such as those that may be encountered in the doctor's surgery, is sometimes inevitable.

The modern patient enters the doctor's surgery at a time when the social climate is permeated by the questioning of professional expertise. A variety of patients' rights are vociferously asserted by sections of the media, encouraged by politicians who sense popular appeal. The ideals of consumerism, whereby patients are encouraged to think of themselves in terms similar to supermarket shoppers, has been enthusiastically promoted in the National Health Service since the 1990s. Authoritarian or 'paternalistic' behaviour by people in the 'helping professions' is now routinely condemned. A new emphasis on listening to the client and being responsive to his or her needs is widespread. Opinion leaders within the professions who promote these ideas draw upon the social sciences to construct new models for professional behaviour.

An example of this trend is the way in which medical thinking about communication between doctors and patients has increasingly become informed by psychology and sociology. Medical students now learn to be conscious of the way they interact with patients, and analysis of videotapes of consultation styles is now an established part of most medical school curricula. Evidence for this shift can also be found in medical textbooks and the writings of social scientists on doctor–patient interaction.

● From your reading of this book so far, can you think of other medical fashions?

■ Collapse therapy for TB and bloodletting may be thought of as 'fashions' if by this it is meant that doctors have at times proceeded without evidence that fulfils modern requirements for proof of efficacy.

The actual practices of doctors, however, may lag behind opinion leaders, for a variety of reasons. One way of characterising the shift in thinking about medical consultations is to contrast a *doctor-centred* style with one that is *patient-centred*.

## 9.2 Doctor-centred and patient-centred styles

You were introduced to the principles of the clinical method in Chapter 7. Its purpose is to identify the meaning of symptoms and signs from the mass of information presented by patients and diagnostic tests, and to summarise this in a diagnosis, perhaps then followed by treatment. The patient, in this model, is the *carrier* of the disease, and the doctor the expert at distinguishing the relevant from the irrelevant. The following quotation is a typical example of this **doctor-centred** model of the clinical method in practice, tape-recorded in a GP's surgery. The consultation concerns Mr Nixon, a supervisor at an engineering plant, who has a rash on his leg.

### A consultation

*Doctor:* Come in please.

*Patient:* Hello.

*Doctor:* Take a seat. I won't be a moment. (pause) Mr Nixon isn't it?

*Patient:* Yes.

*Doctor:* Oh, I recognize you. Haven't seen you for a long time (laughs).

*Patient:* How are you?

*Doctor:* Pretty well thanks.

*Patient:* Are you? Good. Splendid.

*Doctor:* Eh, I shouldn't say how are you? Should I? (laughs) I should say what can I do for you?

Doctor-centred medicine may reduce the patient to being merely the carrier of the disease upon which doctors exercise their skills.

*Patient:* Well, what I've come round about, doctor, on and off from time to time I seem to get like a leg aggravation. It, eh, seems to be like a smarting type of feeling and eh, it aggravates like, it itches.

*Doctor:* Itches, does it?

*Patient:* Yes, and it eh, it's like a smarting kind of thing. Not fiercely but mildly.

*Doctor:* Deep in the leg or on the surface?

*Patient:* No. No. No. On the skin. Surface of the skin. Yes.

*Doctor:* No aching in the leg at all?

*Patient:* Well, what I have found, well, if I have occasion to bend down, you know, (indistinct) eh, it's rather aching on getting up. I know age progresses and so forth but, eh, you know, over the best part of the weekend I wasn't bothered with it and then Sunday it sort of started again. I had it on and off quite a while.

*Doctor:* On and off. I'm still not absolutely sure in my mind what you mean. It's not a skin irritation you're complaining of?

*Patient:* Yes, it's eh.

*Doctor:* Would you call it an itch?

*Patient:* It is. But the, it's also the sensation and feeling of it is, as I say sort of slightly smarting as if the skin is a little sort of taut.

*Doctor:* Raw?

*Patient:* Yes, yes.

*Doctor:* Do you get this all the time or does it vary?

*Patient:* Pardon?

*Doctor:* Do you, is this a constant sensation or does it vary?

*Patient:* Eh, no. Some days I'm not bothered with it.

*Doctor:* No backache at all?

*Patient:* Oh no. No, no.

*Doctor:* You don't feel your leg is less strong than it used to be?

*Patient:* No, not really, I get, as I say, I sort of bend down and you feel a sort of achiness in getting up, sort of thing, but, eh…

*Doctor:* Do your legs ache when you walk?

*Patient:* No, No.

*Doctor:* No pain in the calf if you, um.

*Patient:* (very uncertain and speaking almost inaudibly) No. I didn't know, possibly you know, whether er, blood was a little bit rich or perhaps too much sugar on what I eat, or, you know. It's only a guess on my part, but this, it's not a lot.

*Doctor:* (interrupts) I see you're scratching now. Is this the sort of thing that makes you want to scratch, is it?

*Patient:* Yes it does. It's not a lot to be seen there. It's a little minute sort of blemish, but um.

*Doctor:* Just slip your shoes and socks off. (At this point the doctor began a very careful examination of Mr Nixon which lasted several minutes….)

*Doctor:* Ah ha. Bend your knees. Put your knee up. That's it. No. Everything is fine as far as muscles are concerned. I think its a skin irritation, I'll give you a moisturising cream.

*Patient:* Yes.

(Tuckett *et al.*, 1985, pp. 60–1)

In this extract, after a brief interchange of greetings, business proceeds with the doctor asking a series of questions that require precise answers, followed by a physical examination.

● How are signs and symptoms elicited in this consultation?

■ Mr Nixon's speech contains descriptions of his symptoms, which are the bodily experiences that he knows about. During the physical examination, the doctor is looking for signs, which are disturbances of normal structure or function of which Mr Nixon may not be aware.

The doctor is considering different diagnoses in sifting through the evidence presented to him, and finally arrives at a single one. He does not tell the patient about the different diagnoses that are being considered and ruled out, only the one arrived at. However, there is one interruption to this smooth process of question and answer.

● What is the interruption, and what does the doctor do about it?

■ Mr Nixon starts to talk about his own ideas about what might be wrong: his blood may be too rich, or he may eat too much sugar. The doctor interrupts and asks a question about scratching.

The extract presented above comes from a book, *Meetings Between Experts,* by David Tuckett and his colleagues. Their message was that doctors should listen more to patients' views about their illnesses. They reported a study of some 1 302 tape-recorded consultations and, for a number of these, the patients were also interviewed afterwards. Mr Nixon, when asked by the interviewer why he had gone to see the doctor, said:

> Well, er, the reason being, er that I get a sort of skin aggravation on the legs, you see, and on and off it's playing me up from time to time not over-alarming but enough, um, you know here…It comes and goes, um. I'm not one to analyse these things eh, but, eh, I rather, eh, had the impression it was a bit of flea-bite-us [sic] or something like that. (Tuckett *et al.*, 1985, p. 253)

This was his way of describing *phlebitis* which involves the inflammation of a vein due to circulatory problems, and which Mr Nixon had recently heard about. He thought his diet might have something to do with causing this. What is noticeable is that his attempt to explain this idea in the *consultation* was less coherent than in the *interview* afterwards and was ignored by the doctor. The contrast between the doctor-centred style shown by the doctor interviewing Mr Nixon and the shared, or patient-centred, style advocated by David Tuckett and others is explored more fully in the television programme 'Brief encounters' and audiotape band 'The consultation' made for Open University students and associated with this chapter. (Students should read the Audiocassette Notes and then listen to the tape before answering the following question.)

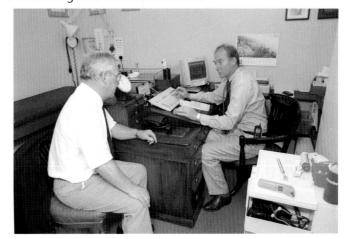

*Doctors differ in their views on whether the consultation is ideally a 'meeting between equals' or an interaction in which a sensitive practitioner decides what is in the patient's best interests to know. (Photo: John Harris/ Report Digital)*

● What are the chief characteristics of the shared or **patient-centred** style of medical practice?

■ Both parties explore each other's ideas about what is wrong and the best course of action. This involves the patient being told the reasons for the doctor's views, and the doctor enabling the patient's ideas to emerge and be explored. Treatment plans are then based on a shared agreement about the nature of the problem which both understand.

## 9.2.1 The influence of psychoanalysis

The ideas put forward by Tuckett are part of a broader medical interest in the patient's view. This has grown since the middle of the twentieth century and has particularly affected general practice in recent years. The work of the GP turned psychoanalyst Michael Balint has been influential. In the 1950s and 1960s Balint argued that the special expertise of GPs lay in their knowledge of their patients' lives, often based on a long-standing relationship in which the same GP saw the whole family. Balint also believed that it was important for GPs to empathise with the emotional aspects of patients' experience of illness. GPs were worried about their status in comparison with hospital specialisms at that time; Balint's ideas became part of a successful strategy to construct a new image of general practice as a specialty with its own theory and unique skills.[1]

In the USA there were similar developments, and these were expressed most clearly in the work of two doctors working in the Institute for Psychoanalysis in Chicago, Thomas Szasz and Marc Hollender. They distinguished three models for **doctor-patient interaction**, and these are presented in Table 9.1.

**Table 9.1**  Three basic models of the physician–patient relationship.

| Model | Physician's role | Patient's role | Clinical application of model | Prototype of model |
|---|---|---|---|---|
| 1 activity–passivity | does something to patient | recipient (unable to respond or inert) | anaesthesia, acute trauma, coma, delirium, etc. | parent–infant |
| 2 guidance–cooperation | tells patient what to do | cooperator (obeys) | acute infectious processes, etc. | parent–child (adolescent) |
| 3 mutual participation | helps patient to help himself | participants in 'partnership' (uses expert help) | most chronic illnesses, psychoanalysis, etc. | adult–adult |

Source: Szasz, T. S. and Hollender, M. H. (1956) A contribution to the philosophy of medicine: the basic models of the doctor–patient relationship, *Archives of Internal Medicine*, **97**, p. 586, Table 1.

● How might the three models fit into the distinction between patient- and doctor-centred interactions used in this chapter?

■ The activity–passivity model is perhaps an extreme example of doctor-centredness, but this is best represented by the guidance–cooperation model. Patient-centredness is represented by the mutual participation model.

Szasz and Hollender do not argue that mutual participation is best in all consultations. They recognise that all three styles have their place; it would clearly be inappropriate to expect an unconscious person to discuss theories of illness causation before treatment progressed. However, they do suggest that the first two models satisfy a psychological need in doctors for a sense of mastery and superiority. In guidance–cooperation this may involve gratification of a 'Pygmalion complex', in which doctors wish to mould patients into their own image, and persuade them of the value of their own aims. The third model which Szasz and

[1] The development of general practice is discussed in *Caring for Health: History and Diversity* (Open University Press, 2nd edn 1993; 3rd edn 2001), Chapter 6.

Hollender, writing in 1955, were keen to point out was 'essentially foreign to medicine', involves the doctor in letting go the reins of control. In a passage that reveals some assumptions that are less acceptable in today's more egalitarian climate, they write that this is a model which is

> ...rarely appropriate for children or for those persons who are mentally deficient, very poorly educated, or profoundly immature. On the other hand, the greater the intellectual, educational, and general experiential similarity between physician and patient the more appropriate and necessary this model of therapy becomes. (Szasz and Hollender, 1956, p. 587)

You will recall from the previous chapter that Talcott Parsons was writing at about the same time about the complementary roles of doctors and patients. What Szasz and Hollender were encouraging, put in Parsons' terms, was a renegotiation of the rights and obligations of both patients and doctors. The degree to which patients cooperated with the doctor, or patient *compliance* (as discussed in Chapter 2) became something to be negotiated by doctors, rather than readily assumed. Szasz and Hollender hoped that medical authority would lose its mystery if doctors exposed their medical reasoning to patients.

This type of approach has had its critics from within the medical profession. An example of such a critic is Thurstan Brewin, whose 1985 article on 'Truth, trust and paternalism' is in the Reader.[2] (Open University students should read it now.)

●   What arguments does Brewin put forward in favour of paternalism?

■   It is based on trust. Some patients need more information than others, and a sensitive doctor will recognise that some patients do not want to know everything. The function of the doctor is then to hold the patient's hand in reassurance. Explaining everything can also take an inordinate amount of time.

## 9.3  Breaking bad news

Perhaps the most difficult situation for doctors and patients to encounter is one when it is thought that the patient may die of his or her disease. This is commonly and dramatically experienced in the case of cancer. The following extracts are two contrasting instances of doctors telling women with breast cancer about their test results, derived from a 1988 study of a breast cancer clinic in Canada.

**Breaking bad news 1: the doctor–researcher**

*Patient:* Did you get my report back?

*Doctor:* Yes, as a matter of fact, I have the report here somewhere on my desk. Let me see...Ah yes, it says, 'infiltrating and intraductal lobular carcinoma, well encapsulated in...'

*Patient:* You mean — it is — I've got — cancer?

*Doctor:* Yes.

*Patient:* Are you sure?

*Doctor:* Yes, I went down and checked in the lab and...

[2] *Health and Disease: A Reader* (Open University Press, 2nd edn 1995; 3rd edn 2001).

*Patient:* Am I going to die?

*Doctor:* We have a lot of tools to fight with. Let's talk about the options…

*Patient:* You mean I am going to die? (Patient cries and shakes.)

*Doctor:* Now listen, I was saying there is a lot we can do. We have to make some serious decisions. Pull yourself together…please.

(Taylor, 1988, p. 118)

**Breaking bad news 2: the paternalist**

*Doctor:* You know, my dear, I can see you're upset, but, whether I like it or not, I have lots of women like you come into this office over the last 30 years…Why, you're certainly not alone…

*Patient:* Doctor, tell me…will you have to…operate?

*Doctor:* Well, now, as you've probably guessed, we saw something in your breast that really shouldn't have been there, now should it? Well, I didn't like the looks of it under the microscope, and I must say…it could have looked better.

*Patient:* You mean…I guess I really have to have an operation, oh God no…

*Doctor:* Yes, just to clean up the mess you know…make sure that the nasty lump doesn't give us any more problems. By the way, just today, I had the sweetest little old lady in my office. Why she sat there, just where you are… anyhow… I had operated on her…well it must be 25 or 30 years ago, and she was in for her annual check-up… well, I said to her, how have you managed all these years to look so terrific and to feel so chipper? Well, she said… my mother's always told me… don't get mixed up in things you know nothing about. So I didn't… just left everything up to you, doctor. She has done very well. That's what I want you to do… just relax and leave everything to me… okay?

(Taylor, 1988, p. 124)

The first doctor (extract 1) was actively researching into the best treatment for breast cancer, and was anxious to recruit patients to experimental trials of different treatments.[3] He felt that the best policy was one of open disclosure, as this meant that patients would go along with the treatments he was evaluating. The second doctor (extract 2) was similarly concerned that the patient comply with what would be an unpleasant and invasive treatment, as he regarded this as being her best chance of survival. Less involved in scientific research, he appeals to his long experience of treating the condition successfully in order to persuade the patient to trust his authority. He speaks to the patient as if she were a child, using euphemisms to conceal the medical name for the disease, and expressly advises the patient against enquiring into his reasoning too closely. The second patient expressed considerably less distress during the consultation than the first one.

●   Which consultation is patient-centred, and which is doctor-centred?

[3] Clinical trials are discussed further in *Studying Health and Disease* (Open University Press, 2nd edn 1994; colour-enhanced 2nd edn 2001).

- The first doctor openly presents the patient with his medical knowledge, and invites the patient to participate in treatment decisions, although he does have his own agenda, which is to include the patient in a research study. The second doctor conceals his thinking, and presents himself as a paternal figure in whom the patient should place her trust. The first doctor is superficially more patient-centred, yet his cold disclosure of dreadful news seems particularly unsupportive to the patient. In contrast, the concern of the second doctor for the patient's feelings is evident.

Patient-centredness means placing the patient's concerns rather than the doctor's at the centre of things. In fact, doctors doing this sort of work face a difficult balance between disclosing so much that patients feel abandoned to their fears, and in concealing so much that patients, when they later discover the truth, lose their trust in the doctor. Neither of the two doctors in these extracts were able to maintain such a balance.

## 9.3.1  Other cultures

Once again, it is helpful to study other cultures to gain insight into this issue. In the USA and United Kingdom most doctors treating terminally ill people believe it is best to tell patients the truth about their illness or impending death, if the doctor judges they are able to cope with this knowledge. This trend is associated with the view that it is psychologically healthy to come to terms with one's own death. The pressure of lying to patients about their condition is seen as intolerable for medical and nursing staff, and to lead to feelings of fear and abandonment in patients. Although in the 1950s studies showed that few doctors believed in telling dying patients the truth, and few patients learned it from doctors, more recent studies show an almost complete reversal in policy.

However, policy and practice are not always the same thing. In the United Kingdom, at least, research evidence shows that between the late 1960s and 1980s people with terminal cancer were increasingly likely to be told their diagnosis and prognosis by doctors (Seale, 1991). But the same study showed that many patients were still left to find out about their condition for themselves. There remain concerns about the clarity with which doctors give, and patients receive, bad news.

In Italy there is less concern with open disclosure. First, a diagnosis of cancer tends to be associated with the expectation of death. This contrasts with the situation in the United Kingdom or the USA where the medical profession has made strenuous and quite successful efforts to persuade the public that many cancers are curable. Second, the doctor–patient relationship in Italy has not been exposed to the psychoanalytic influence described above. On the whole, the relationship that people expect is one that is hierarchical, paternalistic and protective. Communication is less about the imparting of information, more about the maintenance of this relationship.

Nevertheless, Italian medicine is exposed to foreign influence, and patients are sometimes told that they have cancer. Deborah Gordon, an anthropologist studying women in Florence with breast cancer, found that the few who did learn their diagnosis often hid the news from their families. The diagnosis was associated with a loss of hope, and there was a taboo against the public acknowledgement of cancer. On the whole, doctors feared that disclosure would lead to non-compliance because of the loss of hope. American doctors, by contrast, appeal to the popular

American (and British) idea of 'fighting cancer' in justification of disclosure. Deborah Gordon writes of the Italian perception of the American way:

> In fact, among many, there seems to be little perceived value in 'facing the truth' or in 'telling the truth,' in and of itself. Physicians, in turn, have traditionally been esteemed not in terms of 'honesty,' but whether they serve and protect the patient through their expert charismatic authority and knowledge. (Gordon, 1990, p. 290)

The advocacy of mutual participation and shared consultation is relevant in our own culture, but care needs to be taken in assuming it as a universally desirable model. It may be more relevant in general practice than other medical settings. It may only be appropriate in a culture and at a time when professional expertise has been subject to wider questioning, as is certainly the case at the start of the new millennium in the UK.

## 9.4 Surrounding context

To understand what consultations mean to people it is helpful to consider the context that surrounds consultations. A consultation may be better understood if it is seen as one of a series, an episode in a person's life. Characteristics of patients, such as social class, ethnicity or gender may influence what happens. Features of the setting can also help us understand what is going on. This may include, for example, whether it is public or private health care. These aspects of surrounding context will now be considered.

### 9.4.1 Characteristics of patients

A division that many sociologists feel is important in determining people's experience of consultations is that of social class. Studies commonly show that working-class patients in the United Kingdom ask fewer questions, get fewer explanations, are less likely to express disagreement or doubt about the doctor's advice, and spend less time with the doctor than middle-class patients. It is debatable whether patients' expectations or doctors' perceptions are more important in producing these differences.

Other characteristics of patients have also been found to be related to their experience of consultations, as is shown in Table 9.2, which is taken from the study by Tuckett *et al.*

● What does the table show?

■ Evasion of patients' ideas is more common with women patients than men. Afro-Caribbeans are less likely than other ethnic groups to be given reasons or clear statements of the doctors' views.

You may recall that Szasz and Hollender considered mutual participation to be a style more suitable where there was 'experiential similarity' between doctors and patients. Doctors tend themselves to be drawn from higher social class backgrounds; until recently the majority of entrants to medical school were men, and Afro-Caribbean doctors are not well-represented in the UK's health service. The social status of patients appears to affect their access to medical reasoning when speaking with doctors.

**Table 9.2**   Some differences in doctors' information-giving according to gender and ethnic group of the patient.

| | Gender | |
| --- | --- | --- |
| | Women (%) | Men (%) |
| proportion of consultations in which a patient's ideas were evaded by the doctor | 15 | 6 |

| | Ethnic group | |
| --- | --- | --- |
| | Afro-Caribbean (%) | Others (%) |
| proportion of patients given moderately elaborate reasons on at least one topic | 18 | 32 |
| proportion of patients to whom the doctor clearly stated a view on at least one topic | 36 | 63 |

Source: adapted from Tuckett, D. *et al.* (1985) *Meetings Between Experts: An Approach to Sharing Ideas in Medical Consultations,* Tavistock, London, p. 68, Table 4.9.

● Can you think of an alternative explanation?

■ People in lower social class and ethnic minority groups may not *want* to know as much as other people, and may convey this expectation to the doctor. (In fact several studies have shown little class difference in patients' satisfaction with consultations after the event.)

## 9.4.2  The setting: public or private

In addition to the three models of interaction that Szasz and Hollender present, there is a fourth one that is logically possible, in which the patient dominates. Historically this has been the relationship between aristocratic patients and their doctors who in past times were considered as a type of servant. Here, the doctor defers to the client, who is of superior social status, and on whom he or she depends for livelihood and reputation. Studies of modern private medical practice suggest that this type of relationship can still occur. Consider the five extracts below, taken from tape recordings of consultations between doctors and their patients, the first two from paediatric clinics in the USA, the remainder from an oncology (cancer) clinic in London.

*"It's the Royal physician, Ma'am, and would you slip your things off." It is not often the case that doctors have lower social status than their patients. (Punch, 21 January 1972)*

### Consultations in private medical practice

**1**   *Intern* [a junior doctor who sees the patient before the specialist]: How did you get here?

*Mother:* Well, he's been seeing a psychiatrist and he diagnosed minimal brain dysfunction and prescribed X. But we also want to get Dr Stein's [a neurologist] opinion as we felt we ought not just to have a psychiatric opinion.

**2**   *Mother:* We liked him [Dr Levy] particularly because he was critical of schools and said, 'Don't believe what they say. That's what got us here.'

*Doctor:* True. It's very important work the Learning Disability Group does in building up consumer appreciation. There's gotta be a dialogue; it's the only way.

**3**   *Mr J:* I'm a member of PPP and so if you send them the account they will pay.... They asked for a report if you can send one.

*Doctor:* What shall I say?

*Mr J:* Whatever you think.

*Doctor:* No, what you say. I'm your agent. I'll write whatever you want.

**4**   *Doctor:* Have you had occasion to see Smith at all?

*Mrs E:* He's very good.

*Doctor:* I thought you were seeing Jones. He thought Smith didn't have anything to contribute.

**5**   *Mrs B:* Now where do we go from here?

*Doctor:* May I ask you something...?

[After a further ten minutes]

*Mrs B:* (standing up) Thank you for your kind attention.

(Extracts 1 and 2, Strong, 1979, pp. 78 and 80; extracts 3 to 5, Silverman, 1984, pp. 196, 198 and 201)

● How do the patients in these extracts demonstrate their dominance?

■ In extract 1, the patient indicates that she is seeking a second opinion, and in extract 5 the patient decides when the consultation is over. In extracts 1, 2 and 4 there is an assumption that there may be good doctors and bad ones, or at least that professional opinions may differ, and that open discussion of this fact is allowed in the consultation.

● How do the doctors demonstrate their willingness to allow patients this power?

■ By going along with the discussion of the merits of other doctors, and in extracts 3 and 5 behaving in a particularly deferential manner. In extract 3 the doctor explicitly assumes the role of the patient's agent.

In private practice doctors are in competition with each other, so their reputation is the guarantee of their expertise and income; patients may also have greater incomes and social status than the doctors. By contrast, in NHS consultations lay challenges to professional expertise are more likely to be resisted.

## 9.4.3 Off-stage behaviour

However, although patients' behaviour in NHS consultations is likely to appear more deferential than in these private settings, this may be deceptive. The consultation is but one point in a continuing relationship, where deferential behaviour may be used tactically by the patient, to achieve certain ends. During the consultation the patient is 'on stage'. *Off-stage behaviour* may reveal attitudes considerably at variance with this, and studies of how people talk about medical encounters before and after the event support this view. Sociologists Gerry Stimson and Barbara Webb, in a study of patients in South Wales, showed that this is the point at which patients evaluate doctors' advice:

> As soon as I saw the pills I knew they were no good. I said to Terry when he brought them in 'I've had them before and they were no good'.... I didn't know that's what the doctor was giving me when he wrote out the prescription, otherwise I would have told him then that I'd had them before and they were no good. (Stimson and Webb, 1975, pp. 71–2)

People may join together in planning strategies for consultations:

> The last time I went about bronchitis, he [the doctor] gave me these new pills. 'Just come out,' he said, and you know, they did work, they were better than the ones I had before. And so, there's this other lady I know also gets it badly, so I told her to tell the doctor to give her these ones. (Stimson and Webb, 1975, p. 86)

People may compensate for their lack of power in face-to-face interaction by ridiculing the doctor in stories that redress the balance. Stimson and Webb found one woman who had missed some periods and had previously been told she was infertile:

> When I went back for the results a fortnight later I knew what he was going to tell me because there he was, this doctor, pooving around the room, sort of hopping from one foot to another like a nervous rabbit. And he finally said: 'Eh — I'm afraid to have to tell you Miss Brown our tests have shown you're three months pregnant' — I was two months pregnant when they told me I was infertile! (Stimson and Webb, 1975, p. 106)

Another person giving a critical account said:

> I called him in. She had what I thought was chicken pox. And he stood there with his backside in front of the fire, and she was on the settee. 'Well it could be chicken pox' he said.
>
> (Stimson and Webb, 1975, p. 107)

● In the audiotape 'Why me? Why now?',[4] in which Jocelyn Cornwell interviews Wendy about her hysterectomy, there are a number of instances where Wendy presents herself as using doctors to suit her own ends. What were they?

---

[4] The audiotape, 'Why me? Why now?' is specially made for Open University students studying this book and was listened to in Chapter 2.

■ She rejects the family planning doctor's proposal that she give up smoking if she wants to continue with the pill, and finds another doctor who will prescribe the pill without conditions. After one gynaecologist refused her, she found another one who would do her bidding and take out her womb.

Thus it is important to examine the surrounding context in order to understand the meaning of consultations.

## 9.5   Different styles for different needs

It is also likely that different consulting styles are appropriate for different types of condition. Szasz and Hollender (Table 9.1) argued that the mutual participation model was more suitable in cases of chronic illness or psychological problems. Here, definitions of what counts as good health are rather less clear-cut than in curable physical conditions. Negotiation about what is to count as success, recognition of the patient's contribution to healing and of the doctor's relative lack of expertise, are more appropriate.

There is some evidence to support this view. In 1990 Richard Savage, a general practitioner, and David Armstrong, the doctor and sociologist referred to in Chapter 8, published a paper that compared groups of patients who had been randomly allocated to receive two different styles of consultation: a 'shared' or patient-centred approach, and a 'directed' or doctor-centred approach. The patients were asked whether they had felt able to discuss their problem well, whether they received an excellent explanation, whether the GP seemed to understand their problem and whether they felt helped or better. On the whole, patients preferred the directed approach. However, there were exceptions to this general rule with patients who suffered from psychological or chronic conditions showing no significant preference.

● What might the objections be to evaluating the patient-centred style according to whether patients felt it met their needs?

■ It might be argued that patients have been trained to expect a directed approach, and that although a shared approach might be beneficial in the long term, it might at first produce feelings of confusion and difficulty as patients reluctantly learned to take responsibility for their own health.

## 9.6   Conclusion

Preferences for different styles of consultation are influenced by a large number of things. It is not easy to arrive at once-and-for-all answers about what is right. It is important to recognise that the advocacy of a particular style — as in the case of patient-centredness — should be assessed in its cultural context. Patient-centredness had a particular appeal in late-twentieth-century American and British health care because of a complex mixture of factors. These included broader social movements that reflected on issues like democracy in client–professional relationships, and changes in popular views of authority and psychological health. Different styles may be applied in different contexts, and may be judged appropriate or inappropriate depending on the illness presented. The most fundamental issue may be the generation of a feeling of trust, however that is achieved.

# 9.7  Postscript

We began this book by inviting you to think of yourself as a traveller in a strange land, journeying around different kinds of medical knowledge with this book as your guide. It may be that, by now, you feel you have made some advances in your understanding of medical knowledge. If not in possession of all the answers to questions of health and disease, you may at least be able to see what some of the questions are and why they are significant.

A main aim of this book has been to increase your sense of the strangeness of the health beliefs and medical practices current in the society we live in. In particular, the study of how other societies, and of how our own society in the past, have viewed the workings of the body, the naming and treating of disease, can help us see that our own ways of doing these things are only one way, particular to a place and time in history. Achieving a position of *anthropological strangeness* involves increasing one's doubt about things which otherwise appear fixed as 'common sense,' or 'expert knowledge'.

We might, then, choose to adopt the view that modern medical knowledge is but one way of doing things; that it could have been different if history had earlier taken a slightly different course; that it could be overthrown at the pronouncement of some future genius; or that it might have been different for us had we been born into a different society. The implication of this view is profoundly disturbing. It seems to abandon any attempt to distinguish true from false knowledge, or to create areas of certainty in a landscape of doubt. This book has outlined some aspects of the historical development of the scientific method, which many in the medical profession propose as an objective way of establishing truth. It has shown the variety of some of the medical knowledge that has been produced. But it has also introduced you to critiques of the medical claim to scientific objectivity.

Your task now is to chart your own course as you travel further. To help you in this, we propose in the next book in this series[5] to show you the different methods used by those concerned with creating medical knowledge. This should provide you with some of the equipment you will need to study further accounts of health and disease that emanate from a variety of academic disciplines.

## OBJECTIVES FOR CHAPTER 9

When you have studied this chapter, you should be able to:

**9.1** Define and use, or recognise definitions and applications of, each of the terms printed in **bold** in the text.

**9.2** Describe the characteristics of doctor-centred and patient-centred consultations and the strengths and weaknesses of each.

**9.3** Demonstrate that criteria for judging the appropriateness of different consultation styles depend on cultural assumptions.

**9.4** Assess the importance of surrounding context in interpreting the meaning of doctor–patient interactions.

---

[5] *Studying Health and Disease* (Open University Press, 2nd edn 1994; colour-enhanced 2nd edn 2001).

## QUESTIONS FOR CHAPTER 9

**1** (*Objective 9.2*)

The following conversations are between nurses and their patients.

**Extract 1**

*Nurse:* Right…Apart from feeling tired, you've been feeling alright?

*Patient:* Well, I've got tingling sensations in my toes and finger ends.

*Nurse:* Are you sleeping alright?

*Patient:* I never do.

*Nurse:* Appetite, is that OK?

*Patient:* No, not really. I don't feel like food.

*Nurse:* Good. Right then, you know what's going on, don't you? Can I put your wrist label on?

*Patient:* I don't know which wrist you want.

*Nurse:* I'll have it on this one then? Right, that's all I need to know. Thanks.

(Source: Wilkinson, 1991, p. 683)

**Extract 2**

*Nurse:* Can you tell me what you think is causing the pain?

*Patient:* The cancer. It's come back in my bones and that's why he [the doctor] wants to do some X-ray treatment to relieve the pain.

*Nurse:* Mr W. has told you it's in your bones, has he?

*Patient:* Yes, love.

*Nurse:* What do you think about that?

*Patient:* Well, I'm not pleased. I was very upset when he told me as I realize that I may not get better. But if he can get rid of this pain I shall be so thankful as my grandchildren are coming from Canada for a holiday and I just want to be able to enjoy their visit and be able to go out for days with them. (Source: Wilkinson, 1991, p. 682)

What characteristics of these interactions identify one as more patient-centred, and the other as more centred on the concerns of the nurse?

**2** (*Objective 9.3*)

There are several stages to the transformation of one regime of truth into another. First there is the recognition that silence can be construed as a lie, then there is the defence of the lie as a form of truth, and finally as the boundary between lying and truth-telling is redrawn the lie is revealed as truly a lie. (Armstrong, 1987, p. 653)

How might this analysis be applied to the gradual shifts in medical opinion about telling the truth to cancer patients, in the United Kingdom, the USA and Italy?

**3**   (*Objective 9.4*)

David Silverman reports the following interaction between doctor and patient at a private oncology clinic.

> *Patient:* One interesting thing about the cause of cancer — is it changes of temperature?
>
> *Doctor:* I don't close my mind to your suggestion.
>
> *Patient:* What about blood cancer — could it be a knock?
>
> *Doctor:* Well there is so much evidence that there's a viral origin... (The patient talks for five minutes. Then the doctor closes the topic.)
>
> *Doctor:* Now with regard to yourself...
>
> (Source: Silverman, 1984, p. 129)

Why would this be unlikely to occur in an NHS clinic?

# References and further sources

## References

Ackerknecht, E. H. (1967) *Medicine at the Paris Hospital 1794–1848*, Johns Hopkins Press, Baltimore.

Anderson, E. and Anderson, P. (1987) General practitioners and alternative medicine, *Journal of the Royal College of General Practitioners*, **37**, pp. 52–5.

Armstrong, D. (1983) *Political Anatomy of the Body: Medical Knowledge in Britain in the Twentieth Century*, Cambridge University Press, Cambridge.

Armstrong, D. (1987) Silence and truth in death and dying, *Social Science and Medicine*, **24**(8) pp. 651–7.

Asher, R. (1972) *Talking Sense*, a collection of papers edited by Jones, F. A., Pitman Medical; and extract 'Malingering' appears in Davey, B., Gray, A. and Seale, C. (eds) *Health and Disease: A Reader*, (1995) 2nd edn and (2001) 3rd edn, Open University Press, Buckingham.

Atkinson, P. (1981) *The Clinical Experience: The Construction and Reconstruction of Medical Reality*, Gower, Farnborough.

Balint, M. (1956) *The Doctor, his Patient and the Illness*, Pitman, London.

Behring, E. von, and Kitasato, S. (1890) Über das Zustandekommen der Diptherie-Immunitä und der Tetanus-Immunität bei Thieren, *Deutsche Medizinische Wochenschrift*, **16**, pp. 1113–4.

Bhopal, R. S. (1986) The inter-relationship of folk, traditional and western medicine within an Asian community in Britain, *Social Science and Medicine*, **22**(1), pp. 99–105.

Blane, D. (1991) Health professions, in Patrick, D. and Scambler, G. (eds) *Sociology As Applied to Medicine*, Baillière-Tindall, London.

Blaxter, M. (1983) The causes of disease: women talking, *Social Science and Medicine*, **17**(2), pp. 59–69.

Blaxter, M. (1990) *Health and Lifestyles*, Tavistock/Routledge, London.

Brewin, T. (1985) Truth, trust and paternalism, *Lancet*, 31 August 31, pp. 490–2; reproduced in Davey, B., Gray, A. and Seale, C. (eds) *Health and Disease: A Reader*, (1995) 2nd edn and (2001) 3rd edn, Open University Press, Buckingham.

Briquet, P. (1859) *Treatise on Hysteria* (Traité Clinique et Thérapeutique de l'Hystérie), Baillière, Paris.

British Holistic Medical Association (1986) *Report of the British Medical Association Board of Science Working Party on Alternative Therapy*, British Holistic Medical Association, London.

British Medical Association (1986) *Alternative Therapy*, BMA, London.

Brown, P. (1992) The return of the big killer, *New Scientist*, 10 Oct.

Bryder, L. (1988) *Below the Magic Mountain: A Social History of Tuberculosis in Twentieth-Century Britain*, Oxford University Press, Oxford.

Buckley, T. and Gottlieb, A. (1988) *Blood Magic: Explorations in the Anthropology of Menstruation*, University of California Press, Berkeley and London.

Bury, M. (1986) Social constructionism and the development of medical sociology, *Sociology of Health and Illness*. **8**(2), pp. 137–69.

Charcot, J.-M. (1878) De la choréthmique hystérique, *Progres Medical*, **6**(6).

Charcot, J.-M. (1889) *Lectures on Diseases of the Nervous System*, New Sydenham Society, trans. and ed. by George Sigerson, 3 vols, London, 1877–89.

Clarétie, J. (1882) *La Vie à Paris—1881*, V. Howard, Paris.

Clark, J. M. (1981) Communication in nursing, *Nursing Times*, 1 January, pp. 12–18.

Conrad, P. (1985) The meaning of medication: another look at compliance, *Social Science and Medicine*, **20**, pp. 29–37.

Cornwell, J. (1984) *Hard-earned Lives*, Tavistock, London.

Cousins, M. and Hussain, A. (1984) *Michel Foucault*, Macmillan Education Ltd., London.

Crofton, J. (1960) Tuberculosis undefeated, *British Medical Journal*, **ii**, p. 679.

Crojé, G. (1984) Tuberculosis and mortality decline in England and Wales, 1851–1900, in Woods, R. and Woodward, J. (eds) *Urban Disease and Mortality in Nineteenth-Century England*, Croom Helm, London.

Descartes, R. (1637) *Discourse on Method*, trans. Veitch, J. (1912), Dent, London (Everyman edition).

Descartes, R. (1651) *Treatise of Man*, trans. Hall, T. S. (1972), Harvard University Press, Cambridge, Mass.

Egger, J., Stolla, A. and McEwen, L. M. (1992) Controlled trial of hyposensitisation in children with food-induced hyperkinetic syndrome, *Lancet*, **339**, pp. 1150–4.

Eisenburg, L. (1977) Disease and illness: distinctions between professional and popular ideas of sickness, *Culture, Medicine and Psychiatry*, **I**, pp. 9–23.

Epsom, J. (1978) The mobile health clinic: report on the first year's work, in Tucket, D. and Kaufert, J. (eds) *Basic Readings in Medical Sociology*, Tavistock, London.

Fabrega, H. (1979) Elementary systems of medicine, *Culture, Medicine and Psychiatry*, **3**, pp. 167–98.

Feldman, W. H. (1946) The chemotherapy of tuberculosis—including the use of streptomycin, *Journal of the Royal Institute of Public Health and Hygiene*, **9**, pp. 267–363.

Foucault, M. (1967) Madness and Civilization: A History of Insanity in the Age of Reason, Tavistock, London.

Fox, N. J. (1992) *The Social Meaning of Surgery*, Open University Press, Buckingham.

Freidson, E. (1970a) *Profession of Medicine*, Harper & Row, New York and London.

Freidson, E. (1970b) *Professional Dominance*, Russell Sage, New York.

Freud, S. and Breuer, J. (1980) *Studies on Hysteria, 1883–1895*, The Pelican Freud Library, vol. 3, Penguin Books, Harmondsworth, Middx (1st edn 1895).

Fulder, S. J. (1986) A new interest in complementary (alternative) medicine: towards pluralism in medicine? *Impact of Science on Society*, **143**, pp. 235–43.

Fulder, S. J. and Munro, R. E. (1985) Complementary medicine in the United Kingdom: patients, practitioners, and consultations, *Lancet*, 7 September, pp. 542–5.

Giddens, A. (1991) *Modernity and Self-Identity: Self and Society in the Late Modern Age*, Polity Press, Cambridge.

Gordon, D. R. (1990) Embodying illness, embodying cancer, *Culture, Medicine and Psychiatry*. **14**, pp. 275–97.

Greenwood, M. (1928) Tuberculosis, *British Medical Journal*, **i**, p. 793.

Hart, D'Arcy and Wright, Payling G. (1939) *Tuberculosis and Social Conditions in England with Special Reference to Young Adults, a Statistical Study*, National Association for the Prevention of Tuberculosis, London.

Harvey, W. (1628) Exercitatio Anatomica de Motu Cordis et Sanguinis in trans. Franklin, K. J. (1907) *William Harvey, the Circulation of the Blood and Other Writings*, Dent and Dutton, London (Everyman edition).

Heath, S. (1982) *The Sexual Fix*, The Macmillan Press Ltd., London and Basingstoke.

Helman, C. G. (1990) *Culture, Health and Illness*, Butterworth-Heinemann, London; an extract 'Feed a cold, starve a fever' appears in Davey, B., Gray, A. and Seale, C. (eds) *Health and Disease: A Reader*, (1995) 2nd edn and (2001) 3rd edn, Open University Press, Buckingham.

Hippocrates, *Epidemics*, trans. Jones, W. H. S. (1957) *Hippocrates with an English Translation* (The Loeb Edition), Harvard University Press, Boston.

Hunt, L. M., Jordan, B., Irwin, S. and Browner, C. H. (1989) Compliance and the patient's perspective: controlling symptoms in everyday life, *Culture, Medicine and Psychiatry*, **13**(3), pp. 315–34.

Illich, I. (1976) *Limits to Medicine*, Marion Boyars, London; an extract 'The epidemics of modern medicine' appears in Davey, B., Gray, A. and Seale, C. (eds) *Health and Disease: A Reader*, (1995) 2nd edn and (2001) 3rd edn, Open University Press, Buckingham.

James, M. (1994) Hysteria and demonic possession, originally published for Open University students; reprinted in Davey, B., Gray, A. and Seale, C. (eds) *Health and Disease: A Reader*, (1995) 2nd edn and (2001) 3rd edn, Open University Press, Buckingham.

Jorden, E. (1603) *Briefe Discourse of a Disease Called the Suffocation of the Mother*, John Windet, London.

Katz, P. (1981) Ritual in the operating room, *Ethnology*, **20**, pp. 335–50.

Katz, P. (1985) How surgeons make decisions, in Hann, R. A. and Gaines, A. D. (eds) *Physicians of Western Medicine*, D. Reidel, Holland.

Keers, R. Y. (1978) *Pulmonary Tuberculosis: A Journey down the Centuries*, Baillière-Tindall, London.

Kitzinger, S. (1982) The social context of birth, in MacCormack, C. P. (ed.) *An Ethnography of Fertility and Birth*, Academic Press, London.

Kleinman, A. (1980) *Patients and Healers in the Context of Culture*, University of California Press, Berkeley.

Kleinman, A., Eisenberg, L. and Good, B. (1978) Culture, illness and care: clinical lessons from anthropologic and cross-cultural research, *Annals of Internal Medicine*, **88**, pp. 251–8.

Kramer, H. and Sprenger, J. (1486) *Malleus Maleficarum*, translated with an introduction, bibliography and notes by Summers, M. (1951), Pushkin Press, London.

Lancet (1986) Notes and news: alternative medicine, *Lancet*, 12 July, pp. 116–17.

Larkin, G. V. (1978) Medical dominance and the control of radiographers, *Sociological Review*, **26**, pp. 843–58.

Larkin, G. V. (1992) Orthodox and osteopathic medicine in the inter-war years, in Saks, M. (ed.) *Alternative Medicine in Britain*, Clarendon Press, Oxford, pp. 112–23.

Lewis, O. (1955) Medicine and politics in a Mexican village, in Paul, B. D. (ed.) *Health, Culture and Community*, Russell Sage, New York.

Locke, J. (1690) *Essay Concerning Human Understanding*, ed. Nidditch, P. H. (1975) Clarendon Press, Oxford.

Long, E. R. (1965) *A History of Pathology*, Dover, New York.

Lower, R. (1666) The method observed in transfusing the blood of one animal into another, *Philosophical Transactions*, **2**, pp. 323–8.

Lower, R. (1669) *Tractatus de Corde* Jacob Allestry, London, translated by Franklin, K. J. in Gunther, R. T. (1932) *Early Science in Oxford*, vol. 9 (privately printed), Oxford.

Macintosh, J. M. (1944) *The Nation's Health*, Pilot Press, London.

Maclean, I. (1980) *The Renaissance Notion of Women*, Cambridge University Press, Cambridge.

Manning, H. (1775) *A Treatise on Female Disease*, 2nd edn, R. Baldwin, London (first published 1717).

Martin, E. (1989) *The Woman in the Body: A Cultural Analysis of Reproduction*, Open University Press, Buckingham.

McPherson, K., Wennberg, J. E., Hovind, O. B. and Clifford, P. (1982) Small area variations in the use of common surgical procedures: an international comparison of New England, England and Norway, *New England Journal of Medicine*, **307**, pp. 1310–14.

Merskey, H. and Potter, P. (1989) The womb lay still in ancient Egypt, *British Journal of Psychiatry*, **cliv**, pp. 751–3.

Micale, M. (1990) Hysteria and its historiography: the future perspective, *History of Psychiatry*, **i**, pp. 33–124.

Miner, H. (1956) Body ritual amongst the Nacirema, *American Anthropologist*, **58**, pp. 503–7.

Ministry of Health (1947) *Report of the Chief Medical Officer for the Year 1946*, HMSO, London.

Ministry of Health (1949) *Report of the Chief Medical Officer for the Year 1948*, HMSO, London.

Montaigne, M. E. de (1952 trans.) *Essais*, Book 2, Essay 37.

Morgagni, G. B. (1761) *On the Seats and Causes of Diseases Investigated by Anatomy*, trans. Alexander, B. (1769), 3 vols, London.

Navarro, V. (1976) *Medicine Under Capitalism*, Prodist, New York; an extract 'The mode of state intervention in the health sector' appears in Davey, B., Gray, A. and Seale, C. (eds) *Health and Disease: A Reader*, (1995) 2nd edn and (2001) 3rd edn, Open University Press, Buckingham.

Nettleton, S. (1988) Protecting the vulnerable margin: towards an analysis of how the mouth came to be separated from the body, *Sociology of Health and Illness*, **10**(2), pp. 156–69; an edited version with the same title appears in Davey, B., Gray, A. and Seale, C. (eds) *Health and Disease: A Reader*, (1995) 2nd edn and (2001) 3rd edn, Open University Press, Buckingham.

Office of Health Economics (1962) *Progress against Tuberculosis*, OHE, London.

Palis, J., Rossopoulos, E. and Triarkou, L.-C. (1985) The Hippocratic concept of hysteria: a translation of the original texts, *Integrative Psychiatry*, **iii**, pp. 226–8.

Parish, H. J. (1965) *A History of Immunization*, Livingstone, Edinburgh.

Parsons, T. (1951) *The Social System*, Free Press, Glencoe, Illinois.

Payer, L. (1990) *Medicine and Culture*, Victor Gollancz, London.

Rabinow, P. (ed.) (1984) *The Foucault Reader*, Penguin, London.

Reiach, A. and Hurd, R. (1944) *Building Scotland*, The Saltire Society, Edinburgh.

Rose, G. (1981) Strategy of prevention: the lessons from cardiovascular disease, *British Medical Journal*, **282**, pp. 1847–51.

Roth, J. (1957) Ritual and magic in the control of contagion, *American Sociological Review*, **22**, pp. 310–14.

Rousseau, J.-J. (1974 edition) *Emile*, trans. Foxley, B., Dent, London.

Sadler, J. (1636) *The Sicke Woman's Private Looking Glass*, printed by Anne Griffin, London.

Saks, M. (ed.) (1992) *Alternative Medicine in Britain*, Clarendon Press, Oxford.

Savage, R. and Armstrong, D. (1990) Effect of a general practitioner's consulting style on patients' satisfaction: a controlled study, *British Medical Journal*, **301**, pp. 968–70.

Scambler, A., Scambler, G. and Craig, D. (1981) Kinship and friendship networks and women's demand for primary care, *Journal of the Royal College of General Practitioners*, **26**, pp. 746–50.

Scambler, G. (ed.) (1991) *Sociology as Applied to Medicine*, 3rd edn, Baillière-Tindall, London.

Scarre, G. (1987) *Witchcraft and Magic in 16th and 17th Century Europe*, Macmillan Education, Hampshire and London.

Schulzer, M., Fitzgerald, J. M., Enarson, D. A. and Grzybowsky, S. (1992) An estimate of the future size of the tuberculosis problem in sub-Saharan Africa resulting from HIV infection, *Tubercle and Lung Disease*, **73**, pp. 52–8.

Seale, C. F. (1991) Communication and awareness about death: a study of a random sample of dying people, *Social Science and Medicine*, **32**(8), pp. 943–52.

Sharma, U. M. (1990) Using alternative therapies: marginal medicine and central concerns, in Abbott, P. and Payne, G. (eds) *New Directions in the Sociology of Health*, Falmer Press, Brighton, pp. 140–52; an edited version appears in Davey, B., Gray, A. and Seale, C. (eds) *Health and Disease: A Reader*, (1995) 2nd edn and (2001) 3rd edn, Open University Press, Buckingham.

Shorter, E. (1992) *From Paralysis to Fatigue: A History of Psychosomatic Illness*, Free Press, New York.

Showalter, E. (1987, new edn 1991) *The Female Malady: Women, Madness and English Culture, 1830–1980*, Virago Press, London (first published 1985, Pantheon Books, New York).

Silverman, D. (1984) *Communication and Medical Practice: Social Relations in the Clinic*, Sage, London.

Smith R. (1991) Where is the wisdom…? The poverty of medical evidence, *British Medical Journal*, **303**, pp. 798–9.

Smith-Rosenberg, C. (1972) The hysterical woman: sex roles and role conflict in nineteenth century America, *Social Research*, **39**, pp. 652–78.

Sontag, S. (1978) *Illness as Metaphor*, Penguin, Harmondsworth.

Stacey, M. (1988) *The Sociology of Health and Healing*, Unwin Hyman, London.

Stevens, R. (1976) The evolution of the health care systems in the United States and the United Kingdom: similarities and differences, in *Priorities in the Use of Resources in Medicine*, No. 40 in Fogarty International Center Proceedings, US Dept of Health, Education and Welfare.

Stimson, G. and Webb, B. (1975) *Going to See the Doctor: The Consultation Process in General Practice*, Routledge and Kegan Paul, London.

Strong, P. M. (1979) *The Ceremonial Order of the Clinic*, Routledge and Kegan Paul, London.

Summers, M. (trans. and ed.) (1971) *The Malleus Maleficarum of Heinrich Kramer and James Sprenger*, Dover Publications, New York.

Szasz, T. S., and Hollender, M. H. (1956) A contribution to the philosophy of medicine: the basic models of the doctor–patient relationship, *Archives of Internal Medicine*, **97**, pp. 585–92.

Tahzib, F. and Daniel, S. O. (1986) Traditional medicine and the modern medical curriculum, *Lancet*, 26 July, pp. 203–4.

Taylor, K. M. (1988) 'Telling bad news': physicians and the disclosure of undesirable information, *Sociology of Health and Illness*, **10**(2), pp. 109–31.

Taylor, S. (1944) *Battle for Health: A Primer of Social Medicine*, Nicholson and Watson, London.

Thorogood, N. (1990) Caribbean home remedies and their importance for black women's health care in Britain, in Abbott, P. and Payne, G. (eds) *New Directions in the Sociology of Health*, Falmer Press, Brighton, pp. 140–52.

Titmuss, R. M. (1970) *The Gift Relationship: From Human Blood to Social Policy*, George Allen and Unwin, London.

Tuckett, D., Boulton, M., Olson, C. and Williams, A. (1985) *Meetings Between Experts: An Approach to Sharing Ideas in Medical Consultations*, Tavistock, London.

U205 Course Team (1985) *Experiencing and Explaining Disease*, Open University Press, Milton Keynes.

Vander, H. J., Sherman, J. H. and Luciano, D. S. (1980) *Human Physiology: Mechanisms of Body Function*, 3rd edn, McGraw-Hill, New York.

Vander, H. J., Sherman, J. H. and Luciano, D. S. (1985) *Human Physiology: Mechanisms of Body Function*, 4th edn, McGraw-Hill, New York.

Veith, I. (1965) *Hysteria: the History of a Disease*, Phoenix Books, The University of Chicago Press, Chicago and London.

Waitzkin, H. and Waterman, B. (1973) *The Exploitation of the Sick Role in Capitalist Society*, Prentice Hall, New Jersey.

Waksman, S. A. (1965) *The Conquest of Tuberculosis*, Robert Hale, London.

Wender, P. H. (1971) *Minimal Brain Dysfunction in Children*, New York, Wiley.

Wheeler Robinson, H. (1909) 'Blood' in Hastings, J. (ed.) *Encyclopaedia of Religion and Ethics*, Clark, Edinburgh.

Wilkinson, S. (1991) Factors which influence how nurses communicate with cancer patients, *Journal of Advanced Nursing*, **16**, pp. 677–88.

Williams, L. (1908) The worship of Moloch, *British Journal of Tuberculosis*, **2**, pp. 56–62.

Wollstonecraft, M. (1986) *Vindication of the Rights of Woman*, Penguin Books Ltd., Harmondsworth, Middx. (1st edn 1792).

World Health Organisation (1964), Expert Committee on Tuberculosis, Technical Report Series, **290**, WHO, Geneva.

World Health Organisation (1982) Expert Committee on Tuberculosis, *Tuberculosis Control*, Technical Report Series, **671**, WHO, Geneva.

World Health Organisation (1988) *WHO/87 Press Release*, 23 November 1998; available from http://www.who.int/inf-pr-1998/en/pr98–87.html [accessed May 2000].

World Health Organisation (2000a) *Tuberculosis*, WHO Factsheet No.104, revised April 2000, available from http://www.who.int/inf-fs/en/fact104.html [accessed May 2000].

World Health Organisation (2000b) *WHO Global Tuberculosis Control, 4th Report* (2000), WHO, Geneva; or available from http://www.who.int/gtb/publications/globrep00 [accessed May 2000].

Wren, C. (1750) Parentalia, or: Memoirs of the Family of the Wrens, London.

Wright, P. and Treacher, A. (1982) *The Problem of Medical Knowledge*, Edinburgh University Press, Edinburgh.

Wunderlich, C. A. (1871) *On the Temperature in Diseases: A Manual of Medical Thermometry*, first German edition 1868; English trans., The New Sydenham Society, London.

Young, A. (1976) Internalising and externalising medical belief systems: an Ethiopian example, *Social Science and Medicine*, **10**(3/4), pp. 147–56.

Zola, I. K. (1973) Pathways to the doctor: from person to patient, *Social Science and Medicine*, **7**, pp. 677–89.

Zollman, C. and Vickers, A. (1999) Users and practitioners of complementary medicine, *British Medical Journal*, **319**, pp. 836–8.

## Further sources

### Sociology of health and illness

If you want to keep up to date with research and thinking in health-related sociology, then two academic journals — *Social Science and Medicine* and *Sociology of Health and Illness* — are considered the leaders in this field. You could also check the website of the Medical Sociology Group of the British Sociological Association, where details of conferences and publications are posted (http://medsocbsa.swan.ac.uk). Textbooks we recommend include *Health and Illness in a Changing Society*, by Michael Bury (1997, Routledge, London), which is probably the most accessible for readers new to the subject area; *Medical Power and Social Knowledge*, by Bryan S. Turner and Colin Samson (1995, Sage, London); *The Sociology of Health and Illness*, by Sarah Nettleton (1995, Polity Press, Cambridge); *The Sociology of Health and Medicine*, by Ellen Annandale (1998, Polity Press, Cambridge); and *Medicine as Culture: Illness, Disease and the Body in Western Societies*, by Deborah Lupton (1994, Sage, London).

### History of medicine

For those interested in learning more about the history of medicine in its social context *The Greatest Benefit to Mankind*, by Roy Porter (1997, HarperCollins Publishers, London), and *History of the Human Sciences*, by Roger Smith, in the 'Norton History' series (1997, W. W. Norton and Co., USA) are both highly recommended accounts. *A Short History of Medicine*, by Erwin H. Ackerknecht (revised edition 1982, Johns Hopkins Paperbacks, Baltimore and London), provides a general map of medical developments down the centuries, and is still in print. Many of the chapters in *Medicine in Society: Historical Essays*, edited by Andrew Wear (1992, Cambridge University Press, Cambridge), are useful on particular topics such as madness and its treatment and changing views of the patient. Two frequently-cited but out of print books are available on loan through libraries: *The Development of Modern Medicine*, by Richard Harrison Shryock (1979, University of Wisconsin Press, Madison and London), gives a succinct and critical account of modern medicine in its social context from 1600 to the middle of the twentieth century. Those interested in the development of ideas about disease, its identification and classification, will find an introduction in *Medical Thinking*, by Lester S. King (1982, Princeton University Press, Princeton and London). See also the Wellcome Trust's website (http://www.wellcome.ac.uk).

### Complementary health care

Books that explore the developing social position of alternative or complementary medicine, discuss the legal, political and scientific aspects, and consider why people in Western cultures increasingly choose complementary remedies or consult non-orthodox healers, are: *Complementary and Alternative Medicines: Knowledge in Practice*, edited by Sarah Cant and Ursula Sharma (1996, Free Association Books); *A New Medical Pluralism: Alternative Medicine, Doctors, Patients and the State*, also by Sarah Cant and Ursula Sharma (1998, UCL Press, London); and *Handbook of Alternative and Complementary Medicine*, edited by Stephen Fulder (1996, Oxford University Press, Oxford).

### Chapters 1–3

In addition to the titles listed in all the sections above, we also recommend the following: *Culture, Health and Illness*, by Cecil Helman (1990, Butterworth-Heinemann, London), is a good introduction to the field of medical anthropology (Chapter 4 on 'Caring and curing:

the sectors of health care' is of particular relevance). On the moral connotations of illness and disease see especially two essays by Susan Sontag, now published as a single volume: *Illness as Metaphor* and *AIDS and its Metaphors* (1991, Penguin, Harmondsworth). *Illness as Metaphor* gives an account of the variety of moral connotations attached to tuberculosis and cancer, with examples taken largely from literature. *AIDS and its Metaphors* discusses the moral metaphors attached to AIDS, following up the ideas of the earlier work. Here Sontag stresses that the scientific view of AIDS is less moralising, and has therefore been welcomed by people with the disease.

## Chapter 4 Tuberculosis

*Below the Magic Mountain: A Social History of Tuberculosis in Twentieth-Century Britain*, by Linda Bryder (1988, Oxford University Press, Oxford), is a comprehensive, accessible and balanced introduction from the health and health-care perspectives, concentrating on the period 1900–1950. Several recent books on the history of TB have been published in the USA, where the upsurge in cases in the 1990s has created major public interest; they are all readily available: *Living in the Shadow of Death: Tuberculosis and the Social Experience of Illness in American History* by Sheila M. Rothman (1995, Johns Hopkins University Press); *Disease and Class: Tuberculosis and the Shaping of Modern American Society*, by Georgina Feldberg (1995, Rutgers University Press); *Fevered Lives: Tuberculosis in American Culture since 1870*, by Katherine Ott (paperback edition, 1999, Harvard University Press); and *From Chaos to Coercion: Detention and Control of Tuberculosis*, by Richard J. Coker (2000, St. Martin's Press). *The White Death: A History of Tuberculosis*, by Thomas Dormandy (1999, Hambledon Press, London) is strong on stories of the famous victims of TB (the Brontes, Keats, Chopin, Chekhov, D. H. Lawrence, Kafka, among others), but tends to ignore the mass of disease among the working poor. An introduction to modern medical research, written for a medical audience, can be found in *Current Topics in Microbiology and Immunology, Volume 215, Tuberculosis*, edited by T. M. Shinnick (1996, Springer-Verlag, Berlin and Heidelberg). You can keep track of developments in the global epidemiology of TB on the World Health Organisation's Tuberculosis website (http://www.who.int/health-topics/tb.htm).

## Chapter 5 Blood

The best single resource on issues related to the chapter on blood is *Blood, Pure and Eloquent: A Story of Discovery, of People, and of Ideas*, edited by Maxwell M. Wintrobe (1980, McGraw Hill, New York). *Circulation of the Blood: Men and Ideas*, by Alfred P. Fishman and Dickinson W. Richards (1964, Oxford University Press, New York), is an old but classic account of important ideas and developments in the history of the discovery of the circulation of the blood. At a more popular level, Andrew Cunningham's article 'William Harvey: The discovery of the circulation of the blood', in *Man Masters Nature*, edited by Roy Porter (1987, BBC Publications, London), develops and extends some of the material about Harvey considered in Cunningham's chapter in the course book. An extensive and approachable account can be found in *Blood Transfusion*, edited by Geoffrey Keynes (1949, Simpkin Marshall (1941) Ltd, London). The sociological and ethical aspects of blood donation are explored in *The Gift Relationship: From Human Blood to Social Policy*, by Richard Titmuss (1970, George Allen and Unwin, London).

## Chapter 6 Hysteria

In *Approaching Hysteria: Disease and its Interpretations* (1995, Princeton University Press, USA), Mark Micale reviews a range of representations and understandings of the disease by historians of medicine, art and gender studies, doctors, psychoanalysts and scientists. *Hysteria: the History of a Disease*, by Ilza Veith (1965, The University of Chicago Press, Chicago and London), is out of print but provides a detailed, informative and well-written account of the varied manifestations of hysteria from ancient Egypt to the evolution of psychoanalysis and examines the changing approach of physicians to this condition. *The Female Malady: Women, Madness and English Culture, 1830–1980* by Elaine Showalter (1987, Virago Press, London; new edition 1991) provides a broad feminist social history of psychiatry. Two chapters deal with hysteria, offering a lucid interpretation of this condition as a consequence of the traditional female role. A good general account of witchcraft is to be found in *The Witch-Hunt in Early Modern Europe* by Brian P. Levack (1987, Longman, London). For an excellent discussion of the relations between hysteria, witchcraft, possession, insanity and medicine at the beginning of the seventeenth century see *Witchcraft and Hysteria in Elizabethan London: Edward Jorden and the Mary Glover Case*, by Michael MacDonald (1991, Routledge, London). *In Dora's Case: Freud, Hysteria and Feminism*, edited by Charles Bernheimer and Claire Kahane (1985, Virago Press, London), is a collection of essays which combines feminist and psychoanalytic perspectives with avant-garde literary theory. The first of two lengthy introductory essays provides a brief history of hysteria.

### Chapter 7 Medical knowledge and medical practice

An article by Michael Bury, 'Social constructionism and the development of medical sociology' (1986, *Sociology of Health and Illness*, **8**(2), pp. 137–69), gives a clear account of social constructionism and the problems it poses. Some chapters in *Culture, Health and Illness*, by Cecil Helman (1990, Butterworth-Heinemann, London), are also particularly relevant; Chapter 6 looks at gender and reproduction, and Chapter 9 at ritual and the management of misfortune.

### Chapter 8 Medicalisation and surveillance

*Political Anatomy of the Body: Medical Knowledge in Britain in the Twentieth Century*, by David Armstrong (1983, Cambridge University Press, Cambridge), applies Foucault's ideas about disciplinary power and surveillance to twentieth-century British medical knowledge. For the Marxist approach to medicine, *The Political Economy of Health*, by Lesley Doyal with Imogen Pennell (1979, Pluto Press, London), provides a comprehensive statement and review, and is still in print. *Limits to Medicine: Medical Nemesis — The Expropriation of Health*, by Ivan Illich (1995, Marion Boyars Publishers), is a full account of Illich's ideas about the negative effects of medicine, while 'Medicine as an institution of social control' by Irving Kenneth Zola in John Ehrenreich (ed.) *The Cultural Crisis of Modern Medicine* (1978, Monthly Review Press, New York and London), gives further details and information about the medicalisation thesis.

### Chapter 9 Doctor–patient interaction

Peter Maguire and Ann Faulkner train doctors and other health-care staff in how to communicate with cancer patients. In 'Barriers to psychological care of the dying', by Peter Maguire (1985, *British Medical Journal*, **291**, pp. 1 711–13), there is an account of common difficulties that staff experience in working with dying people. 'How to do it: communicate with cancer patients: Handling bad news and difficult questions', by Peter Maguire and Anne Faulkner (1988, *British Medical Journal*, **297**, pp. 907–9), is a statement of their approach to helping people cope in this situation, and their book *Talking to Cancer Patients and their Relatives* (1994, Oxford University Press) refers to a particularly difficult area of communication. *Meetings Between Experts: An Approach to Sharing Ideas in Medical Consultations*, by David Tuckett, Mary Boulton, Coral Olson and Anthony Williams (1985, Tavistock, London), argues for a shared, patient-centred consulting style on the basis of analysis of actual consultation styles and interviews with patients. A sociological view of doctor–patient interaction drawn from the analysis of a variety of settings can be found in *Communication and Medical Practice: Social Relations in the Clinic*, by David Silverman (1987, Sage, London). This is dense but worthwhile reading.

### Internet database (ROUTES)

A large amount of valuable information is available via the Internet. To help OU students and other readers of books in the *Health and Disease* series to access good quality sites without having to search for hours, the OU has developed a collection of Internet resources on a searchable database called ROUTES. All websites included in the database are selected by academic staff or subject-specialist librarians. The content of each website is evaluated to ensure that it is accurate, well presented and regularly updated. A description is included for each of the resources.

The URL for ROUTES is: http://routes.open.ac.uk/

Entering the OU course code U205 in the search box will retrieve all the resources that have been recommended for *Health and Disease*. Alternatively if you want to search for any resources on a particular subject, type in the words which best describe the subject you are interested in.

Here is one of the main websites: ROUTES will have many more.

The Wellcome Trust's website (http://www.wellcome.ac.uk) has links to news and reviews of its research programmes in the History of Medicine and the Biomedical Sciences, links to the resources held in its huge free reference library in Euston Road, London (some of which are accessible on-line), and recent news stories of major public interest on a wide range of topics in health and medicine.

# Answers to questions

## Chapter 2

1    Humoral theory saw disease as the result of a disturbance in the whole system, or an imbalance of natural forces. The 1911 text claims to 'impart a vigour to the whole system'. The 1984 tin refers to a 'natural sparkle' that has been overrun, perhaps by imbalanced behaviour the night before. The use of the remedy as a laxative is reminiscent of the purges recommended for medieval patients.

2    There is good evidence (see, for example, Table 2.1) to show that most health care is dealt with in the lay sector, with doctors only seeing the tip of the 'clinical iceberg', so the large size of that circle is appropriate. However, in the United Kingdom, the alternative sector is much smaller than the professional sector, so the relative sizes of these two sectors are misleading. (This might not be true in countries with large numbers of traditional healers: India, for example.)

Alternative and professional sectors overlap where doctors, for example, practise therapies such as acupuncture, or adopt a 'holistic' philosophy. Helman shows how doctors sometimes compromise with patients' lay health beliefs, and patients are influenced by and apply aspects of biomedical knowledge every time they follow their doctors' advice, so these would be examples of overlap between professional and lay sectors. Overlap between alternative and lay sectors might be represented by self treatment with homeopathic or herbal remedies bought over the counter.

3    The candles are described as 'non-invasive'. Ursula Sharma's study showed that fear of invasive treatment was one factor motivating people to consult alternative practitioners. The emphasis on both physical and mental effects invokes the appeal of holistic remedies.

4    Claims are made to stimulate blood circulation, strengthen the immune system and enhance the lymphatic system, all suitably 'scientific' sounding terms. The material about 'reflex zones' and 'energy points' are not derived from any system that most doctors would recognise to be true, but are suitably pseudo-scientific and thus have an indirect appeal.

## Chapter 3

1    An historical overview of the development of medical knowledge, however brief, immediately reveals that aspects of ancient traditions persist in the present day, even in modern medical practice (as described by Helman in Chapter 2). The emphasis on experimentation, the use of animals as 'models' for human disease, and mechanistic concepts of the body are accepted today as part of modern scientific medicine, but have their ancestry in antiquity. Laboratory medicine has resurfaced several times and in different places from antiquity to the present day. Moreover, in all times and places, including the United Kingdom, rival theories were and are hotly debated, specialists in centres of elite knowledge espouse different views about causes and treatments from those of provincial practitioners just a few miles away, and different cultures produce different medical solutions for the same health problem.

**2**    The women in Blaxter's analysis are expressing a view of disease causation that most closely resembles the paradigm of bedside medicine. Disease is an expression of the accumulated experience of their whole lives: a consequence of interactions between their personal constitution, past events and the external environment, rather than a random breakdown of one particular part of the body.

## Chapter 4

**1**    In the seventeenth century an insight into the importance of tuberculosis was provided by the London *Bills of Mortality*, which suggested that up to 25 per cent of deaths in the capital were due to consumption. However, sources of data from outside London were less adequate, until the nineteenth century when city authorities began to collect death statistics. Lemuel Shattuck in 1850 was able to estimate figures for pulmonary TB alone ranging between 14 and 24 per cent of deaths in various American and European cities in the early nineteenth century (Table 4.1). Figure 4.1 presents data that include all forms of tuberculosis, suggesting that, by 1882, when Koch gave his lecture, deaths from TB had declined from earlier higher levels. One-seventh (14%) of all deaths might therefore have been an accurate estimate by then.

**2**    It is noticeable that before the 1840s the major advances in understanding were made by anatomists and pathologists using naked-eye observation or simple instruments. These observers (for example, Morgagni, Bayle, Laënnec) depended on access to post-mortem materials. The experimental approach derived from the chemist Louis Pasteur, who used the equipment of chemistry and evolved special experimental techniques. Pasteur's pupil Villermin established by experiment that TB was a specific agent which could be passed from animal to animal by injection. Confirmation of these findings required the combination of even more rigorous experiments involving the culture of bacteria in Petri dishes, as well as tissue-staining techniques and sophisticated microscopes capable of a high level of magnification. This combination of experiment and microscopy by Robert Koch enabled him to reach definitive conclusions that all forms of TB were caused by the same bacteria.

**3**    British scientists operated in a situation in which TB was gradually but perceptibly in decline. They and their associates in the large and well-established sanatorium system naturally attributed this decline to the success of their methods. It seemed better to pursue well-tried practices, providing the pace of improvement was maintained. Also the use of a vaccine carried an element of risk which might lead to embarrassing public health scandals, such as had occurred during the 1920s with some rival vaccines. Anti-vaccination organisations were vociferous, and there was also a distinct element of chauvinism in attitudes to BCG on the part of British scientists who had their own vaccines to promote.

**4**    It is necessary to employ combinations of drugs in 'multiple drug therapy' in a long course of treatment in order to finally eradicate the TB bacterium from the body. Lax administration of these regimes has led to the emergence of multi-drug-resistant strains. Optimism concerning global eradication programmes was quickly dispelled when it was appreciated that health-care systems in the developing world were unable to sustain elaborate treatment regimes. These difficulties have been compounded by the emergence of AIDS, which has caused TB to escalate out of control and has contributed to the problem of drug-resistant strains. Poverty and homelessness in a world hit by recession in the late 1980s, and by a succession of conflicts and natural disasters, has accelerated the spread of TB.

## Chapter 5

1   The gift of blood has been characterised in government advertising as the 'greatest gift of all'. This view of blood as containing the essence of life harks back to Aristotle and Harvey, who believed the soul to reside in the blood. This contrasts with the modern scientific view of blood as a neutral fluid. The beliefs of Jehovah's Witnesses give explicitly religious significance to blood.

2   These techniques aimed to extend the senses of the doctor to the interior of the patient's body. This was felt to be important in identifying the location of pathological lesions that were understood to be causing symptoms of disease, which were defined in terms of *syndromes*: constant and characteristic sets of symptoms, signs, and post-mortem findings.

3   Descartes saw the body as a machine, with the heart being a pump for an inanimate fluid (blood) made up from tiny particles, that were selectively sieved off to make up different body fluids. The vitalist view, represented by Harvey amongst others, saw blood as alive, indeed as being the repository of the soul. Thus vitalists thought that by transferring blood from one person's body to another's, they might be able to transfer qualities of character or temperament whose essence was contained in blood.

4   Laboratory medicine made possible the investigation and identification of micro-organisms that cause disease, whose existence had previously only been theoretically deduced. Vaccines had been developed before the mechanisms of immunity were known, by Jenner and Pasteur for instance. The microscope enabled direct observation of the white cells involved in an immune response to infection, and laboratory cultivation of pathogens and analysis of bacterial toxins led to the idea of antibodies. All of these discoveries inform the modern understanding of immunity.

## Chapter 6

1   Through Thomas Willis's theory of hysteria in the seventeenth century as the result of a delicate nervous system, this disease came to be associated with sensitivity and delicacy generally. For middle- and upper-class women in the eighteenth century, who lived soft and luxurious lives, femininity and delicacy went hand in hand. The refinement of mind and body that these women cultivated was thought to be confirmed by a propensity to hysteria. This served to reinforce the medical formulation of the condition.

2   While not denying the existence of witchcraft, Johann Weyer and Edward Jorden in the late sixteenth and early seventeenth centuries argued that natural medical causes were responsible for certain cases of hysteria. Weyer and Jorden were influenced by the growth in scepticism and free thought associated with the Renaissance.

3   The doctors were all male, they were socially important and they aimed to please Charcot, the powerful leader of their School. The patients were usually female, poor and socially unimportant, and they too had reason to wish to

please Charcot. In addition, they were isolated from other influences on the grounds that this was therapeutic, and financial and status rewards were attached to appropriate hysterical displays, particularly if these could be reproduced in Charcot's public lectures.

4   Willis located the source of hysteria in the brain, rejecting earlier attempts to locate it in a wandering uterus. He also referred to notions of general physical constitution which were a precursor of more psychological explanations. Charcot sought for explanations that were located in the nervous system, reasoning that the distinct stages that he and Briquet had described must have some underlying physiological correlate. Freud rejected the search for physical causes, developing instead a general theory of the role of early psychological trauma in causing mental illness.

5   Two explanations are offered in the text. First, women now have more control over their lives, so may not resort to this avenue of self expression. Second, other disease categories (for example chronic fatigue syndrome (CFS), anorexia, schizophrenia) may now be applied to patients whom doctors might formerly have diagnosed as suffering from hysteria.

## Chapter 7

1   The virus is characterised as a military invader, attacking an industrial complex and taking over the cell processes by force of arms. The body is presented as the site of conflict between opposing forces. This metaphor underlies the aggressive approach to fighting disease that is a particular feature of American medical practice.

2   The doctor *takes a history* by asking the patient questions about what had led to the hospital admission, and about previous medications taken. *Symptoms* of pain, gas and hiccoughing are reported by the patient. The doctor examines the patient by palpating the abdomen (a *physical examination*), during which he is looking for *signs*. Previously taken X-rays reveal signs of abnormal structure. The students try to guess at what might be wrong; their guesses show them learning the skill that leads to a diagnosis, as the doctor teaches them how evidence and logic rule out some hypotheses. The eventual *diagnosis* is that of a suspected ruptured diverticulum.

3   Different systems of medical thought would describe this patient's trouble in different ways. However, the reality of his pain and other bodily experience seems incontrovertible. Two hundred and fifty years ago, however, his problems might have been ascribed to an imbalance in his bodily humours, or a misalignment of his astrological signs. The students are learning to construct the modern view of the body of the patient and the underlying pathological lesion as the physical cause of his symptoms.

4   The idea of ritual depends on a notion of technical effectiveness. Actions which are done repeatedly and serve a non-technical purpose are often called rituals. Whether toothbrushing is a ritual depends on whether there is evidence that it is effective in preserving the teeth and gums from decay. To the extent that it serves other functions, such as instilling a sense of discipline and obedience, or encouraging a view of the mouth as an entry point for mysterious contagions, it is ritual.

## Chapter 8

1   Parsons' ideas arose from study of American society in the 1940s. In both the examples cited by Friedson, entry into the sick role is enforced on the patient, and reciprocity with a healer designated to make the patient well again is not involved. Even though social order is maintained, the functioning of the social system is entirely disadvantageous to the patient, as the sick role becomes a form of execution.

2   In all four regions of the USA, fewer blacks were judged unfit for military service than whites, and the difference between the two ethnic groups was greatest in the South. There are three possible explanations for the pattern. First, blacks may have been fitter than whites, which seems unlikely given their poorer economic circumstances. Second, blacks and whites might have varied in their ability to feign illness in order to avoid being conscripted; perhaps white conscripts had a greater insight into how to fool white doctors. Third, white doctors might have been racially prejudiced and therefore more likely to consider blacks as expendable in war.

If the last explanation is true, doctors might be seen as acting against the interests of blacks and for the interests of whites, particularly in the Southern States where blacks were once kept as slaves. However, this interpretation is only possible if entering the army at a time of war is agreed to be undesirable, something with which patriotic army generals might disagree. Whatever the explanation, the study illustrates the power given to doctors to act as gatekeepers to the sick role and the potential for medical surveillance to become an instrument of social control.

3   Ivan Illich is similarly scathing about the negative consequences of medical efforts, arguing that medicine harms people both directly through unwelcome side-effects (medical iatrogenesis), and indirectly through removing people's natural ability to take care of themselves (social iatrogenesis).

4   Just as the mad people whom Tuke and Pinel released from their chains were subjected to a new moral regime, which they internalised and carried with them in their thoughts, so the Lahontans make themselves believe they are ill by internalising the medical view of what is normal. Things become significant that were never before perceived in that way, just as the state of one's teeth is now the subject of commentary in the light of dental theory.

## Chapter 9

1   The first extract shows the nurse eliciting facts for some purpose of her own. The patient's concerns are not followed up or are brushed aside (when the patient complains of not feeling like food, the nurse replies 'Good'). The second demonstrates exploration of the patient's concerns. The second extract is the more patient-centred.

2   In Italy silence about the diagnosis of cancer, or the likelihood of death, is generally considered protective of patients. This is appropriate given Italian perceptions of the meaning of cancer, and expectations of doctors. The same was true in the USA and the United Kingdom in the 1950s. Only gradually was this 'construed as a lie' as changing views about medical authority, patients' rights, and the curability of cancer gained sway in the USA and the United

Kingdom. Thurstan Brewin's argument in favour of medical paternalism in this area represents 'the defence of the lie in the form of truth.' The increasing acceptance by doctors of a policy of open truth-telling wherever possible represents the final stage, where 'the lie is revealed as truly a lie'.

3    The patient is presenting the doctor with his lay theories about the causes of cancer. The doctor allows him considerable time to expound them and does not contradict the patient directly. This is unlikely to happen in an NHS clinic where doctors are more likely to feel pressure of time and less likely to be dealing with patients of high social status upon whose opinion of them their fee depends.

# Acknowledgements

Grateful acknowledgement is made to the following sources for permission to reproduce material in this book:

## Figures

*Figures 1.1a, b, d, 2.3, 8.3* Mike Levers/Open University; *Figure 1.1c* Jim Holmes/Panos Pictures; *Figures 3.1, 3.2, 3.3, 3.4, 3.5, 4.3, 4.4, 6.1b, 6.1c, 6.1d, 6.1e* The Wellcome Library, © The Trustee of the Wellcome Trust, London; *Figure 4.1* Bryder, L. (1988) *Below the Magic Mountain: A Social History of Tuberculosis in Twentieth-Century Britain*, by permission of Oxford University Press; *Figures 4.2, 4.5, 5.1, 5.3, 6.3, 6.5, 6.7, 6.8, 6.9* The British Library; *Figure 4.6* Macintosh, J. M. (1944) *The Nation's Health*, The Pilot Press; *Figure 4.7* Taylor, S. (1944) *The Battle for Health: A Primer of Social Medicine*, Nicholson and Watson, London; *Figure 4.8* Brown, P. (1992) 'The return of the big killer', *New Scientist*, 10 October 1992; *Figure 5.2* Philadelphia Museum of Art; *Figure 6.1a* The Royal Society of Medicine; *Figure 6.4* Rijksmuseum-Stichting, Amsterdam; *Figure 6.6* Achille Beltrane/Mary Evans Picture Library; *Figure 6.10* Mary Evans Picture Library; *Figure 7.1* Guyton, A. C. (1981) *Textbook of Medical Physiology*, 6th edn, W. B. Saunders Company; *Figure 7.2* Warwick, R. and Williams, P. L. (1973) *Gray's Anatomy*, 35th edn, Churchill Livingstone; *Figure 7.3 Time* magazine, 30 April 1984, vol 67, Figure 6, p. 38. Reprinted by permission from Time; *Figure 8.1* Roger-Viollet, Paris; *Figure 8.2* © University College London Library, 115/44, Bentham Papers; *Figure 8.4* Reprinted from *Social Science & Medicine*, **5**, (67), Waitzkin, H., 'Latent functions of the sick role in various institutional settings'. Copyright 1971, with kind permission from Pergamon Press Ltd, Headington Hill Hall, Oxford OX3 0BW.

## Tables

*Table 2.1* Scambler, A., Scambler, G. and Craig, D. (1981) Kinship and friendship networks and women's demand for primary care, *Journal of the Royal College of General Practitioners*, **26**, p. 748, Royal College of General Practitioners; *Table 2.2* MORI (1989) *Alternative Medicine*, 21–25, MORI, London; *Table 4.1* Waksman, S. A. (1965) *The Conquest of Tuberculosis*, Robert Hale, London; *Table 4.2* Bryder, L. (1988) *Below The Magic Mountain: A Social History of Tuberculosis In Twentieth-Century Britain*, by permission of Oxford University Press; *Table 4.3* Hart, P. D. and Wright, P. G. (1939) *Tuberculosis and Social Conditions in England with Special Reference to Young Adults, A Statistical Study*, National Association for the Prevention of Tuberculosis; *Table 7.1* Reprinted by permission of *The New England Journal of Medicine*, **307**, p. 1311, 1982; *Tables 7.2 and 7.3* Roth, J. (1957) Ritual and magic in the control of contagion, *American Sociological Review*, **22**, pp. 310–314, American Sociological Association; *Table 9.1* Szasz, T. S. and Hollender, M. H. (1956) A contribution to the philosophy of medicine: the basic models of the doctor–patient relationship, *Archives of Internal Medicine*, **97**, p. 586, Copyright 1956, American Medical Association; *Table 9.2* Tuckett, D., Boulton, M., Olson, C. and Williams, A. (1985) *Meetings Between Experts*, Tavistock Publications, London.

## Text/box

*Box 8.1* Scambler, G. (1991) *Sociology As Applied To Medicine*, Baillière-Tindall; *pp. 171–2* Tuckett, D., Boulton, M., Olson, C. and Williams, A. (1985) *Meetings Between Experts*, Tavistock Publications.

## Un-numbered photographs/illustrations

*pp. 15, 16, 19 (right), 29, 40, 41, 108, 141, 142, 147 (right)* Mike Levers/Open University; *p. 19 (left), 98, 163* The Wellcome Library, © The Trustee of the Wellcome Trust, London; *p. 31* Rex Features; *pp. 39, 152* Hulton Getty Picture Collection; *pp. 57, 94* Mary Evans Picture Library; *p. 62* Sigerist, H. (1965) *Grosse Ärzte*, J. F. Lehmanns Verlag, Munich; *p. 66* Reproduced by courtesy of Professor Paul Weindling; *p. 72 (top)* Reiach, A. and Hurd, R. (1944) *Building Scotland*, The Saltire Society, Edinburgh; *p. 72 (bottom)* Bodleian Library, Oxford; *p. 74* W. Suschitzky, Photo by Edith Tudor Hart; *p. 82* A. Crump/WHO/TDR; *p. 87* Mansell/Katz Pictures Ltd.; *p. 88* © The British Library, 17738, folio 187; *p. 102* Hamish Wilson/Panos Pictures; *pp. 103, 112 (right)* The British Library; *p. 106* © Private Collection/Bridgeman Art Library; *p. 112 (left)* Bibliothèque Nationale, Paris; *p. 124 Nouvelle Iconographie de la Salpêtrière*, Vol II, 1898, Masson, Paris; *p. 147 (left)* David Mercado/Reuters/Popperfoto; *pp. 148, 156, 162* Science Photo Library Ltd.; *p. 157* Courtesy of the Institute of Alcohol Studies, London; *p. 159* Kevin Kallaugher; *p. 173* John Harris/Report Digital; *p. 179 Punch*, 21 January 1972.

## Cover

*Background* Photograph by David Malin © Anglo Australian Observatory; *Middleground* Mountain High Map™, © 1993 Digital Wisdom, Inc; *Foreground* Warwick, R. and Williams, P. L. (1973) *Gray's Anatomy*, 35th edn, by permission of Churchill Livingstone.

# Index

Entries and page numbers in orange type refer to key words which are printed in **bold** in the text. Indexed information on pages indicated by *italics* is carried mainly or wholly in a figure or table.